Diagnostic Pathology: Gastrointestinal

Diagnostic Pathology: Gastrointestinal

Editor: Joanna Bell

AMERICAN
MEDICAL PUBLISHERS
www.americanmedicalpublishers.com

AMERICAN
MEDICAL PUBLISHERS
www.americanmedicalpublishers.com

Cataloging-in-Publication Data

Diagnostic pathology : gastrointestinal / edited by Joanna Bell.
p. cm.
Includes bibliographical references and index.
ISBN 978-1-63927-135-1
1. Gastrointestinal system--Diseases--Diagnosis. 2. Diagnosis. 3. Pathology. I. Bell, Joanna.
RC803 .D53 2022
616.330 75--dc23

American Medical Publishers,
41 Flatbush Avenue,
1st Floor, New York,
NY 11217, USA

ISBN 978-1-63927-135-1 (Hardback)

Contents

Preface

This book aims to highlight the current researches and provides a platform to further the scope of innovations in this area. This book is a product of the combined efforts of many researchers and scientists, after going through thorough studies and analysis from different parts of the world. The objective of this book is to provide the readers with the latest information of the field.

Gastrointestinal pathology is the sub-specialty of surgical pathology. It primarily focuses on the diagnosis, treatment and characterization of neoplastic and non-neoplastic diseases of the digestive tract and other accessory organs. The digestive tract or the gastrointestinal (GI) tract is the passage for the transport of food and absorption of nutrients. Gastrointestinal pathology involves the diagnostic evaluation of surgical organs and biopsy pathology of gastrointestinal tissues. Its physiology, disease mechanisms and histomorphology also fall under its focus areas. The two major symptoms associated with it are abdominal pain and gastrointestinal hemorrhage. The diagnosis of abdominal pain depends on the length of the time of the pain. The causes of this pain are inflammation, perforation, obstruction and vascular diseases. The diagnosis of upper gastrointestinal bleeding is possible with endoscopy, while the diagnosis of a lower gastrointestinal bleeding requires colonoscopy or sigmoidoscopy. This book provides significant information of this discipline to help develop a good understanding of gastrointestinal pathology and related fields. It will also provide interesting topics for research which interested readers can take up. Those in search of information to further their knowledge will be greatly assisted by this book.

I would like to express my sincere thanks to the authors for their dedicated efforts in the completion of this book. I acknowledge the efforts of the publisher for providing constant support. Lastly, I would like to thank my family for their support in all academic endeavors.

Editor

1

Faecal short-chain fatty acids - a diagnostic biomarker for irritable bowel syndrome?

Per G. Farup[1,2*], Knut Rudi[3] and Knut Hestad[1,4,5]

Abstract

Background: The diagnosis of irritable bowel syndrome (IBS) relies on symptom-based criteria. A valid and reliable biomarker that could confirm the diagnosis is desirable. This study evaluated the properties of faecal short-chain fatty acids (SCFA) as diagnostic biomarkers for IBS.

Methods: Twenty-five subjects with IBS and 25 controls were included in this explanatory case–control study. Stool samples were analysed for SCFA (acetic acid, propionic acid, butyric acid, isobutyric acid, valeric acid, and isovaleric acid) with gas chromatography and reported as mmol/l and molar%. In the search for the best way to distinguish between subjects with and without IBS, the total amount and the amount of each of the SCFA were measured, and the proportions and differences between the SCFA were calculated.

Results: In the IBS and control group, the mean age was 46.2 (SD 12.9) and 49.2 (SD 14.6), and the number of females was 13/25 (52 %) and 15/25 (60 %) respectively. The difference between propionic and butyric acid (mmol/l) had the best diagnostic properties, the area under the Receiver Operating Characteristic curve was 0.89 (95 % CI: 0.80–0.98) ($p < 0.001$). With a cut-off value > 0.015 mmol/l indicating IBS, the sensitivity, specificity, positive and negative likelihood ratio, and diagnostic odds ratio were 92 %, 72 %, 3.29, 0.11 and 29.6 respectively. Similar diagnostic properties were shown for all the IBS subgroups.

Conclusions: The study indicated that faecal SCFA could be a non-invasive, valid and reliable biomarker for the differentiation of healthy subjects from subjects with IBS.

Background

Irritable bowel syndrome (IBS) is a common functional gastrointestinal disorder [1, 2]. The diagnosis is based on internationally accepted symptom-based criteria (the Rome criteria) after exclusion of organic diseases [3]. Since multiple disorders have similar symptoms, a valid and reliable diagnostic biomarker for IBS has been highly demanded. Physicians often avoid setting a positive diagnosis of IBS without extensive investigations. Clarke et al.'s statement in 2009 has the same actuality today: "The successful identification of biomarkers is critical to progressing our understanding of IBS and addressing the unmet therapeutic needs of this debilitating condition" [4].

Extensive research has been carried out to find valid and reliable biomarkers for IBS. Several biomarkers separate IBS from organic diseases (e.g. Inflammatory Bowel Disease) and healthy volunteers, but so far none has been judged as satisfactory for the use in daily practice [5, 6].

The association between IBS and the gut microbiota has been demonstrated in several studies and efforts have been made to characterise the abnormal microbiota in patients with IBS [7, 8]. So far, the results have been inconsistent. For the human health and disease, the function of the microbiota might, therefore, be as important as the phylotype. It has been argued that "the phylotype provides the environmentally selected interface for the functions"[9]. The function could be measured as chemicals and metabolites in the faeces. The microbiota metabolises non-digestible food constituents into short-chain fatty acids (SCFA) that have extensive immunological and regulatory functions and appear to be the link in the host-microbe interactions [10–13].

* Correspondence: per.farup@ntnu.no
[1]Department of Research, Innlandet Hospital Trust, N-2381 Brumunddal, Norway
[2]Unit for Applied Clinical Research, Department of Cancer Research and Molecular Medicine, Faculty of Medicine, Norwegian University of Science and Technology, N-7491 Trondheim, Norway
Full list of author information is available at the end of the article

The relation between functional characteristics, such as SCFA and functional bowel disorders has not been extensively investigated. The immunological activation often seen in subjects with IBS could be associated with the changes in SCFA [11, 14–17]. In one study, volatile organic metabolites showed promising diagnostic properties for IBS [16].

The aims of this case–control study were to compare faecal SCFA in subjects with and without IBS and search for biomarkers that could aid in differentiating patients with IBS from healthy subjects.

Methods

Design

This study was an add-on to a previous study comparing patients with depression and unspecified neurological symptoms [18, 19]. Fifty patients, 25 with IBS and 25 without, were arbitrarily selected for this case–control study.

Participants

In the previous study, patients above 17 years of age with the diagnosis of idiopathic depression (according to ICD-10; F 32–34 spectre) were included in the "depression group". Patients admitted to an inpatient neurological clinic with unexplained neurological symptoms were included in the "neurological group". In both groups, organic diseases were excluded after comprehensive clinical, laboratory, and supplementary investigations according to the doctors' discretion. In the neurological group, the examinations included a thorough neurological examination, analysis of the cerebrospinal fluid and either a cerebral CT or MRI scan. Subjects with excessive alcohol intake were excluded. Inclusion and exclusion criteria, design and methods have been described in detail in previous papers [18, 19].

Variables

Demographics: Gender; Age (years); education (number of years in school).

Abdominal complaints: IBS (yes/no) according to the Rome III criteria was assessed with a validated Norwegian translation of the Rome-questionnaire [3].

Depression: Beck Depression Inventory v. II (BDI II) (minimal, mild, moderate and severe depression; scores 0–13, 14–19, 20–28 and 29–63 respectively) [20]. Montgomery-Åsberg Depression Scale (MADRS): (symptom absent, mild, moderate and severe depression; scores 0–6, 7–19. 20–34 and 35–60 respectively) [21].

Faecal samples: Stool samples were analysed for short-chain fatty acids (acetic acid, propionic acid, butyric acid, isobutyric acid, valeric acid, and isovaleric acid) with gas chromatography as described by Szczesniak et al. [22]. The amounts of SCFA have been reported as mmol/l and molar%. In the search for the best way to distinguish subjects with and without IBS, the amount of SCFA and the proportion and differences between the SCFA were used.

Statistics

The exact chi-square test and Student *t*-test were used for the comparisons between the groups, and non-parametric statistics was used in addition for variables without normal distribution. Linear multiple regression was used to study independent predictors. The diagnostic properties were assessed with Receiver Operating Characteristics (ROC) curves, sensitivity, specificity, positive- and negative Likelihood Ratio (LR) and Diagnostic Odds Ratio (DOR). *P*-values below 0.05 were judged as statistically significant.

Ethics

The study was approved by the Norwegian Regional Committees for Medical and Health Research Ethics, PB 1130, Blindern, 0318 Oslo, Norway (reference number 2009/2196a) and performed in accordance with the Declaration of Helsinki. Written informed consent was given by all participants before inclusion.

Results

Participants

Twenty-five Caucasian subjects with IBS and 25 without were included in the study. Table 1 gives the characteristics of the subjects. No patients were excluded from the study due to an organic disorder that could explain the IBS-like symptoms, and none used antibiotics. The number of subjects with constipation-predominant IBS (IBS-C), diarrhoea-predominant IBS (IBS-D), mixed IBS (IBS-M) and undefined IBS (IBS-U) was 8, 9, 7 and 1 respectively. Except for higher scores for depression in the IBS group than in the control group, the groups were well balanced. The imbalance in the degree of depression occurred by chance and was due to a higher proportion of subjects from the "depression group" in the IBS group (19/25; 76 %) than in the control group (14/25; 56 %).

SCFA

Table 2 gives the results of the SCFA with comparisons between subjects with and without IBS. Butyric acid (molar%) was statistically significantly higher in the control group, and there was a non-significant trend toward a higher concentration of propionic acid (mmol/l and molar%) in the IBS group. Therefore, the propionic/butyric ratio and the differences between propionic acid and butyric acid (Prop-But) were calculated. They showed highly statistically significant differences between the groups. The best one for the discrimination between subjects with and without IBS turned out to be Prop-But (mmol/l). This variable also showed statistically

Table 1 The participants' characteristics

Characteristics	IBS (no 25)	Control (no 25)	Statistics (p-values)
Gender (female/male)	13 (52 %)/12 (48 %)	15 (60 %)/10 (40 %)	ns ($p = 0.78$)
Age (years)	46.2 (12.9)	49.2 (14.6)	ns ($p = 0.45$)
Group (depression/neuro)	19 (76 %)/6 (24 %)	14 (56 %)/11 (44 %)	ns ($p = 0.23$)
Education (years)	13.0 (2.8)	13.1 (2.5)	ns ($p = 0.83$)
BDI II (score)	26.7 (15.6)	14.2 (9.5)	$p = 0.001$
MADRS (score)	24.8 (11.4)	15.5 (9.4)	$p = 0.003$

The results are given as the number with proportion (%) in brackets and mean with SD in brackets
BDI II Beck Depression Inventory v. II
MADRS Montgomery-Åsberg Depression Scale

significant differences between the three subgroups of IBS (IBS-C, IBS-D and IBS-M) and the control group (Table 3).

The imbalance between the groups concerning depression made it necessary to control for confounding. A linear regression analysis with Prop-But as the dependent variable, and group (IBS/control) and BDI II as covariates was performed. IBS, but not BDI II was an independent predictor of Prop-But; standardised beta and p-values were 0.55, $p < 0.001$; and - 0.01, $p = 0.92$; respectively.

Diagnostic properties of SCFA

The differences between subjects with and without IBS were highly statistically significant for the "Propionic acid/Butyric acid ratio" and "Propionic acid minus Butyric acid (mmol/l and molar%)" (Prop-But) (Tables 2 and 3). Prop-But (mmol/l) showed the best diagnostic properties. Figure 1 shows the diagnostic property of Prop-But (mmol/l) presented as the Receiver Operating Characteristics (ROC) curve. The area under the curve (AUC) was 0.89 (95 % CI 0.80: 0.98), $p < 0.001$. A Prop-But value > 0.015 was judged as a well-suited cut-off for a positive test for IBS and was used in the calculation of the diagnostic properties. Table 4 gives the diagnostic properties of Prop-But (mmol/l) (AUC, sensitivity, specificity, positive- and negative likelihood ratio and diagnostic odds ratio) for all patients and for each of the IBS subgroups. A Prop-But value < - 0.13 excluded IBS (the sensitivity was 100 %), and a value > 0.46 confirmed the diagnosis of IBS (the specificity was 100 %).

Discussion

There is a pressing need for a good biomarker for IBS. The list of attempts to find a suitable biomarker is long

Table 2 Faecal short-chain fatty acids in subjects with and without IBS with comparisons between the groups

Short-chain fatty acids (SCFA)	IBS (no 25)	Control (no 25)	Statistics (p-values)
The sum of SCFA (mmol/l)	10.54 (9.14)	8.36 (7.57)	ns ($p = 0.36$)
Acetic acid (mmol/l)	6.42 (6.29)	4.81 (4.98)	ns ($p = 0.32$)
Propionic acid (mmol/l)	1.93 (1.43)	1.34 (0.98)	ns ($p = 0.10$)
Butyric acid (mmol/l)	1.56 (1.25)	1.67 (1.56)	ns ($p = 0.80$)
Iso-Butyric acid (mmol/l)	0.17 (0.10)	0.15 (0.12)	ns ($p = 0.52$)
Valeric acid (mmol/l)	0.19 (0.13)	0.17 (0.13)	ns ($p = 0.42$)
Iso-Valeric acid (mmol/l)	0.25 (0.13)	0.22 (0.14)	ns ($p = 0.34$)
Acetic acid (molar%)	56.26 (7.56)	55.48 (8.23)	ns ($p = 0.73$)
Propionic acid (molar%)	20.20 (4.95)	17.85 (3.94)	ns ($p = 0.07$)
Butyric acid (molar%)	15.58 (2.75)	19.00 (4.55)	$p = 0.003$
Iso-Butyric acid (molar%)	2.21 (1.07)	2.10 (1.42)	ns ($p = 0.75$)
Valeric acid (molar%)	2.25 (0.74)	2.08 (1.00)	ns ($p = 0.49$)
Iso-Valeric acid (molar%)	3.50 (2.04)	3.50 (1.98)	ns ($p = 0.99$)
Propionic – Butyric acid (mmol/l)	0.36 (0.34)	- 0.32 (0.69)	$p < 0.001$
Propionic – Butyric acid (molar%)	4.61 (5.22)	- 1.15 (5.46)	$p < 0.001$
Propionic/Butyric mmol/l ratio (%)	132 % (37 %)	98 % (27 %)	$p < 0.001$

The results are given as mean values with SD in brackets. The Student *T*-test was used for the comparisons between the groups. Several of the variables were not normally distributed. Analyses with non-parametric statistics (Mann–Whitney *U*-test) showed principally identical results (data not shown)

Table 3 The "Propionic minus Butyric acid (mmol/l)" values in the subgroups of subjects with IBS and comparisons with the control group

IBS subtype	Propionic minus Butyric acid		Statistics *p*-value
	IBS	Control	
IBS-C (no 8)	0.21 (0.24)	- 0.32 (0.69)	$p = 0.04$
IBS-D (no 9)	0.51 (0.37)	- 0.32 (0.69)	$p = 0.002$
IBS-M (no 7)	0.37 (0.37)	- 0.32 (0.69)	$p = 0.016$
IBS-U (no 1)	0.24 (---)	- 0.32 (0.69)	ns ($p = 0.43$)

Abbreviations: IBS-C: Constipation-predominant IBS; IBS-D: Diarrhoea-predominant IBS; IBS-M: Mixed IBS; IBS-U: Undefined IBS. No: Number of subjects

The results are given as mean values with SD in brackets. The Student *T*-test was used for the comparisons between the groups. Several of the variables were not normally distributed. Analyses with non-parametric statistics (Mann–Whitney *U*-test) showed principally identical results (data not shown)

and has increased the understanding of IBS, but not resulted in a tool for use in daily practice [5, 6]. It was recently stated that no tool has surpassed the symptom-based criteria [5]. This study indicated that faecal SCFA could be a valuable diagnostic biomarker for IBS. With the chosen cut-off value, a negative test nearly excluded IBS.

The evidence for an association between the gut microbiota and IBS is increasing, at least in a subpopulation of the patients [7, 8, 23]. The microbiota is presumed to induce pathophysiological reactions such as activation of the mucosal immune system, increased intestinal permeability, activation of sensory pathways, and modulation of the enteric motility. Several studies show differences, but not the same differences, between the microbiota in patients with IBS and healthy volunteers and between subgroups of patients with IBS [8]. The findings indicate an imbalance of the microbiota (dysbiosis) in subjects with IBS, but a precise description of the imbalance has so far not been successful.

Knowledge of the function of the microbiota might be as relevant as knowledge of the microbiota itself and might add diagnostic and mechanistic insight to the study of the composition of the microbiota [12, 13, 23]. SCFA are produced by the microbiota trough fermentation of ingestible polysaccharides and proteins, and have been described as the link between the microbes and the host [10, 11]. SCFA have anti-inflammatory effects by modulation of the immune cell chemotaxis, and the release of reactive oxygen species (ROS) and cytokines [10]. The effects are mediated mainly by inhibition of histone deacetylases (HDACs) and stimulation of G-protein-coupled receptors (GPCRs), particularly GPR43 [10, 12]. IBS might be an inflammatory disorder. Studies in subjects with IBS have shown an activation of the immune system and an imbalance in the cytokine pattern [14, 15]. The lack of association between the total amount of SCFA in subjects with and without IBS seen in this and other studies could be due to different and opposite effects of the SCFA [11, 23–26]. The exact pathophysiology of IBS is unknown, and the absolute and relative amount of each of the SCFA might be more important than the total amount of SCFA. Butyrate, which is a key promoter of colonic health and the main provider of energy for the colonocytes, inhibits Il-12 and increases Il-10 production, and has a beneficial effect in various disorders [11, 13, 27]. Propionate is a potent activator of GPR43 that is present in immune, nervous and endocrine cells along the entire gastrointestinal tract [10]. The effects of the SCFA vary significantly, and the variation in absolute and relative amount could explain the seemingly different associations between SCFA and diseases [11–13]. The unfavourable effect of propionic acid in subjects with IBS, and the reverse effects of propionic and butyric acid have been reported in some but not all studies [23–26]. The discrepancies between the studies could be caused by dietary variations such as variation in the intake of FODMAPs [17]. The findings in this study and other studies indicate that SCFA, particularly the relation between propionate and butyrate, could be a diagnostic biomarker of IBS.

In this study, SCFA showed very satisfactory diagnostic properties for the diagnosis of IBS. The best parameter was Prop-But (mmol/l) with AUC = 0.89, sensitivity 92 % and specificity 72 %. The results seem to be as good as other diagnostic tools, but comparisons are difficult [5, 6].

A test's diagnostic properties depends on the reference standard (the gold standard), the aim of the test, and the population. No gold standard exists. In this study, the reference standard was the Rome III criteria after exclusion of organic diseases. Most studies have used symptom-based criteria (e.g. Manning, Rome I, II and III) with a more or less complete exclusion of organic diseases [16, 28–31]. Other studies (like the one that validated the Rome III criteria) have used a not standardised definition [32]. The use of different reference standards makes comparisons of diagnostic tests for IBS nearly impossible.

Also, the aims of other studies have varied. Some studies aimed at separating patients with IBS-symptoms and organic diseases (like IBD) from patients with true IBS, some aimed at separating patients with IBS from healthy subjects, and some aimed at distinguishing subtypes of IBS [16, 28–31, 33]. The test results with one diagnostic marker vary depending on the aim of the study, as clearly shown by Ahmed et al. [16]. Most markers only differentiate IBS from organic diseases and not from healthy volunteers. At last, the participants in other studies have been selected from different populations, e.g. the general population, primary, secondary and

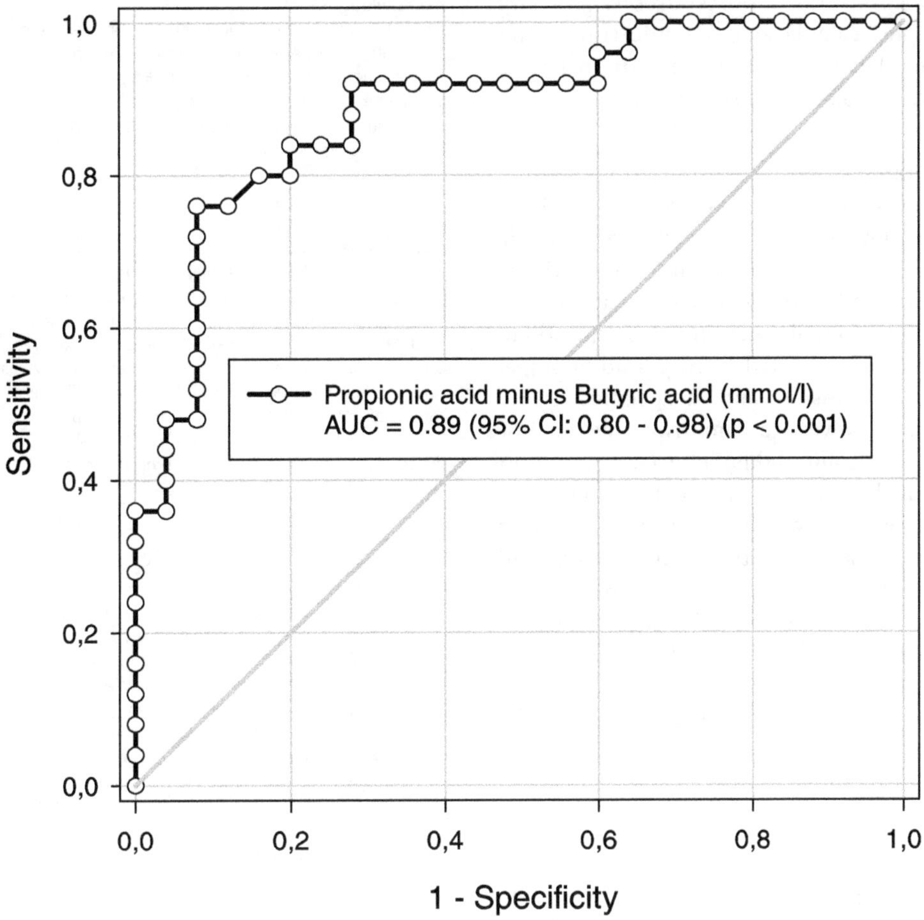

Fig. 1 The diagnostic properties of Propionic – Butyric acid (mmol/l) presented as the Receiver Operating Characteristic curve

tertiary care; healthy volunteers; different types of IBS and degree of symptoms; and patients with various organic disorders [16, 29, 31]. Comparisons of the results from studies of tests for the diagnosis IBS are unreliable without a strict control for the gold standard, the aims of the studies and the populations in the studies. Heterogeneity and design-related bias make comparisons of studies of diagnostic tests difficult [34, 35].

Ahmed et al. have studied the diagnostic accuracy of faecal volatile organic metabolites in IBS and showed that the results depended on the aim [16]. When the aim was to differentiate IBS from healthy individuals, as it was in the actual study, the sensitivity and specificity of the test were 90 and 80 % respectively. In the actual study, the marker was a simple difference between two SCFA, whereas Ahmed et al. used a complex discriminatory model [16]. Tests

Table 4 The diagnostic properties of "Propionic acid minus Butyric acid (mmol/l)" for the diagnosis of IBS in all subjects and the subgroups of IBS

IBS group	AUC (95 % CI)	Significance	Sens	Spec	Pos. LR	Neg. LR	DOR
IBS (all subjects)	0.89 (0.80:0.98)	$p < 0.001$	92 %	72 %	3.29	0.11	29.6
IBS-C (no 8)	0.83 (0.67:0.99)	$p = 0.006$	87.5 %	72 %	3.13	0.17	18.0
IBS-D (no 9)	0.92 (0.78:1.00)	$p < 0.001$	89 %	72 %	3.17	0.15	20.6
IBS-M (no 7)	0.91 (0.81:1.00)	$p = 0.001$	100 %	72 %	3.57	0.00	NA
IBS-U (no 1)	0.92 (0.81:1.00)	ns ($p = 0.16$)	100 %	72 %	3.57	0.00	NA

Abbreviations: IBS-C: Constipation-predominant IBS; IBS-D: Diarrhoea-predominant IBS; IBS-M: Mixed IBS; IBS-U: Undefined IBS; AUC: Area Under the Curve; CI: Confidence interval; Sens.: Sensitivity; Spec: Specificity; Pos. LH: Positive Likelihood Ratio; Neg. LR: Negative Likelihood Ratio; DOR: Diagnostic Odds Ratio

requiring resource consuming procedures (e.g. a large test battery, complex calculations, colonic transit time and faecal bile acid) have not been proven to be better than the more simple ones [16, 28–31].

Strengths and limitations

The results of this small study were promising. If the measurement of SCFA in faeces turns out to be a valuable biomarker for IBS, it will be a simple test without invasive procedures and complicated calculations. The external validity of the actual study might be questioned since the subjects were recruited from a study comparing subjects with depression and unspecified neurological symptoms. However, the multivariable analyses did not indicate any confounding effects. Information about the diet, which has been shown to influence on the faecal microbiota, could have improved the study [17]. Neither was smoking habits recorded. The study evaluated only the diagnostic ability to differentiate IBS from healthy volunteers, and not IBS from organic diseases. Because the study had an exploratory design and a limited number of participants, the results need confirmation in a new, larger and hypotheses driven validation study.

Conclusions

The study indicated that faecal SCFA could be a non-invasive, valid and reliable biomarker for the differentiation of IBS from healthy volunteers, particularly for the exclusion of the diagnosis.

Availability of data and material

Case report forms (CRFs) on paper were used for collection of the clinical data, and all the CRFs are safely stored. The data were transferred manually to SPSS for statistical analyses. The data files are stored by Innlandet Hospital Trust, Brumunddal, Norway, on a server dedicated to research and with security according to the rules given by The Norwegian Data Protection Authority, P.O. Box 8177 Dep. NO-0034 Oslo, Norway. The data are available on request to the authors.

Competing interests

KR: Ownership interest (stocks) and Board Membership in Genetic Analysis AS, Oslo, Norway. PGF and KH have no competing interests.

Authors' contributions

PGF has participated in the planning of the study and has the responsibility for the gastroenterological part of the study. He analysed the data and were the person in charge for the preparation of the manuscript. KR has been responsible for analyses of SCFA. KH is the guarantor and project leader and has the responsibility for the integrity of the work from inception to published article. He designed the study, wrote the main protocol, and has been responsible the inclusion and follow-up of the patients. All authors have participated in the preparation of the manuscript and approved the final version.

Acknowledgements

The authors thank Inge Christa Kristiansen (Registered Nurse, Research Assistant), Innlandet Hospital Trust for conscious help with the collection of data; Michel Brunes Berg (Graduate Engineer) Norwegian University of Life Sciences for performing the analyses of SCFA; the study participants and participating institutions for their co-operation; and Innlandet Hospital Trust for the funding.

Author details

[1]Department of Research, Innlandet Hospital Trust, N-2381 Brumunddal, Norway. [2]Unit for Applied Clinical Research, Department of Cancer Research and Molecular Medicine, Faculty of Medicine, Norwegian University of Science and Technology, N-7491 Trondheim, Norway. [3]Department of Chemistry, Biotechnology and Food Science, Norwegian University of Life Sciences, P.O. Box 5003, N-1432 Ås, Norway. [4]Department of Psychology, Faculty of Social Sciences and Technology Management, Norwegian University of Science and Technology, N-7491 Trondheim, Norway. [5]Department of Public Health, Hedmark University College, N-2418 Elverum, Norway.

References

1. Vandvik PO, Lydersen S, Farup PG. Prevalence, comorbidity and impact of irritable bowel syndrome in Norway. Scand J Gastroenterol. 2006;41:650–6.
2. Lovell RM, Ford AC. Global prevalence of and risk factors for irritable bowel syndrome: a meta-analysis. Clin Gastroenterol Hepatol. 2012;10:712–21.
3. Longstreth GF, Thompson WG, Chey WD, Houghton LA, Mearin F, Spiller RC. Functional bowel disorders. Gastroenterology. 2006;130:1480–91.
4. Clarke G, Quigley EM, Cryan JF, Dinan TG. Irritable bowel syndrome: towards biomarker identification. Trends Mol Med. 2009;15:478–89.
5. Sood R, Gracie DJ, Law GR, Ford AC. Systematic review with meta-analysis: the accuracy of diagnosing irritable bowel syndrome with symptoms, biomarkers and/or psychological markers. Aliment Pharmacol Ther. 2015;42: 491–503.
6. Plavsic I, Hauser G, Tkalcic M, Pletikosic S, Salkic N. Diagnosis of Irritable Bowel Syndrome: Role of Potential Biomarkers. Gastroenterol Res Pract. 2015;2015:490183.
7. Dupont HL. Review article: evidence for the role of gut microbiota in irritable bowel syndrome and its potential influence on therapeutic targets. Aliment Pharmacol Ther. 2014;39:1033–42.
8. Bennet SM, Ohman L, Simren M. Gut microbiota as potential orchestrators of irritable bowel syndrome. Gut Liver. 2015;9:318–31.
9. Avershina E, Rudi K. Is it who you are or what you do that is important in the human gut? Benef Microbes. 2013;4:219–22.
10. Tan J, McKenzie C, Potamitis M, Thorburn AN, Mackay CR, Macia L. The role of short-chain fatty acids in health and disease. Adv Immunol. 2014;121:91–119.
11. Vinolo MA, Rodrigues HG, Nachbar RT, Curi R. Regulation of inflammation by short chain fatty acids. Nutrients. 2011;3:858–76.
12. Natarajan N, Pluznick JL. From microbe to man: the role of microbial short chain fatty acid metabolites in host cell biology. Am J Physiol Cell Physiol. 2014;307:C979–85.
13. Furusawa Y, Obata Y, Fukuda S, Endo TA, Nakato G, Takahashi D, et al. Commensal microbe-derived butyrate induces the differentiation of colonic regulatory T cells. Nature. 2013;504:446–50.
14. Bashashati M, Rezaei N, Shafieyoun A, McKernan DP, Chang L, Ohman L, et al. Cytokine imbalance in irritable bowel syndrome: a systematic review and meta-analysis. Neurogastroenterol Motil. 2014;26:1036–48.
15. Bashashati M, Rezaei N, Andrews CN, Chen CQ, Daryani NE, Sharkey KA, et al. Cytokines and irritable bowel syndrome: where do we stand? Cytokine. 2012;57:201–9.
16. Ahmed I, Greenwood R, Costello BL, Ratcliffe NM, Probert CS. An investigation of fecal volatile organic metabolites in irritable bowel syndrome. PLoS One. 2013;8:e58204.
17. Halmos EP, Christophersen CT, Bird AR, Shepherd SJ, Gibson PR, Muir JG. Diets that differ in their FODMAP content alter the colonic luminal microenvironment. Gut. 2015;64:93–100.
18. Farup PG, Hestad K. Cognitive Functions and Depression in Patients with Irritable Bowel Syndrome. Gastroenterol Res Pract. 2015;2015:438329.

19. Naseribafrouei A, Hestad K, Avershina E, Sekelja M, Linlokken A, Wilson R, et al. Correlation between the human fecal microbiota and depression. Neurogastroenterol Motil. 2014;26:1155–62.
20. Beck AT, Steer RA, Brown GK. BDI-II, Beck depression inventory: manual. San Antonio, Tex: Psychological Corp: Boston: Harcourt Brace; 1996.
21. Montgomery SA, Asberg M. A new depression scale designed to be sensitive to change. Br J Psychiatry. 1979;134:382–9.
22. Szczesniak O, Hestad K, Hanssen JF, Rudi K. Isovaleric acid in stool correlates with human depression. Nutr Neurosci. 2015. http://dx.doi.org/10.1179/1476830515Y.0000000007.
23. Tana C, Umesaki Y, Imaoka A, Handa T, Kanazawa M, Fukudo S. Altered profiles of intestinal microbiota and organic acids may be the origin of symptoms in irritable bowel syndrome. Neurogastroenterol Motil. 2010;22:512–5.
24. Hurst NR, Kendig DM, Murthy KS, Grider JR. The short chain fatty acids, butyrate and propionate, have differential effects on the motility of the guinea pig colon. Neurogastroenterol Motil. 2014;26:1586–96.
25. Uchiyama K, Yasukawa Z, Tokunaga M, Okubo T, Mizushima K, Tanaka M. Various Effects to Intestinal Epithelial Wound Healing by Partially Hydrolyzed Dietary Fiber and Its Intestinal Metabolites Such As Short Chain Fatty Acids. Gastroenterology. 2015;148:S-921.
26. Ringel-Kulka T, Choi CH, Temas D, Kim A, Maier DM, Scott K, et al. Altered Colonic Bacterial Fermentation as a Potential Pathophysiological Factor in Irritable Bowel Syndrome. Am J Gastroenterol. 2015;110:1339–46.
27. Zaleski A, Banaszkiewicz A, Walkowiak J. Butyric acid in irritable bowel syndrome. Prz Gastroenterol. 2013;8:350–3.
28. Jones MP, Chey WD, Singh S, Gong H, Shringarpure R, Hoe N, et al. A biomarker panel and psychological morbidity differentiates the irritable bowel syndrome from health and provides novel pathophysiological leads. Aliment Pharmacol Ther. 2014;39:426–37.
29. Camilleri M, Shin A, Busciglio I, Carlson P, Acosta A, Bharucha AE, et al. Validating biomarkers of treatable mechanisms in irritable bowel syndrome. Neurogastroenterol Motil. 2014;26:1677–85.
30. Lembo AJ, Neri B, Tolley J, Barken D, Carroll S, Pan H. Use of serum biomarkers in a diagnostic test for irritable bowel syndrome. Aliment Pharmacol Ther. 2009;29:834–42.
31. Bouin M, Plourde V, Boivin M, Riberdy M, Lupien F, Laganiere M, et al. Rectal distention testing in patients with irritable bowel syndrome: sensitivity, specificity, and predictive values of pain sensory thresholds. Gastroenterology. 2002;122:1771–7.
32. Ford AC, Bercik P, Morgan DG, Bolino C, Pintos-Sanchez MI, Moayyedi P. Validation of the Rome III criteria for the diagnosis of irritable bowel syndrome in secondary care. Gastroenterology. 2013;145:1262–70.
33. Pimentel M, Morales W, Rezaie A, Marsh E, Lembo A, Mirocha J, et al. Development and validation of a biomarker for diarrhea-predominant irritable bowel syndrome in human subjects. PLoS One. 2015;10:e0126438.
34. Dinnes J, Deeks J, Kirby J, Roderick P. A methodological review of how heterogeneity has been examined in systematic reviews of diagnostic test accuracy. Health Technol Assess. 2005;9:1–113. iii.
35. Lijmer JG, Mol BW, Heisterkamp S, Bonsel GJ, Prins MH, van der Meulen JH, et al. Empirical evidence of design-related bias in studies of diagnostic tests. JAMA. 1999;282:1061–6.

2

Real life results in using 5-ASA for maintaining mild to moderate UC patients in Japan, a multi-center study, OPTIMUM Study

Masakazu Nagahori[1*], Shuji Kochi[2], Hiroyuki Hanai[3], Takayuki Yamamoto[4], Shiro Nakamura[5], Soji Omuro[6], Mamoru Watanabe[1], Toshifumi Hibi[7] and OPTIMUM Study Group

Abstract

Background: Efficacy of maintenance therapy in ulcerative colitis (UC) in the remission stage has been reported to depend on release profile or dosing regimen of oral 5-aminosalicylic acid (5-ASA) products used. Aim of this study is to investigate real life results in using oral 5-ASA products for maintaining mild to moderate UC patients in Japan.

Methods: Adult UC outpatients treated with oral 5-ASA products were enrolled from 379 sites in Japan between July 2012 and July 2013, and followed for 52 weeks. Remission maintenance rate was evaluated by products and dosages. Factors affecting recurrence were also examined.

Results: A total of 5695 UC patients were registered. Among the 4677 patients in whom remission maintenance was observed, remission maintenance rate at week 52 was 80.2%. As for disease duration and dosage, Pentasa® 4000 mg/day in 2 divided doses was administered to 480 (21.0%) patients in remission and 341 (46.6%) patients in active stage, and Asacol® 3600 mg/day in 3 divided doses was administered to 696 (46.4%) patients in remission and 473 (67.3%) patients in active stage.

The remission maintenance rate at week 52 by dosage and frequency did not significantly differ between Pentasa® Tablets at 4000 mg/day in 2 divided doses (76.5%) and Asacol® Tablets at 3600 mg/day in 3 divided doses (76.1%, $P = 0.7868$).

Factors affecting the risk of relapse in UC were identified. Significantly persistent remission maintenance was noted in patients in whom duration of remission maintenance until enrollment was 12 to <24 months or ≥24 months relative to the reference category of <3 months (12 to <24 months: HR 0.600 [0.486–0.740], $p < 0.0001$]; ≥24 months: HR 0.352 [0.289–0.431], $p < 0.0001$).

Conclusions: Efficacy of real life results in using oral 5-ASA products for maintaining mild to moderate UC patients was favorable. Maintaining remission for 12 months or longer after induction therapy was shown to reduce recurrence risk thereafter.

Keywords: Ulcerative colitis, Observational study, Oral 5-ASA products, Remission maintenance rate

* Correspondence: nagahori.gast@tmd.ac.jp
[1]Department of Gastroenterology, Tokyo Medical and Dental University, 1-5-45, Yushima, Bunkyoku, Tokyo 113-8519, Japan
Full list of author information is available at the end of the article

Background

Ulcerative colitis (UC) is a diffuse non-specific inflammatory bowel disease of unknown cause, characterized by erosions and ulcers in the large intestine. Since designation in 1973 as a specified disease (intractable disease) by the Ministry of Health and Welfare (at that time) in Japan, the patient population has been growing and exceeded 160 thousand patients in 2013, as estimated based on the number of medical care certificates and registration certificates issued [1].

The medical therapy for UC involves remission induction in the active stage and remission maintenance after induction has been achieved. The Guidelines for Treatment of Ulcerative Colitis 2014 (internal medicine) [2] recommend remission maintenance with 5-aminosalycilic acid (5-ASA) products (oral agent, enema, suppository), as well as immunomodulators (azathioprine, 6-MP), infliximab infusion, and adalimumab subcutaneous injection. Among these drugs, 6-MP has not been approved UC in Japan. For infliximab and adalimumab, scheduled maintenance therapy is recommended only for cases that achieved remission induction with the drug.

In Japan, the following 5-ASA products are approved and widely used as first-line drugs for treatment of mild to moderate UC: Salazopyrin® (salazosulfapyridine) tablets, approved in 1969; Salazopyrin® suppositories, in 1981; Pentasa® tablets, 1996; Pentasa® enema, 2002; Asacol® tablets, 2009; Pentasa® suppositories, 2013; and Pentasa® granules, approved in 2015. After remission induction has been achieved, 5-ASA products are continued for remission maintenance. 5-ASA products are superior to placebo for maintenance therapy [3]. Regarding doses of 5-ASA products in remission maintenance, one study has reported that continued use of the same dose as used for remission induction led to long-term remission maintenance [4], while another has reported that remission maintenance rate and patient satisfaction with prescription differed depending on the dosage and frequency [5].

Aim of this study is to investigate real life results in using oral 5-ASA products for maintaining mild to moderate UC patients in Japan. In addition, risk factors for relapse during the observation period were also investigated.

Methods

Study population

Among UC outpatients who visited 379 medical institutions in Japan between July 2012 and July 2013, those diagnosed with mild to moderate active-stage UC or remission-stage UC based on the Diagnostic Criteria in Ulcerative Colitis (revised on February 13, 2010) [6] and receiving remission induction therapy or remission maintenance therapy with oral 5-ASA products (Pentasa® Tablets, Asacol® Tablets, Salazopyrin® Tablets, and generics of these drugs) were included in the study. The patients were enrolled in sequential order at site visit. The following patients were excluded from the study: severe/fulminant active-stage UC patients, patients undergoing total/subtotal proctocolectomy, patients complicated with a malignancy, pregnant or potentially pregnant patients; and others judged ineligible by the investigator or subinvestigators.

Patient observation and evaluation

The efficacy for remission maintenance was evaluated during the observation period, at enrollment, week 26, and week 52. Patients observed for longer than 52 weeks were included in the analysis of evaluation at week 52.

At enrollment, patients were examined for the following demographics: age, sex, height, weight, month and year of diagnosis, classification of disease type based on the extent of lesion (total colitis, left-sided colitis, proctitis, others), classification by clinical course (first onset type, relapse-remitting type, chronic continuous type), smoking habit, drinking habit, employment status, and complications. Clinical course was classified as follows: one attack only; relapse-remitting type, in which the relapse and the remission are repeated; chronic continuous type, in which the symptoms persist for >6 months from the onset. Drinking habit was classified as follows; No habit; once a week and less, Habit; twice a week and more. Smoking habit was classified as follows: No habit; non-smoker, Habit; smoker and ex-smoker. The complications were intended for all diseases. Patients diagnosed with UC in the remission stage at enrollment were also examined for the duration of remission maintenance until enrollment.

At enrollment, week 26, and week 52, patients were evaluated using partial UCDAI (pUCDAI) consisting of stool frequency, bloody stool, and physician's global assessment (PGA), which was designed using the UC disease activity index (UCDAI) by Sutherland, et al. [7] as reference. This was a 4-point scale from 0 to 3 (maximum total: 9), with higher score indicating severer symptom. The results of endoscopy, if performed, were also evaluated on a 4-point scale. The pUCDAI was reported on the case report form. Disease stage (remission, relapse) was judged by attending UC specialist.

If prescription of an oral 5-ASA product was changed during the observation period, the name, dose, and frequency of the drug as well as the reason for the change were recorded. If the disease stage or prescription of an oral 5-ASA product was changed, changes during the observation period from enrollment through week 26 were documented in the evaluation at week 26, and those during the observation period after week 26 were documented in the evaluation at week 52, based on the data in the patient's medical record. The adherence to medication of oral 5-ASA products was investigated using a visual analogue scale (VAS) of a questionnaire on adherence to medication of oral 5-ASA products (Additional file 1). Aim of this study is to investigate real life results in using oral 5-ASA products for maintaining mild to moderate UC patients in Japan. Because We did not acquire the safety data.

Study endpoints

The primary endpoint in the present study was the percentage of patients who maintained remission throughout the observation period until week 52 (remission maintenance rate). Remission maintenance rate was calculated by totaling the percentage of UC patients in the remission stage at enrollment who maintained remission throughout the observation period and the percentage of UC patients in the active stage at enrollment who achieved remission induction by remission induction therapy and maintained remission for the rest of the observation period.

The secondary endpoints were the number of relapses (the number of relapses per year from enrollment of remission-stage cases or from the first remission introduction after enrollment of active-stage cases, as determined by the person-years method), duration of remission maintenance (the number of days from enrollment of remission-stage cases or from remission induction of active cases until the first relapse or discontinuation), and drug adherence rate.

UC patients who were in the active stage at enrollment or who were in the remission stage at enrollment but experienced relapse thereafter were examined for post-induction dose of oral 5-ASA products to calculate remission maintenance rate separately for patients who received the same dose as used in remission induction or patients who received a reduced dose. In addition, risk factors for relapse were also investigated during the observation period.

Statistical analysis

Ito, et al. have reported 1-year remission maintenance of 76 to 80% with oral 5-ASA products [8]. In the present study, which was an observational study, 1-year remission maintenance rate with oral 5-ASA products was assumed to be 80%. The necessary sample size to provide at least 80% power to detect 5% difference in remission maintenance rate as statistically significant difference at a significance level of $\alpha = 0.05$ was calculated to be at least 906 patients per group, or at least 1812 patients for 2 groups. As the Guidelines for Treatment of Ulcerative Colitis recommend various dosing regimens of oral 5-ASA products in remission maintenance for UC patients, it is expected that various dosing regimens are actually used in clinical practice. Therefore, assuming that 1812 patients in the 2 largest study groups account for approximately 2/5 (40%) of the overall study population, enrollment of 4530 patients was considered necessary. Although they were expected to visit study sites regularly, the target sample size was set at 5000, allowing for a dropout rate of approximately 10%. Patient baseline characteristics were expressed as actual number and percentage for categorical variables and as mean ± standard deviation (SD) for continuous variables. The data of the endpoints were expressed as mean (±SD). Comparison of remission maintenance rate by drug group was performed using Cochran-Mantel-Haenszel test [9, 10] for the following adjustment factors: age (≤60 years vs. ≥61 years), classification by the extent of lesion, classification by clinical course, smoking habit, concomitant use of drugs for UC other than probiotics/cytapheresis therapy, duration of disease, and duration of remission maintenance until enrollment (0 for patients in the active stage at enrollment). Note that analyses by the extent of lesion and by clinical course were conducted after exclusion of classification by the extent of lesion and classification by clinical course, respectively, from adjustment factors. To identify factors affecting relapse, the following items were analyzed by stepwise selection in the Cox regression model: age, sex, BMI, duration of disease, classification by the extent of lesion, classification by clinical course, smoking habit, drinking habit, complications, concomitant use of infliximab or adalimumab, concomitant use of tacrolimus, concomitant use of an immunomodulator, concomitant use of probiotics, concomitant use of a 5-ASA enema or suppository, drug adherence at enrollment, type of oral 5-ASA products used, daily dose of oral 5-ASA products, duration of remission maintenance until enrollment (0 for patients in the active stage at enrollment), and stool frequency score, bloody stool score, and PGA score at enrollment.

Results

Enrolled patients

A total of 5695 UC patients were enrolled from 379 sites in Japan. Of these, 4155 patients were in the remission stage, and 1540 patients were in the active stage. Of all patients enrolled, 4677 patients were included in the observational study of remission maintenance, and 1018 patients were excluded (Fig. 1).

Baseline characteristics

The patient baseline characteristics of 5695 patients enrolled and 4677 patients included in the observational study of remission maintenance are shown in Table 1. Among the 5695 patients enrolled, oral 5-ASA products used was Pentasa® Tablets in 3023 patients (53.1%), Asacol® Tablets in 2202 patients (38.7%), Salazopyrin®

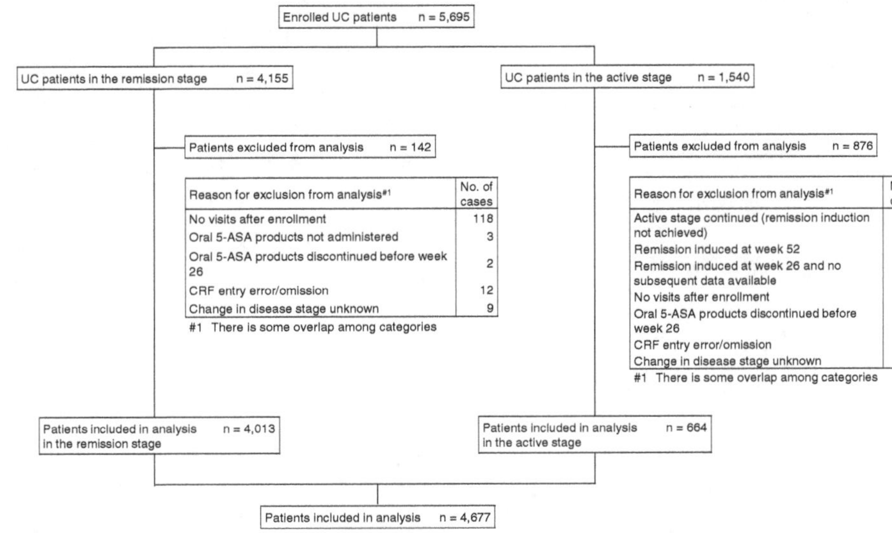

Fig. 1 Patient Disposition

Tablets in 419 patients (7.4%), a generic of any of these drugs in 20 patients (0.4%), combination of oral 5-ASA drugs in 28 patients (0.5%), and not indicated in 3 patients (0.1%). Daily dose of each drug was 250 mg/day to 6000 mg/day for Pentasa® Tablets, 400 mg/day to 4800 mg/day for Asacol® Tablets, and 500 mg/day to 8000 mg/day for Salazopyrin® Tablets.

By stage/dosage, the most frequently used dose of Pentasa® Tablets was >2250 mg/day in both remission stage and active stage (937 patients in the remission stage, 520 patients in the active stage), with 4000 mg/day particularly commonly used (505 patients in the remission stage, 357 patients in the active stage). Asacol® Tablets was administered most commonly at 3600 mg/day both in the remission stage and active stage (741 patients in the remission stage, 488 patients in the active stage). Salazopyrin® Tablets was administered most commonly at 3000 mg/day both in the remission stage and active stage (331 patients in the remission stage, 88 patients in the active stage) (Fig. 2).

Further analysis by stage/dosage and frequency revealed that Pentasa® Tablets was most frequently administered at 4000 mg/day in 2 divided doses (480 patients [21.0%] in the remission stage, 341 patients [46.6%] in the active stage), and Asacol® Tablets at 3600 mg/day in 3 divided doses (696 patients [46.4%] in the remission stage, 473 patients [67.3%] in the active stage), showing use of a high dose regardless of disease stage.

Results of the overall patients included in the observational study of remission maintenance

Among the 4677 patients included in the observational study of remission maintenance, the remission maintenance rate at week 52 was 80.2% (95% confidence interval [CI]: 79.0–81.3). The remission maintenance rate at week 52 by patients who were diagnosed within two years was 78.4%. The time-course of cumulative remission maintenance rate is shown in Fig. 3. The number of relapses was 0.2 ± 0.5 times/person-year, and the duration of remission maintenance was 311.6 ± 103.5 days.

Remission maintenance rates by concomitant drugs, duration of disease

The remission maintenance rate at week 52 by drug was 82.1% for oral 5-ASA alone, 78.7% for oral 5-ASA + probiotics, and 77.1% for oral 5-ASA + topical 5-ASA. The time-course of cumulative remission maintenance rate for oral 5-ASA alone, oral 5-ASA + probiotics, and oral 5-ASA + topical 5-ASA is shown in Fig. 3.

The remission maintenance rate at week 52 by patient which was diagnosed within 2 years was 82.0% for oral 5-ASA alone, 73.1% for oral 5-ASA + probiotics, and 74.3% for oral 5-ASA + topical 5-ASA.

Remission maintenance rates by drugs, by dosage and frequency, by the extent of lesion, and by clinical course in real life

The remission maintenance rate at week 52 by drug was 81.9% for Pentasa® Tablets, 78.0% for Asacol® Tablets, and 77.6% for Salazopyrin® Tablets, and 3-group comparison after adjustment for adjustment factors showed no significant difference among the 3 groups ($p = 0.1426$, Fig. 4a).

The remission maintenance rate at week 52 by dosage and frequency did not significantly differ between Pentasa® Tablets at 4000 mg/day in 2 divided doses and Asacol® Tablets at 3600 mg/day in 3 divided doses which were bases of the case setting of the present

Table 1 Patient Baseline Characteristics

Item			No. of enrolled patients ($n = 5,695$)[a]		No. of patients receiving remission maintenance ($n = 4,677$)[b]	
			No. of patients	(%)	No. of patients	(%)
Sex	Male		3188	(56.0)	2610	(55.8)
	Female		2505	(44.0)	2065	(44.2)
	Unknown		2	(0.0)	2	(0.0)
Age (years)	<20		8	(0.1)	4	(0.1)
	20–30		713	(12.5)	538	(11.5)
	31–40		1327	(23.3)	1063	(22.7)
	41–50		1371	(24.1)	1114	(23.8)
	51–60		1010	(17.7)	869	(18.6)
	61 - 70		826	(14.5)	713	(15.2)
	≥71		435	(7.6)	373	(8.0)
	Not indicated		5	(0.1)	3	(0.1)
BMI	<18.5		609	(10.7)	485	(10.4)
	18.5–<25.0		4061	(71.3)	3354	(71.7)
	≥25.0		975	(17.1)	801	(17.1)
	Not indicated		50	(0.9)	37	(0.8)
Disease stage	Disease stage		No. of patients	(%)	No. of patients	(%)
	Active stage	Mild	1303	(22.9)	574	(12.3)
		Moderate	236	(4.1)	89	(1.9)
		Not indicated	1	(0.0)	1	(0.0)
	Remission stage		4155	(73.0)	4013	(85.8)
Extent of lesion	Total colitis type		2378	(41.8)	1942	(41.5)
	Left-sided colitis type		1951	(34.3)	1391	(34.0)
	Proctitis type		1243	(21.8)	1043	(22.3)
	Other		121	(2.1)	99	(2.1)
	Not indicated		2	(0.0)	2	(0.0)
Clinical course	First onset type		953	(16.7)	838	(17.9)
	Relapse-remitting type		3995	(70.1)	3427	(73.3)
	Chronic continuous type		745	(13.1)	410	(8.8)
	Not indicated		2	(0.0)	2	(0.0)
Drinking habit	No		3250	(57.1)	2631	(56.3)
	≤1 day/week		1201	(21.1)	992	(21.2)
	2 - 5 days/week		712	(12.5)	595	(12.7)
	≥6 days/week		513	(9.0)	443	(9.5)
	Not indicated		19	(0.3)	16	(0.3)
Smoking habit	No		4207	(73.9)	3442	(73.6)
	Yes		1473	(25.9)	1222	(26.1)
	Not indicated		15	(0.3)	13	(0.3)
Complications	Yes		1166	(20.5)	966	(20.7)
	No		4529	(79.5)	3711	(79.3)
Employment status	Student		136	(2.4)	108	(2.3)
	Part-time worker		645	(11.3)	534	(11.4)
	Full-time worker		3242	(56.9)	2632	(56.3)

Table 1 Patient Baseline Characteristics *(Continued)*

	Other	1666	(29.3)	1401	(30.0)
	Not indicated	6	(0.1)	1	(0.0)
Use of oral 5-ASA agent	Pentasa®	3023	(53.1)	2528	(54.1)
	Asacol®	2202	(38.7)	1743	(37.3)
	Salazopyrin®	419	(7.4)	368	(7.9)
	Other (generic)	20	(0.4)	16	(0.3)
	Concomitant use (oral products)	28	(0.5)	22	(0.5)
	Not indicated	3	(0.1)	0	(0.0)
concomitant medication	Yes	2669	(46.9)	2076	(44.4)
	No	3026	(53.1)	2601	(55.6)
	probiotics	960	(16.9)	789	(16.9)
	topical 5-ASA	810	(14.2)	593	(12.7)
	topical steroid	259	(4.5)	170	(3.6)
	systemic steroid	401	(7.0)	275	(5.9)
	immunomodulator	870	(15.3)	699	(14.9)
	anti-TNF	169	(3.0)	129	(2.8)
	tacrolims	52	(0.9)	26	(0.6)
	cyclosporine	1	(0.0)	0	(0.0)
	leukocyte apheresis	37	(0.6)	21	(0.4)
pUCDAI and score of each category (Mean ± SD)	pUCDAI	0.9 ± 1.5 (n = 5694)		0.6 ± 1.2 (n = 4677)	
	Stool frequency	0.4 ± 0.7 (n = 5694)		0.3 ± 0.6 (n = 4677)	
	Bloody stool	0.2 ± 0.5 (n = 5695)		0.1 ± 0.4 (n = 4677)	
	PGA	0.3 ± 0.5 (n = 5695)		0.2 ± 0.4 (n = 4677)	
Duration of disease (mean ± SD) (months)		108.2 ± 93.5 (n = 5670)		110.5 ± 95.0 (n = 4658)	
Duration of remission maintenance until enrollment (mean ± SD) (months)		31.4 ± 40.3 (n = 4107)		31.6 ± 40.5 (n = 3958)	
Drug adherence (mean ± SD)		90.5 ± 14.2% (n = 5648)		90.7 ± 13.7% (n = 4646)	

[a]%: Percentage of a total of 5695 patients
[b]Subjects other than those remaining in the active stage throughout the observation period from enrollment. %: Percentage of a total of 4677 patients

study, or between Pentasa® Tablets at 2000 mg/day in 1 dose and Asacol® Tablets at 2400 mg/day in 3 divided doses, regardless of use of concomitant drugs (other than probiotics) (Fig. 4b, c).

Comparisons of the remission maintenance rate at week 52 by the extent of lesion and by clinical course also revealed no significant difference between Pentasa® Tablets at 4000 mg/day in 2 divided doses and Asacol® Tablets at 3600 mg/day in 3 divided doses, or between Pentasa® Tablets at 2000 mg/day in 1 dose and Asacol® Tablets at 2400 mg/day in 3 divided doses for either comparison (Fig. 4d, e).

Remission maintenance rate by the presence or absence of dose reduction after remission had been induced in real life

The number of cases in the active stage at enrollment that achieved remission induction by remission induction therapy and the number of cases in the remission stage at enrollment that had relapse during the observation period and then achieved remission induction by remission induction therapy totaled 1373. Of these cases, dose was not reduced after remission had been induced in 1181 cases (86.0%), supporting the general practice of not reducing dose immediately after remission induction. In the group receiving reduced dose after remission had been induced (dose reduction group) and the group receiving maintained dose (non-dose reduction group), the remission maintenance rate was 83.0 and 81.8%, respectively, showing almost the same values (p = 0.7823, Fig. 5).

Factors affecting relapse

The following factors were identified to affect relapse, for patients with those factors at enrollment having a higher subsequent risk for relapse: left-sided colitis

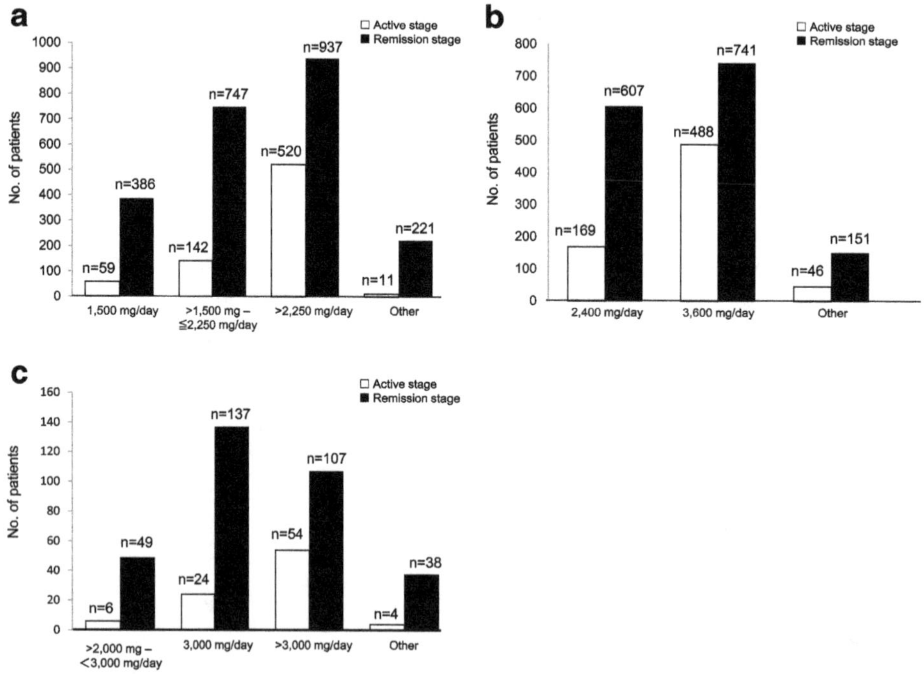

Fig. 2 Number of Patients by Disease Stage at Enrollment and by Drug. **a** Daily dose of Pentasa® **b** Daily dose of Asacol® **c** Daily dose of Salazopyrin®

relative to the reference category of total colitis as the extent of lesion (hazard ratio [HR] = 1.159 [1.001–1.341], $p = 0.0487$); relapse-remitting type relative to the reference category of first onset type as disease stage (HR = 1.456 [1.198–1.770]; $p = 0.0002$); and bloody stool score 2 relative to the reference category of score 0 as symptom (HR 1.721 [1.126–2.628], $p = 0.0120$). In contrast, significantly persistent remission maintenance was noted in patients in whom duration of remission maintenance until enrollment was 12 to <24 months or ≥24 months relative to the reference category of <3 months (12 to <24 months: HR 0.600 [0.486–0.740], $p < 0.0001$]; ≥24 months: HR 0.352 [0.289–0.431], $p < 0.0001$) (Table 2).

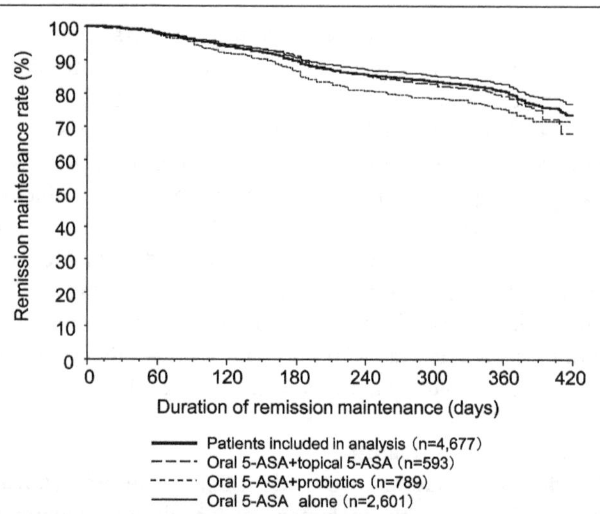

Fig. 3 Cumulative remission maintenance rate

Drug adherence

Drug adherence was 90.5% ± 14.2% ($n = 5648$) at enrollment, 90.8% ± 13.8% ($n = 5, 332$) at week 26, and 91.0% ± 13.8% ($n = 4984$) at week 52, confirming extremely favorable adherence. The drug adherence by dosage and frequency at enrollment was 91.2% ± 13.5% ($n = 409$) for one dose/day, 90.8% ± 14.6% ($n = 2324$) for 2 divided doses/day, 90.2% ± 14.0% ($n = 2848$) for 3 divided doses/day, and 86.6% ± 14.2% ($n = 65$) for 4 divided doses/day, showing favorable adherence regardless of dosage and frequency.

Discussion

In the present study, 5695 patients were enrolled from 379 sites in Japan. It was confirmed that the distributions of the residential area classification, age, and sex of enrolled patients were almost consistent with those of the Report on Public Health Frequency and Services FY2012 by the Ministry of Health, Labour and Welfare [11]. Compared with the Results of Tabulation of Personal Health Records FY2007 [12], enrolled patients showed a distribution by classification of clinical course with a slightly higher proportion of the relapse-remitting type and a similar distribution by disease type classification based on the extent of lesion. Furthermore, as

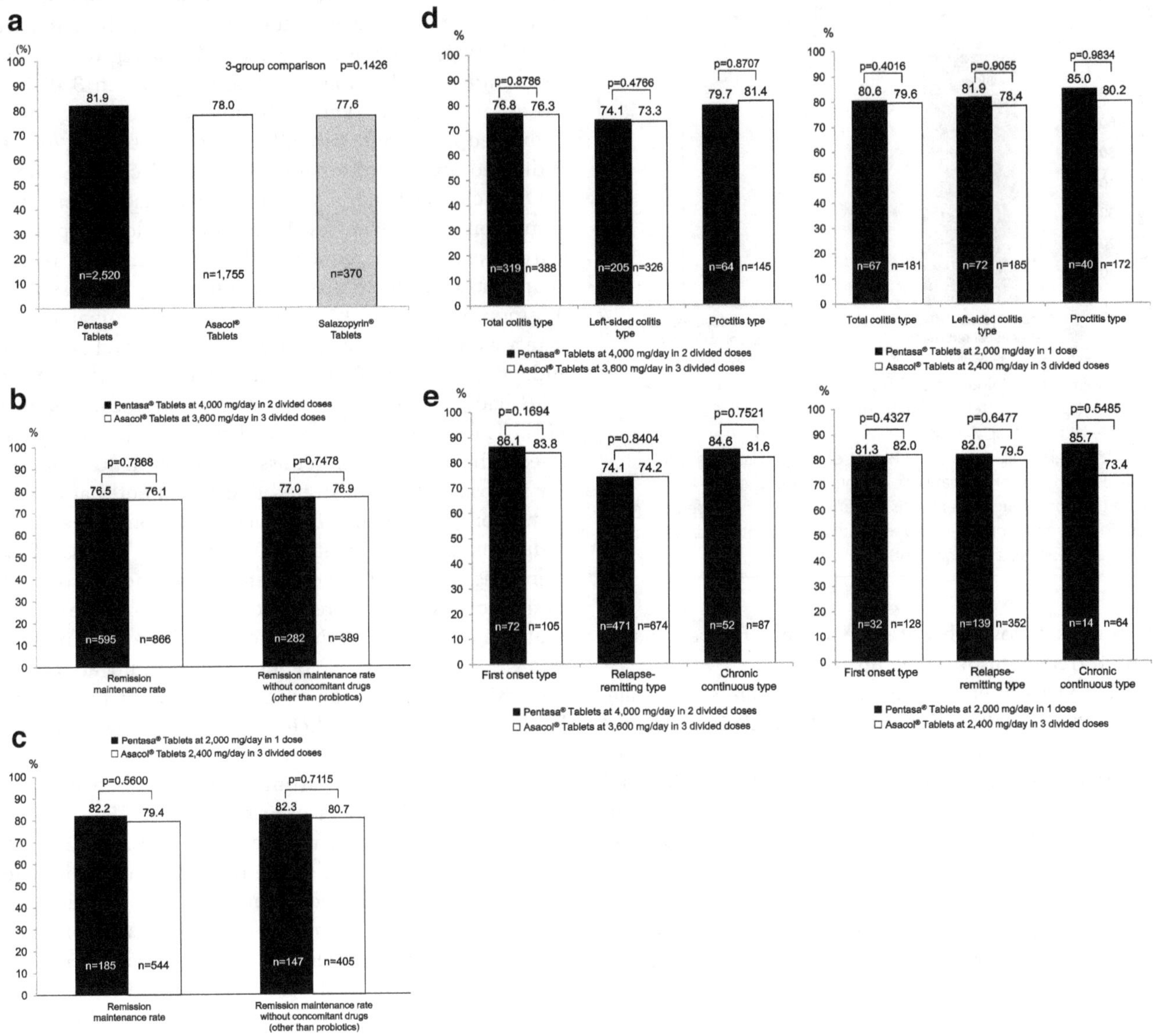

Fig. 4 Remission maintenance rates. **a** Comparison by drug. Cochran-Mantel-Haenszel test. Adjustment factors: age (≤60 years, ≥61 years), classification by the extent of lesion, classification by clinical course, smoking habit, concomitant use of drugs for UC other than probiotics/cytapheresis therapy, duration of disease, duration of remission maintenance until enrollment (0 for patients in the active stage at enrollment). **b** Comparison between Pentasa® Tablets at 4000 mg/day in 2 divided doses and Asacol® Tablets at 3600 mg/day in 3 divided doses. Cochran-Mantel-Haenszel test. Adjustment factors: age (≤60 years, ≥61 years), classification by the extent of lesion, classification by clinical course, smoking habit, concomitant use of drugs for UC other than probiotics/cytapheresis therapy, duration of disease, duration of remission maintenance until enrollment (0 for patients in the active stage at enrollment). **c** Comparison between Pentasa® Tablets at 2000 mg/day in 1 dose and Asacol® Tablets 2400 mg/day in 3 divided doses. Cochran-Mantel-Haenszel test. Adjustment factors: age (≤60 years, ≥61 years), classification by the extent of lesion, classification by clinical course, smoking habit, concomitant use of drugs for UC other than probiotics/cytapheresis therapy, duration of disease, duration of remission maintenance until enrollment (0 for patients in the active stage at enrollment). **d** Comparison by the extent of lesion. Cochran-Mantel-Haenszel test. Adjustment factors: age (≤60 years, ≥61 years), classification by clinical course, smoking habit, concomitant use of drugs for UC other than probiotics/cytapheresis therapy, duration of disease, duration of remission maintenance until enrollment (0 for patients in the active stage at enrollment). **e** Comparison by clinical course. Cochran-Mantel-Haenszel test. Adjustment factors: age (≤60 years, ≥61 years), classification by the extent of lesion, smoking habit, concomitant use of drugs for UC other than probiotics/cytapheresis therapy, duration of disease, duration of remission maintenance until enrollment (0 for patients in the active stage at enrollment)

compared with the CARE study, conducted in Germany, enrolled patients had longer duration of disease regardless of the classification of disease stage and higher percentage of total colitis in disease type classification based on the extent of lesion; however, the tendency was generally similar [13]. Accordingly, the study population was considered to be representative of the UC patient populations both in Japan and overseas.

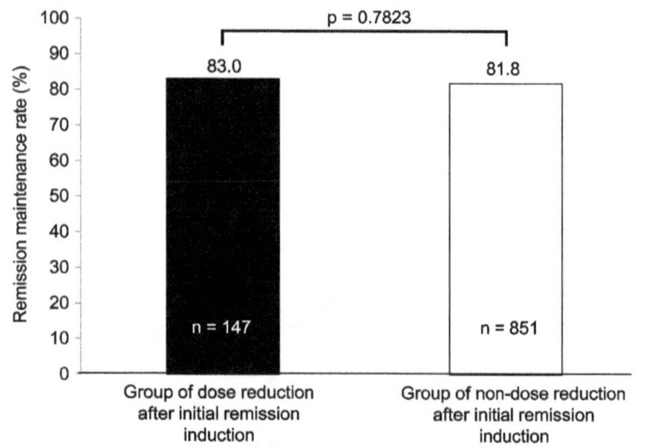

Fig. 5 Remission Maintenance Rate by the Presence or Absence of Dose Reduction after Remission has been Induced. Cochran-Mantel-Haenszel test. Adjustment factors: age (≤60 years, ≥61 years), classification by the extent of lesion, classification by clinical course, smoking habit, concomitant use of drugs for UC other than probiotics/cytaphresis therapy, duration of disease, duration of remission maintenance until enrollment (0 for patients in the active stage at enrollment)

It was as follows that it was thought for reasons of drop off treatment or follow up.

(1) No visits after enrollment: in the remission stage, self-interruption of the treatment with remission continuing and custom having occurred, in the active stage, self-interruption by the symptom improvement, the hospital transfer by a symptom not being improved, (2) Remission induced at week 26 and no subsequent data available: self-interruption by the symptom improvement, (3) Oral 5-ASA products discontinued before week 26: changing to treatment except the oral 5-ASA product prescription.

Among 4677 patients included in the analysis population (patients in the remission stage at enrollment and those in the active stage at enrollment who had achieved remission induction), remission maintenance rate at week 52 was 80.2%. A remission maintenance rate of oral 5-ASA alone was slightly high as a result of real life. It was thought that these results had more oral 5-ASA alone the calm patients with symptom.

Also, remission maintenance rate of real life, oral 5-ASA alone, oral 5-ASA + probiotics, oral 5-ASA + topical 5-ASA were higher than the patients which were diagnosed within two years. It was thought to be many ratios of patients that the activity was higher in the patients which were as diagnosed within two years.

By drug, the remission maintenance rate was 81.9% ($n = 2520$) for Pentasa®, 78.0% ($n = 1755$) for Asacol® Tablets, and 77.6% ($n = 370$) for Salazopyrin® Tablets, showing high values for all the drugs. The absence of significant difference in remission maintenance rate among the 3 groups suggests that the type of drug hardly affects efficacy in clinical practice despite the difference in release profile. The lack of significant difference in remission maintenance rate in the comparisons between Pentasa® Tablets at 2000 mg/day in one dose and Asacol® Tablets at 2400 mg/day in 3 divided doses, and between Pentasa® Tablets at 4000 mg/day in 2 divided doses and Asacol® Tablets at 3600 mg/day in 3 divided doses further supported the discussion above.

On the other hand, it was confirmed that patients with remission maintained for 12 months or longer prior to enrollment have a reduced subsequent risk for relapse than those with remission maintained for less than 12 months. Green, et al. reported that annual relapse rate was 35% in patients who newly achieved remission induction after enrollment, compared with 21% in those who had maintained remission since before enrollment [14]. The present study also identified relationship between the duration of remission maintenance and risk for relapse and demonstrated that treatment that enables remission maintenance for at least 12 months leads to a reduction in subsequent risk for relapse. This is of extreme significance in that it determined the approximate desirable duration of remission induction. The reason that female patients tended to be relapse did not unknown. Bitton A, et al. reported that multivariate Cox regression analysis retained greater number of prior relapses in women as predictors of shorter time to clinical relapse. However, there was no significant effect of medication use on the strong interaction between gender (female) and number of prior relapses [15].

The results of the present study suggested that 12-month or longer continued use of the dose that successfully introduces remission would be an approach to reducing a risk for relapse in treatment with oral 5-ASA products. The comparison between the group receiving reduced dose after remission had been first induced (dose reduction group) and the group receiving maintained dose (non-dose reduction group), however, failed to show definite difference in remission maintenance rate. This is explained as follows: In the present study, the duration of observation was set at 52 weeks from the time of enrollment; therefore, for example, for patients in the active stage at enrollment, the duration required for remission induction was to be included in the duration of observation, resulting in the duration of remission maintenance shorter than 52 weeks. Nevertheless, if in the remission stage at week 52, the cases were judged to have maintained remission, resulting in a failure to demonstrate the difference between the presence and absence of dose reduction after remission had been induced. And we did not conduct sub analysis of endoscopic evaluation. A future long-term observational study starting from the time of remission induction involving endoscopic evaluation will reveal a difference in remission maintenance rate between the presence and absence of dose reduction.

Table 2 Factors Affecting Relapse

		Univariate analysis				Multivariate analysis[#1]		
		No. of patients	Hazard ratio	Confidence interval of hazard ratio	P-value for Wald test statistics	Hazard ratio	Confidence interval of hazard ratio	P-value for Wald test statistics
Age (years)	<20	4						
	20–30	538	0.778	0.109–5.563	$p = 0.8028$			
	31–40	1063	0.611	0.086–4.358	$p = 0.6233$			
	41–50	1114	0.545	0.076–3.887	$p = 0.5450$			
	51–60	869	0.491	0.069–3.504	$p = 0.4777$			
	61–70	713	0.414	0.058–2.966	$p = 0.3802$			
	≥71	373	0.336	0.046–2.435	$p = 0.2807$			
Sex	Male	2610						
	Female	2065	1.165	1.024–1.326	$p = 0.0201$	1.126	0.988–1.282	$p = 0.0744$
BMI	<18.5	485						
	18.5–<25.0	3354	0.883	0.718–1.087	$p = 0.2411$			
	≥25.0	801	0.837	0.653–1.074	$p = 0.1630$			
Duration of disease (months)	<12	344						
	12–<60	1424	0.808	0.631–1.034	$p = 0.0900$			
	60–<120	1238	0.738	0.573–0.950	$p = 0.0186$			
	≥120	1652	0.692	0.541–0.885	$p = 0.0034$			
Classification by the extent of lesion	Total colitistype	1942						
	Left-sided colitis type	1591	1.204	1.042–1.393	$p = 0.0121$	1.159	1.001–1.341	$p = 0.0487$
	Proctitis type	1043	0.910	0.762–1.086	$p = 0.2937$	0.957	0.800–1.144	$p = 0.6271$
	Other	99	0.773	0.461–1.295	$p = 0.3282$	0.858	0.512–1.439	$p = 0.5618$
Classification by linical course	First onset type	838						
	Relapse-remitting type	3427	1.608	1.325–1.952	$p < 0.0001$	1.456	1.198–1.770	$p = 0.0002$
	Chronic continuous type	410	1.379	1.024–1.859	$p = 0.0344$	1.133	0.837–1.534	$p = 0.4175$
Smoking habit	Yes	1222						
	No	3442	1.036	0.893–1.201	$p = 0.6421$			
Drinking habit	No	2631						
	≤1 day/week	992	1.060	0.900–1.247	$p = 0.4865$			
	2–5 days/week	595	1.058	0.867–1.289	$p = 0.5797$			
	≥6 days/week	443	1.050	0.842–1.309	$p = 0.6670$			
Complications	Yes	965						
	No	3712	1.094	0.930–1.286	$p = 0.2788$			
Employment status	Student	108						
	Part-time worker	534	0.751	0.497–1.135	$p = 0.1740$			
	Full-time worker	2632	0.705	0.482–1.031	$p = 0.0714$			
	Other	1401	0.626	0.424–0.925	$p = 0.0186$			
Concomitant use of infliximab/adalimumab	Yes	129						
	No	4548	1.319	0.847–2.054	$p = 0.2205$			
Concomitant use of tacrolimus	Yes	26						
	No	4651	0.722	0.300–1.738	$p = 0.4674$			

Table 2 Factors Affecting Relapse *(Continued)*

Concomitant use of immunomodulator	Yes	602						
	No	4075	0.874	0.727–1.051	$p = 0.1517$			
Concomitant use of probiotics	Yes	789						
	No	3888	0.919	0.777–1.086	$p = 0.3208$			
Concomitant use of 5-ASA enema/suppository	Yes	594						
	No	4083	0.757	0.631–0.909	$p = 0.0028$			
Drug adherence at enrollment	<80%	705						
	≥80%	3941	1.132	0.939–1.364	$p = 0.1926$			
Type of oral 5-ASA products at enrollment	Pentasa® Tablets	2528						
	Asacol® Tablets	1744	1.301	1.136–1.490	$p = 0.0001$			
	Salazopyrin® Tablets	368	1.273	1.007–1.608	$p = 0.0435$			
	Other (generic)	16	0.000	0.000 > 999.999	$p = 0.9351$			
	Concomitant use (oral products)	22	1.092	0.408–2.921	$p = 0.8615$			
Daily dose of oral 5-ASA products at enrollment (mg)	<1500	287						
	≥1500–<2500	1982	1.190	0.864–1.640	$p = 0.2874$			
	≥2500	2408	1.780	1.301–2.436	$p = 0.0003$			
Duration of remission maintenance prior to enrollment[#2] (months)	<3	1074						
	≥3–<12	1013	0.854	0.721–1.011	$p = 0.0662$	0.928	0.772–1.115	$p = 0.4236$
	≥12–<24	824	0.542	0.445–0.661	$p < 0.0001$	0.600	0.486–0.740	$p < 0.0001$
	≥24	1703	0.316	0.263–0.380	$p < 0.0001$	0.352	0.289–0.431	$p < 0.0001$
Stool frequency score at enrollment	0	3539						
	1	874	1.331	1.132–1.564	$p = 0.0005$	1.129	0.952–1.339	$p = 0.1642$
	2	195	1.788	1.351–2.366	$p < 0.0001$	1.334	0.986–1.806	$p = 0.0618$
	3	69	0.882	0.439–1.772	$p = 0.7243$	0.618	0.303–1.262	$p = 0.1864$
Bloody stool score at enrollment	0	4159						
	1	413	1.693	1.371–2.090	$p < 0.0001$	1.249	0.988–1.578	$p = 0.0631$
	2	98	2.712	1.845–3.987	$p < 0.0001$	1.721	1.126–2.628	$p = 0.0120$
	3	7	0.000	0.000–>999.999	$p = 0.9476$	0.000	0.000–>999.999	$p = 0.9446$
PGA score at enrollment	0	3830						
	1	770	1.564	1.324–1.847	$p < 0.0001$			
	2	76	1.212	0.668–2.200	$p = 0.5275$			
	3	1	0.001	0.000–>999.999	$p = 0.9535$			

#1 Factors affecting relapse in terms of the duration until relapse were investigated using a Cox regression model (multivariate) with the items having $p < 0.05$ in univariate analysis as explanatory variables

#2 Duration of remission maintenance was counted as 0 month for the patients in active stage at enrollment

The study of possible relationship between relapse and adherence in remission-stage UC patients by Kane, et al. reported that all of the patients with relapse at month 6 of follow-up (12%) and 68% of patients with relapse at month 12 months were non-adherent patients (adherence < 80%) [16]. In addition, Kawakami, et al. reported twice higher risk for relapse in non-adherent patients than in adherent patients [17], suggesting relationship between reduced adherence and increased risk for relapse. Furthermore, as for the reasons for drug adherence, Kane, et al. cited skipped doses (50%), the large number of tablets (30%), and no need felt (20%) [16], and Hawthorne, et al. reported involvement of frequent dosing (3 times daily) [18]. Meanwhile, the survey by Kawakami, et al. reported extremely high adherence in Japanese UC patients [17], and the study by Watanabe, et al. did not provide evidence for the effect of the number of doses [19]. As the reason for high adherence in Japanese patients, Japanese temperament and direct consultation with IBD expert as well as lack of financial concerns thanks to financial support system for UC patients (Research on Measures for Intractable Diseases) have been cited [17].

The present study confirmed high remission maintenance rate at week 52, which is considered to be attributable to Japanese-unique favorable drug adherence. It would therefore be fundamental to UC treatment to fully convince patients of the importance of drug adherence for reduction in relapse risk even in the asymptomatic remission stage, thereby pursuing enhancement of adherence.

The data of the concomitant medication describe the drug which they used together at enrollment.

Conclusions

The present study demonstrated consistently high drug adherence and favorable remission-maintaining effect of real life results in using oral 5-ASA products for maintaining mild to moderate UC patients in Japan. This study also suggested the importance of continuing remission maintenance for at least 12 months for a reduction in a risk for relapse.

Abbreviations

5-ASA: 5-aminosalicylic acid; 6-MP: 6-Mercaptopurine; BMI: Body Mass Index; CI: Confidence interval; HR: Hazard ratio; IBD: Inflammatory bowel disease; PGA: Physician's global assessment; SD: Standard deviation; UC: Ulcerative colitis; UCDAI: UC disease activity index; VAS: Visual analog scale.

Acknowledgements

We thank all patients and investigators for their enthusiastic participation in this study.

Funding

This study was funded by Kyorin Pharmaceutical Co., Ltd. The funding body had a role in the study design and data collection, but not in the data analysis. Data were collected by the sponsor and entrusted to a contract research organization (Bell Medical Solutions Inc.). The contract research organization performed statistical analyses.

Authors' contributions

SO, MW, TH made substantial contributions to conception and design. MN, SK, HH, TY, SN made substantial contributions to acquisition of data. Bell Medical Sulutions Inc. performed statistical analysis. All authors made substantial contributions to interpretation of data. MN drafted and revised the manuscript. All authors gave final approval of the version to be published.

Competing interests

MN have received speaker's fees from Eisai Co., Ltd., AbbVie GK, Mitsubishi Tanabe Pharma Corporation, and Kyorin Pharmaceutical Co., Ltd., and grant/support from AbbVie GK and Mitsubishi Tanabe Pharma Corporation. HH has received speaker's fees from EA Pharma Co., Ltd., Kyorin Pharmaceutical Co., Ltd., AbbVie GK, and Mitsubishi Tanabe Pharma Corporation. SN has received speaker's fees from AbbVie GK, Kyorin Pharmaceutical Co., Ltd., Mitsubishi Tanabe Pharma Corporation, Zeria Pharmaceutical Co.,Ltd., and grant/support from Kyorin Pharmaceutical Co., Ltd., Mitsubishi Tanabe Pharma Corporation, Ajinomoto Pharmaceuticals Co., Ltd., Astellas Pharma Inc., AbbVie GK, Asahi Kasei Medical Co.,Ltd., JIMRO Co.,Ltd., Eisai Co.,Ltd., Otsuka Pharmaceutical Factory Inc., Zeria Pharmaceutical Co.,Ltd., Takeda Pharmaceutical Co.,Ltd., Mochida Pharmaceutical Co.,Ltd. SO is an employee of Kyorin Pharmaceutical Co., Ltd. MW has received speaker's fees from AbbVie GK, Eisai Co.,Ltd., Mitsubishi Tanabe Pharma Corporation, Takeda Pharmaceutical Co.,Ltd., Ajinomoto Pharmaceuticals Co., Ltd., Chugai Pharmaceutical Co.,Ltd., Kyorin Pharmaceutical Co.,Ltd., and Daiichi Sankyo Co., Ltd., and grant/support from AbbVie GK, Eisai Co.,Ltd., Kyorin Pharmaceutical Co.,Ltd., Daiichi Sankyo Co., Ltd., Ono Pharmaceutical Co.,Ltd., GeneCare Research Institute Co.,Ltd., Astellas Pharma Inc., Asahi Kasei Kuraray Medical Co.,Ltd., MSD K.K., Mitsubishi Tanabe Pharma Corporation, Chugai Pharmaceutical Co.,Ltd., Takeda Pharmaceutical Co.,Ltd., Ajinomoto Pharmaceuticals Co., Ltd., Otsuka Pharmaceutical Co.,Ltd., Kyowa Hakko Kirin Co.,Ltd., JIMRO Co.,Ltd., Zeria Pharmaceutical Co.,Ltd., UCB Japan Co.,Ltd., Sumitomo Dainippon Pharma Co.,Ltd., Toray Industries, Inc., and Bristol-Myers Squibb K.K,and consultant fees from AbbVie GK, Eisai Co.,Ltd., Takeda Pharmaceutical Co.,Ltd., Ajinomoto Pharmaceuticals Co., Ltd., Mitsubishi Tanabe Pharma Corporation, Ono Pharmaceutical Co.,Ltd., Daiichi Sankyo Co., Ltd., Gilead Sciences, Inc., Janssen Pharmaceutical K.K., Nippon Kayaku Co.,Ltd., Pfizer Japan Inc., and Celgene K.K. T H have received speaker's fee from Mitsubishi Tanabe Pharma Corporation, AbbVie GK, Eisai Co.,Ltd., JIMRO Co.,Ltd., and Zeria Pharmaceutical Co.,Ltd., and grant/support from Abbie GK, Eisai Co.,Ltd., JIMRO Co.,Ltd., and Zeria Pharmaceutical Co.,Ltd., and consultant fees from Mitsubishi Tanabe Pharma Corporation, Takeda Pharmaceutical Co.,Ltd., and EA Pharma Co.,Ltd. Other authors declare that they have no competing interests.

Author details

[1]Department of Gastroenterology, Tokyo Medical and Dental University, 1-5-45, Yushima, Bunkyoku, Tokyo 113-8519, Japan. [2]Division of Gastroenterology, Matsuyama Red Cross Hospital, 1 Bunkyocho, Matsuyama Ehime, Japan. [3]Center for Gastroenterology and Inflammatory Bowel Disease Research, Hamamatsu South Hospital, 26 Shirowacho, Minamiku, Hamamatsu, Shizuoka, Japan. [4]Inflammatory Bowel Disease Center, Yokkaichi Hazu Medical Center, 10-8 Hazuyamacho, Yokkaichi, Mie, Japan. [5]Department of Inflammatory Bowel Disease, Division of Internal Medicine, Hyogo College of Medicine, 1-1 Mukogawacho, Nishinomiya, Hyogo, Japan. [6]Medical Affairs, Clinical Development Center, Kyorin Pharmaceutical Co., Ltd. 4-6 Kanda Surugadai, Chiyodaku, Tokyo, Japan. [7]Center for Advanced IBD Research and Treatment, Kitasato Institute Hospital, Kitasato University, 5-9-1 Shirokane, Minatoku, Tokyo, Japan.

References

1. Japan Intractable Diseases Information Center home page. http://www.nanbyou.or.jp/entry/62 Assessed 15 April 2013.
2. Ministry of Health, Labour and Welfare: Shared Study Report FY 2014 on "Research on intractable inflammatory bowel disease" (Suzuki Group), p. 383
3. Wang Y, Parker CE, Feagan BG, MacDonald JK. Oral 5-Aminosalicylic acid for maintenance of remission in ulcerative colitis. Cochrane Database Syst Rev. 2016;9:CD000544.
4. Kruis W, Jonaitis L, Pokrotnieks J, Mikhailova TL, Horynski M, Bátovský M, et al. Randomised clinical trial: a comparative dose-finding study of three arms of dual release mesalazine for maintaining remission in ulcerative colitis. Aliment Pharmacol Ther. 2011;33:313–22.
5. Dignass AU, Bokemeyer B, Adamek H, Mross M, Vinter-Jensen L, Börner N, et al. Mesalamine once daily is more effective than twice daily in patients with quiescent ulcerative colitis. Clin Gastroenterol Hepatol. 2009;7:762–9.
6. Ministry of Health, Labour and Welfare: Comprehensive Report of Shared Study FY2009 on "Research on intractable inflammatory bowel disease" (Watanabe Group), pp. 484–488
7. Sutherland LR, Martin F, Greer S, Robinson M, Greenberger N, Saibil F, et al. 5-Aminosalicylic acid enema in the treatment of distal ulcerative colitis, proctosigmoiditis, and proctitis. Gastroenterology. 1987;92:1894–8.
8. Ito H, Iida M, Matsumoto T, Suzuki Y, Aida Y, Yoshida T, et al. Direct comparison of two different mesalamine formulations for the maintenance of remission in patients with ulcerative colitis: a double-blind, randomized study. Inflamm Bowel Dis. 2010;16:1575–82.
9. Cochran WG. Some methods of strengthening the common x2 tests. Biometrics. 1954;10:417–51. http://www,sciepub.com/reference/82589.
10. Mantel N, Haenszel W. Statistical aspects of the analysis of data from retrospective studies of disease. J Natl Cancer Inst. 1959;22:719–48.
11. Ministry of Health, Labour and Welfare: Report on Public Health

Administration and Services FY2012. 'Specified intractable diseases. Number of possessor of certification of medical care for specified intractable diseases.' http://www.mhlw.go.jp/toukei/saikin.

12. Ministry of Health, Labour and Welfare: Document on Tabulation of Personal Health Records FY. 2007.
13. Kruis W, Leifeld L, Morgenstern J, Pfützer R, Reimers B, Ceplis-Kastner S, CARE study group. The effect of third-party reporting on adoption of evidence-based mesalazine regimens in ulcerative colitis: an observational study. J Crohns Colitis. 2013;7:e125–32.
14. Green JR, Swan CH, Gibson JA, Kerr GD, Swarbrick ET, Thornton PC. Patient-led variable dosing with balsalazide as long-term therapy for maintenance in ulcerative colitis: a 3-year prospective observational study. Aliment Pharmacol Ther. 2004;19:435–42.
15. Bitton A, Peppercorn MA, Antonioli DA, Niles JL, Shah S, Bousvaros A, et al. Clinical, biological, and histologic parameters as predictors of relapse in ulcerative colitis. Gastroenterology. 2001;120:13–20.
16. Kane S, Huo D, Aikens J, Hanauer S. Medication nonadherence and the outcomes of patients with quiescent ulcerative colitis. Am J Med. 2003;114: 39–43.
17. Kawakami A, Tanaka M, Nishigaki M, Naganuma M, Iwao Y, Hibi T, et al. Relationship between non-adherence to aminosalicylate medication and the risk of clinical relapse among Japanese patients with ulcerative colitis in clinical remission: a prospective cohort study. J Gastroenterol. 2013;48: 1006–15.
18. Hawthorne AB, Rubin G, Ghosh S. Review article: medication non-adherence in ulcerative colitis-strategies to improve adherence with mesalazine and other maintenance therapies. Aliment Pharmacol Ther. 2008;27:1157–66.
19. Watanabe M, Hanai H, Nishino H, Yokoyama T, Terada T, Suzuki Y. Comparison of QD and TID oral mesalazine for maintenance of remission in quiescent ulcerative colitis: a double-blind, double-dummy, randomized multicenter study. Inflamm Bowel Dis. 2013;19:1681–90.

3

Using a hypothetical scenario to assess public preferences for colorectal surveillance following screening-detected, intermediate-risk adenomas: annual home-based stool test vs. triennial colonoscopy

Bernardette Bonello[1], Alex Ghanouni[1], Harriet L. Bowyer[1], Eilidh MacRae[2], Wendy Atkin[2], Stephen P. Halloran[3,4], Jane Wardle[1] and Christian von Wagner[1*]

Abstract

Background: To assess public preferences for colorectal cancer (CRC) surveillance tests for intermediate-risk adenomas, using a hypothetical scenario.

Methods: Adults aged 45–54 years without CRC were identified from three General Practices in England (two in Cumbria, one in London). A postal survey was carried out during a separate study on preferences for different first-line CRC screening modalities (non- or full-laxative computed tomographic colonography, flexible sigmoidoscopy, or colonoscopy). Individuals were allocated at random to receive a pack containing information on one first-line test, and a paragraph describing CRC surveillance recommendations for people who are diagnosed with intermediate-risk adenomas during screening. All participants received a description of two surveillance options: annual single-sample, home-based stool testing (consistent with Faecal Immunochemical Tests; FIT) or triennial colonoscopy. Invitees were asked to imagine they had been diagnosed with intermediate-risk adenomas, and then complete a questionnaire on their surveillance preferences.

Results: 22.1 % (686/3,100) questionnaires were returned. 491 (15.8 %) were eligible for analysis. The majority of participants stated a surveillance preference for the stool test over colonoscopy (60.8 % vs 31.0 %; no preference: 8.1 %; no surveillance: 0.2 %). Women were more likely to prefer the stool test than men (66.7 % vs. 53.6 %; $p = .011$). The primary reason for preferring the stool test was that it would be done more frequently. The main reason to prefer colonoscopy was its superiority at finding polyps.

Conclusions: A majority of participants stated a preference for a surveillance test resembling FIT over colonoscopy. Future research should test whether this translates to greater adherence in a real surveillance setting.

Keywords: Cancer surveillance, Faecal immunochemical test, Colonoscopy, Colorectal cancer, Patient preference, Intermediate-risk adenomas

(Continued on next page)

* Correspondence: c.wagner@ucl.ac.uk
[1]Health Behaviour Research Centre, Department of Epidemiology and Public Health, University College London, 1-19 Torrington Place, London WC1E 7HB, UK
Full list of author information is available at the end of the article

(Continued from previous page)

Abbreviations: BCSP, Bowel cancer screening programme; CI, Confidence interval; CRC, Colorectal cancer; CTC, Computed tomographic colonography; FIT, Faecal immunochemical test; gFOBT, Guaiac faecal occult blood test; IMD, Index of multiple deprivation; IQR, Interquartile range

Background

Since 2006, the population of England aged 60–69 years has been invited to take part in the NHS Bowel Cancer Screening Programme (BCSP), which has since been extended to include people up to the age of 75 years. Eligible individuals are offered a biennial guaiac faecal occult blood test (gFOBt), followed by therapeutic colonoscopy if the initial test result is abnormal. Those who have adenomas detected are often referred for surveillance: Per current BCSP guidelines, standard practice is for individuals who have three or more adenomas (one of which is large; ≥1 cm), or five or more smaller (<1 cm) adenomas to be considered high risk of developing CRC and recommended to undergo a colonoscopy in 12 months, followed by colonoscopies at 3-year intervals. Similarly, individuals who have one or more large (≥1 cm) or 3 or 4 smaller adenomas (<1 cm) are considered to be at 'intermediate risk' of developing CRC, and are referred for triennial colonoscopies [1].

Although annual colonoscopy is considered the optimal surveillance test for individuals at high risk of CRC, there are limitations to its use for surveillance of people at intermediate risk. It is resource-intensive and low yield; only approximately 3 % of surveillance colonoscopies detect advanced adenomas in intermediate risk patients [2, 3]. In addition, around 20 % of those at intermediate risk (and even high risk) for CRC do not attend colonoscopic surveillance [4]. Factors associated with non-attendance of screening colonoscopy may include laxative bowel preparation [5], anxiety about the procedure [5], expectations of pain and embarrassment [5, 6], and perceived unpleasantness of the test [7]. Hence, there is interest in the possibility of incorporating alternative tests into surveillance in order to mitigate these issues and improve uptake [8, 9].

One possible option is the faecal immunochemical test for haemoglobin (FIT), which may also be more acceptable to invitees: A previous trial randomised screening-naïve individuals to an offer of first-line screening with either FIT or colonoscopy and reported higher uptake of FIT (34.2 % vs. 24.6 %, respectively) [10]. Similarly, a recent study found that after experiencing both tests, patients at average risk of CRC preferred FIT [11]. Using FIT as the primary surveillance test could also have the advantage of reducing demand on endoscopy services resulting from widespread adoption of population-based CRC screening programmes [12]. However, previous studies on people's preferences for stool tests (not necessarily FIT) vs. colonoscopy have been in the context of first-line screening [11, 13–17] and to our knowledge, only one has been in the context of surveillance [18]. Furthermore, it is uncertain how FIT performs and compares to colonoscopy for follow-up of patients diagnosed with intermediate risk adenomas, in terms of sensitivity and specificity for advanced adenomas and CRC. A large, pragmatic accuracy and efficacy study ('FIT for Follow-Up') is in progress to assess this. Although the accuracy of FIT has been reported to be lower than colonoscopy as a one-off test [19], FIT might perform comparably with triennial colonoscopy when offered on a shorter test interval (annually) and at a low concentration threshold (high FIT sensitivity) [8, 9, 20, 21]. The present study is part of a related strand of research regarding people's preferences for the respective surveillance tests.

In a previous small-scale, qualitative 'FIT for Follow-Up' study we used four focus groups to explore attitudes towards an annual single-sample FIT vs. triennial colonoscopic surveillance of individuals at intermediate risk of CRC. The principal finding was that participants with no experience of colonoscopic surveillance had positive perceptions of FIT [18]. Interestingly, one of the key perceived benefits of annual FIT was the higher frequency of testing; participants believed this might improve detection of advanced lesions. Conversely, participants who preferred triennial colonoscopy often felt that this was the more sensitive test for finding polyps or cancer. However, since the previous study was small-scale, the present study aimed to obtain a more definitive estimate of public preferences for these two potential surveillance tests, in a larger sample of screening- and surveillance-naïve individuals. Each participant was asked to imagine they were at intermediate-risk of CRC, consider the two possible surveillance options, and state an overall preference for one method or another on a questionnaire, along with their underlying reasons using a multiple choice question.

Methods

Participants

The recruitment strategy has previously been reported in full [22]. In summary, 3100 screening- and surveillance-naïve individuals aged 45–54 years from three General Practices in England (two in Cumbria; one in London), were invited to participate in a survey. Exclusion criteria were (i) a previous diagnosis of bowel cancer or recent (i.e., in the past 6 months) diagnosis of any cancer; (ii) receiving regular colonoscopies; (iii) learning disability or significant cognitive decline; (iv) clinically judged to be unsuitable to participate (e.g., due to physical or psychological difficulties). Eligibility was determined by systematic database queries and inspection of patient records by their primary care physician.

Design and measures

This study took place as part of a larger survey that compared people's willingness to undergo four potential first-line screening tests [22]. Eligible individuals were assigned at random by household to receive a study pack, containing a cover letter, a 12-page, double-sided A5 information booklet ('The Facts' booklet) and a three-fold, double-sided A4 leaflet ('Test Information' leaflet). The cover letter asked invitees to read through the information booklet and leaflet. The Facts booklet explained:

- The concept of screening (i.e., primarily prevention of CRC through detection of adenomas which could become cancers over time but could be removed by prophylactic intervention)
- A summary of how one of four first-line screening tests (colonoscopy, flexible sigmoidoscopy, non-laxative computed tomographic colonography [CTC], or full-laxative CTC) would be carried out
- Possible side-effects and complications from the test
- The chances of possible results and how they would be disseminated
- Recommended follow-up testing where applicable (i.e., colonoscopy following an abnormal flexible sigmoidoscopy or CTC result)
- Sensitivity of the first-line screening test ("over 90 %" for colonoscopy and full-laxative CTC; "over 85 %" for non-laxative CTC; "over 65 %" for flexible sigmoidoscopy)
- Treatment options if cancer is detected.

The Test Information leaflet contained a more detailed explanation of how the first-line screening test would be carried out, including preparation requirements, what would happen at the hospital, any medication that would be required (e.g., sedation in the case of colonoscopy, in accordance with typical practice in the BCSP in England), test duration, and possible after-effects.

Information on CRC surveillance

Study packs also included a standardised questionnaire, which gave participants a summary of how and why the results of a colonoscopy could lead to a recommendation of surveillance, and information that possible surveillance tests consisted of triennial colonoscopy (previously described in the information booklets and applicable leaflet) and a stool test resembling FIT (see Additional file 1):

> *"Remember that if any polyps were found during the [first line screening test], people might be offered a colonoscopy. A colonoscopy looks at the large bowel using a tiny camera passed through the back passage, and requires a laxative preparation. If people have one large or several small polyps removed during colonoscopy, they would be considered to be at 'intermediate risk' of developing bowel cancer. People at intermediate risk would be offered a follow-up test in the future to check that no new polyps have grown. This is called 'polyp surveillance'. There are several possible follow-up tests."*

Immediately after the information about surveillance, participants were asked to imagine that they were found to be at intermediate-risk for CRC during their initial screening episode and asked a hypothetical question:

> *'Imagine that you had a large polyp removed during a colonoscopy and were at intermediate risk of developing bowel cancer. If you were offered follow-up testing to check that no new polyps have grown, which option would you prefer?'*

Response options consisted of:

A. 'Another colonoscopy test every 3 years'
B. 'A stool test at home every year. This would require me to take a sample from one of my bowel motions and post it back to a laboratory in a hygienically sealed envelope. If this test result were abnormal, I would be offered a colonoscopy.'
C. 'No follow-up testing'
D. 'No preference for any of these options'

Option B was designed to resemble the form of stool testing that would be offered to surveillance patients (i.e., FIT, requiring only one stool sample, as distinct from the current gFOBT programme which requires three samples). If participants stated a preference (i.e., they had chosen either option A or B), they were asked to select the reason(s) for their preference from the following list of options and they could choose more than one option: 'more frequent'; 'more thorough'; 'less likely to cause side-effects'; 'more familiar to me as I (would) have had the test in the past'; 'better at finding polyps or cancer'; 'less likely to harm me'; 'more convenient'; or 'better at showing me what is happening during the test'. There was also an 'other (please state)' option. Since no validated measure of surveillance preferences could be located, items were designed by members of the study team (AG, HB & CVW; see Additional file 2). Response options were based on recurring themes in the previous qualitative study [18].

Participants were asked to report their gender, age, ethnicity, current employment status, and highest level of education achieved. Postcodes were used to calculate 2010 Index of Multiple Deprivation (IMD) scores (an area-based measure of socioeconomic deprivation) [23]. Participants were also asked whether they knew anyone who had been diagnosed with bowel cancer and whether they had ever had a bowel test themselves (i.e., not limited to screening but any bowel test for any purpose).

Participants were asked to complete the questionnaire and return it in a provided Freepost envelope (which constituted consent), or to return the questionnaire blank if they did not wish to participate. After 2 weeks, a reminder letter and a replacement Freepost envelope was issued to all non-responders. All study materials are available in online appendices [22].

Analysis

Responses were pooled across the four randomised first-line screening test conditions (since surveillance would be recommended following colonoscopy and the closure of a screening episode, irrespective of the pathway to that point). Stated surveillance preferences and underlying reasons were summarised using descriptive statistics. Further analyses tested for differences in preferences between subgroups (e.g., men and women) using Pearson's χ^2 tests for association. Fisher's exact test was used to compare preferences by employment status and education due to expected counts being less than five in some cells. Wilson score 95 % confidence intervals (CI) were calculated for overall preferences, preferences within each subgroup, and reasons for preferences. Responses to the measure of education were divided into three groups: participants with a degree or higher degree were categorised as "high education", those with a lack of formal qualifications were categorised as "low education" and participants responding in other ways (e.g., A-levels or BTECs) were categorised as "medium education".

Results

Out of 3100 invitations, 686 questionnaires were returned across the four conditions (22.1 %; n per condition: 164 to 178), of which 603 participants (19.5 %) were eligible for the main analysis outlined elsewhere [24]. A further 28 (0.9 %) participants who did not answer the question on surveillance preferences and 84 (2.7 %) patients with previous bowel test experience were excluded as the numbers were too small for subgroup analyses, resulting in a final sample of 491 (15.8 %). Demographic characteristics of the sample are shown in Table 1. The median age was 50 years (interquartile range [IQR]: 47

Table 1 Demographic statistics of respondents with a surveillance preference using a hypothetical scenario of being at intermediate risk for CRC ($n = 490$)

	All participants	Prefer colonoscopy		Prefer a home-based stool test[a]		No preference		*p*-value
	($n = 490$)[b]	% ($n = 152$)	[95 % CI]	% ($n = 298$)	[95 % CI]	% ($n = 40$)	[95 % CI]	
Gender								.011
Male	($n = 220$)	35.9 (79)	[29.7, 42.4]	53.6 (118)	[47.0, 60.1]	10.5 (23)	[7.1, 15.2]	
Female	($n = 270$)	27.0 (73)	[22.1, 32.6]	66.7 (180)	[60.8, 72.0]	6.3 (17)	[4.0, 9.9]	
Ethnicity								.151
White-British	($n = 432$)	29.4 (127)	[25.3, 33.9]	62.0 (268)	[57.4, 66.5]	8.6 (37)	[6.3, 11.6]	
Non-White British	($n = 49$)	42.9 (21)	[30.0, 56.7]	51.0 (25)	[37.5, 64.4]	6.1 (3)	[2.1, 16.5]	
Employment status								.960
Employed	($n = 426$)	31.7 (135)	[27.5, 36.3]	60.3 (257)	[55.6, 64.9]	8.0 (34)	[5.8, 10.9]	
Not employed/retired	($n = 34$)	29.4 (10)	[16.8, 46.2]	64.7 (22)	[47.9, 78.5]	5.9 (2)	[1.6, 19.1]	
Highest level of education								.064
High education	($n = 151$)	27.8 (42)	[21.3, 35.4]	61.6 (93)	[53.6, 69.0]	10.6 (16)	[6.6, 16.5]	
Medium education	($n = 234$)	27.8 (65)	[22.4, 33.8]	64.5 (151)	[58.2, 70.4]	7.7 (18)	[4.9, 11.8]	
Low education	($n = 24$)	54.2 (13)	[35.1, 72.1]	45.8 (11)	[27.9, 64.9]	0.0 (0)	[0.0, 13.8]	
Indirect CRC experience								.477
Knows someone with bowel cancer	($n = 247$)	29.6 (73)	[24.2, 35.5]	63.2 (156)	[57.0, 68.9]	7.3 (18)	[4.7, 11.2]	
Does not know someone with bowel cancer	($n = 234$)	32.5 (76)	[26.8, 38.7]	58.1 (136)	[51.7, 64.3]	9.4 (22)	[6.3, 13.8]	

[a]The home-based stool test was comparable to FIT
[b]n varies because of missing data

to 52) and median IMD score was 11.4 (IQR: 8.6 to 14.0). Females were more likely to respond to the questionnaire than males (25.8 % vs. 18.8 %), as were white British individuals compared with those from other ethnic groups (40.4 % vs. 13.4 %).Compared with non-responders, responders were also slightly older (median age: 50 vs. 49 years) and living in less deprived areas (median IMD score: 11.5 vs 14.4; all p-values < .0005).

Only one participant in the final sample preferred no follow-up testing (0.2 %) and so this category was omitted from subsequent analyses. A small proportion of participants had no preference between the options ($n = 40$; 8.1 %; 95 % CI [6.1 %, 10.9 %]). The majority stated a preference for surveillance with the stool test ($n = 298$; 60.8 %; 95 % CI [56.4 %, 65.0 %]) with colonoscopy preferred less frequently ($n = 152$; 31.0 %; [27.1 %, 35.3 %]). We also found evidence of gender differences in surveillance preferences with women more likely to prefer the stool test than men (66.7 % vs. 53.6 %, χ^2 [2, $N = 490$] = 9.028, $p = .011$). We did not find evidence to suggest differences in surveillance preferences by ethnicity, employment status, level of education, or indirect experience of CRC (all p-values > .05).

The majority of the participants who stated a preference for surveillance with the stool test stated that they did so because they would be tested more frequently (62.1 %) and the test was more convenient (51.7 %; Table 2). A large proportion also said they believed that it was less likely to cause side effects (39.9 %) and less likely to cause harm (32.6 %). The majority of participants who stated a preference for colonoscopy said that they believed the test was better at finding polyps or cancer (77.6 %) and also more thorough (53.9 %). Almost one in three who preferred a colonoscopy gave the reason that they would have already had one and so would be more familiar with the test (29.6 %; Table 2).

Discussion

This study assessed public preferences for two viable surveillance tests that could be offered to patients at intermediate-risk of CRC. We found that the majority of participants stated a preference for surveillance with an annual, single-sample, home-based stool test consistent with FIT over triennial colonoscopy. The findings suggest that participants prioritised frequency, convenience, and lower risk of harm or side effects as the reason for their preference for FIT, and test sensitivity and thoroughness as their reasons for preferring colonoscopy. The views of participants who favoured colonoscopy were also influenced by the perspective that they would have already had a colonoscopy as part of the initial screening pathway. These findings are largely consistent with our previous qualitative study comparing attitudes towards an annual FIT versus triennial colonoscopic surveillance among individuals at intermediate risk of CRC [18]. Stated reasons for participants' preferences were also similar to those of a study in which participants preferred to be screened using FIT when considering test preparation and avoiding complications but preferred colonoscopy when considering accuracy [11]. It was more surprising that 16.8 % of participants who stated a preference for FIT did so on the basis that they would have had the test before; this may have been related to awareness that the current BCSP is based on first-line stool testing (which they expect to take up in future) and that stool tests are available in other contexts (e.g., for diagnosis).

There were no differences by ethnicity, employment status, education level, or for participants that knew someone who had bowel cancer but women were more likely than men to prefer the stool test over colonoscopy. This latter observation is in line with previous research showing that women have lower attendance rates for

Table 2 Reasons for surveillance test preferences using a hypothetical scenario of being at intermediate risk for CRC

	Preferred a home-based stool test[a]		Preferred colonoscopy	
	% ($n = 298$)	[95 % CI]	% ($n = 152$)	[95 % CI]
Reason for preference[b]				
More frequent	62.1 (185)	[56.5, 67.4]	21.7 (33)	[15.9, 28.9]
More convenient	51.7 (154)	[46.0, 57.3]	12.5 (19)	[8.2, 18.7]
Less likely to cause side-effects	39.9 (119)	[34.5, 45.6]	7.2 (11)	[4.1, 12.5]
Less likely to harm me	32.6 (97)	[27.5, 38.1]	5.9 (9)	[3.2, 10.9]
Better at finding polyps or cancer	28.9 (86)	[24.0, 34.3]	77.6 (118)	[70.4, 83.5]
More thorough	21.5 (64)	[17.2, 26.5]	53.9 (82)	[46.0, 61.7]
More familiar as I would have had the test before	16.8 (50)	[13.0, 21.4]	29.6 (45)	[22.9, 37.3]
Better at showing what is happening during the test	6.4 (19)	[4.1, 9.8]	17.8 (27)	[12.5, 24.6]
Other reasons	7.0 (21)	[4.5, 10.7]	3.3 (5)	[1.4, 7.5]

[a]The home-based stool test was comparable to FIT
[b]*N.B* participants could select more than one reason

screening colonoscopy than men [24, 25], that they hold more negative expectations about the test (e.g., relating to pain or fear of a cancer diagnosis) [25, 26], and are more concerned about modesty, embarrassment, and risks related to the procedure [25, 26]. In terms of colonoscopy experience, women report poorer tolerance [27], more pain [28], and more discomfort [29] during colonoscopy than men, suggesting that some of their pre-existing concerns are well-founded. The higher proportion of women stating a preference for the stool test is also consistent with a meta-analysis of studies on FIT in the context of screening and another recent study that tested patients' preferences after experiencing both colonoscopy and FIT [11, 30].

As with the previous qualitative study, these findings are most directly applicable to the English BCSP. In organised CRC screening programmes, it is often necessary to offer a default first-line and therapeutic test (e.g., first-line gFOBt and therapeutic colonoscopy) and impractical to offer a range of options. This also applies to surveillance tests when they are offered to a large number of people in a centralised fashion. Previous studies have reported several barriers to colonoscopy attendance [5–7, 24–26] and our findings suggest that a home-based stool test may be a more attractive alternative to colonoscopy. Hence, the present study adds evidence that offering annual FIT as the default surveillance method could be an effective strategy for increasing participation rates in the context of surveillance. Furthermore, it could also lower colonoscopy demand, which is a significant challenge for healthcare systems in several countries [12, 19]. In principle, the BCSP could use a similar system for surveillance of people at intermediate risk of CRC to that used for coordinating first-line screening with gFOBt. Annual, single-sample FIT kits could be posted to eligible individuals, who could then complete the test at home and return it to a laboratory for analysis. However, the preference for a stool test resembling FIT was not universal, with about 1 in 3 participants preferring triennial colonoscopies. One potential method of optimising uptake of CRC surveillance would be to offer FIT as a default test but for colonoscopic surveillance to remain an option for those who persistently decline FIT. These findings also suggest that in healthcare systems that offer a choice of tests, it would be effective to allow patients to select their preferred method.

These possible applications should be considered in the context of current uncertainties regarding the relative sensitivity of annual FIT and triennial colonoscopy. Higher uptake of FIT may not translate to superior health outcomes or cost-effectiveness unless it delivers adequate sensitivity and specificity. The results of the FIT for Follow-Up study will address this important question [8].

An important limitation of this study was that participants were asked to imagine that they were being offered follow-up testing after being diagnosed as intermediate risk of CRC. Therefore, preferences may not be representative of individuals in a real life setting (i.e., with people who had undergone CRC screening, including a diagnostic colonoscopy). For example, one previous study found that a majority of patients undergoing colonoscopy reported that the experience was better than expected [31]. Similarly, patients facing the prospect of surveillance following screening would be older than this sample (and would differ on related demographic characteristics e.g., employment and personal health status). Participants in this study were recruited on the basis of being screening-naïve but approaching the eligible screening age, in order to assess preferences for first-line tests without their perceptions being affected by previous invitations and experience of tests as part of the existing BCSP [22]. However, surveillance preferences may differ to this screening-naïve sample. In addition, although the sample was larger than the previous qualitative study, the response rate was lower than expected, introducing a possible selection bias. Although we observed few differences in preferences between subgroups, the number of participants that were non-white British, not employed or retired, and had a low level of education was lower than in the general population and there may have been differences that could not be detected in this study.

Another important limitation was that participants were only given information about the sensitivity of colonoscopy and not the stool test. In the absence of more definitive estimates, information on the sensitivity of FIT could have been provided using data on its performance as a one-off, first-line test [12] or a biennial test [32]. Estimates of sensitivity for FIT are relatively low compared with colonoscopy in this context. However, they were omitted due to being unlikely to offer a valid approximation of the performance of FIT as a surveillance test repeated over three rounds. Consequently, participants' perceptions of the stool test may have been based primarily on its appearance (e.g., a non-invasive and less thorough test may have also been perceived as less capable of detecting adenomas) and preferences may change in light of additional information [11]. Future research could determine whether preferences are consistent when people are also given this information, once more applicable estimates are available.

Furthermore, the four randomised conditions provided slightly different information about the first-line screening tests. For example, invitees allocated to receive literature about colonoscopy for first-line screening were provided with extra information about the test e.g., that it was *'over 90 % accurate for detecting polyps and cancer*,' whereas invitees in other conditions were given the associated statistic for a different test (either flexible sigmoidoscopy or a form of CTC). This meant that participants receiving information about colonoscopy might have had more knowledge about its capabilities, particularly since information on accuracy of FIT as a diagnostic test was not provided. However, although information and measures relating to preferences for first-line screening tests may have been distracting, when we compared surveillance preferences across the four conditions we did not find statistically significant differences. The numbers were small but this suggests that the type of information participants received regarding screening did not affect their preferences for surveillance tests.

Conclusions

When asked to imagine being at intermediate risk of CRC, individuals aged 45–54 years generally stated a preference for an annual single-sample home-based stool test resembling FIT over triennial colonoscopy for surveillance. FIT may be a viable alternative to colonoscopy, and may be favoured by women in particular. Future research should consider whether this preference translates to improved adherence in a real surveillance setting.

Acknowledgements

We dedicate this Article in memory of Professor Jane Wardle (1950-2015). The authors thank Station House Surgery, Windermere Health Centre, and Oak Lodge Medical Centre for their role in identifying and randomising eligible participants, and mailing out study packs, and First Colour for printing patient information booklets, leaflets, questionnaires and other study materials. The study team acknowledges the support of the National Institute for Health Research through the Primary Care Research Network.

Funding

This article presents independent research funded by the National Institute for Health Research (NIHR) under its Programme Grants for Applied Research funding scheme (RP-PG-0407-10338) and its Health Technology Assessment programme grant (09/22/192). The views expressed in this article are those of the authors and not necessarily those of the NHS, the HTA programme, the NIHR or the Department of Health.

Authors' contributions

AG and CVW conceived the study and participated in its design. AG, BB and HB participated in the acquisition and analysis of the data. BB, AG, HB and CVW participated in interpretation of data and drafting of the manuscript. All authors participated in the critical revision of the manuscript and approved the final version.

Competing interests

The authors declare that they have no competing interests.

Author details

[1]Health Behaviour Research Centre, Department of Epidemiology and Public Health, University College London, 1-19 Torrington Place, London WC1E 7HB, UK. [2]Department of Surgery and Cancer, Imperial College London, London, UK. [3]NHS Bowel Cancer Screening Southern Programme Hub, Guildford, Surrey, UK. [4]Royal Surrey County Hospital NHS Foundation Trust & University of Surrey, Guildford, Surrey, UK.

References

1. Atkin WS, Saunders BP. Surveillance guidelines after removal of colorectal adenomatous polyps. Gut. 2002;51:v6–9. doi:10.1136/gut.51.suppl_5.v6.
2. Winawer S, Zauber A, O'Brien M, Ho M, Gottlieb L, Sternberg S. Randomized comparison of surveillance intervals after colonoscopic removal of newly diagnosed adenomatous polyps. New Engl J Med. 1993;328:901–6.
3. Van Stolk R, Beck G, Baron J, Haile R, Summers R. Adenoma characteristics at first colonoscopy as predictors of adenoma recurrence and characteristics at follow-up. Gastroenterology. 1998;115:13–8.
4. Lund JN, Scholefield JH, Grainge MJ, et al. Risks, costs, and compliance limit colorectal adenoma surveillance: lessons from a randomised trial. Gut. 2001; 49(1):91–6.
5. McLachlan S-A, Clements A, Austoker J. Patients' experiences and reported barriers to colonoscopy in the screening context—A systematic review of the literature. Patient Educ Couns. 2012;86(2):137–46.
6. Ely JW, Levy BT, Daly J, Xu Y. Patient Beliefs About Colon Cancer Screening. J Cancer Education. Epub ahead of print 27 January 2015; doi: 10.1007/s13187-015-0792-5.
7. de Wijkerslooth TR, de Haan MC, Stoop EM, et al. Reasons for participation and nonparticipation in colorectal cancer screening: a randomized trial of colonoscopy and CT colonography. Am J Gastroenterol. 2012;107(12):1777–83.
8. National Institute for Health Research. HTA - 09/22/192: Faecal immunochemical testing (FIT) for adenoma surveillance. FIT for Follow-up. 2011. http://www.nets.nihr.ac.uk/projects/hta/0922192. Accessed 09 Sept 2015.
9. Lane JM, Chow E, Young GP, et al. Interval fecal immunochemical testing in a colonoscopic surveillance program speeds detection of colorectal neoplasia. Gastroenterology. 2010;139:1918–26.
10. Steele RJC, McDonald P, Digby J, et al. Clinical outcomes using a faecal immunochemical test for haemoglobin as a first-line test in a national programme constrained by colonoscopy capacity. United European Gastroenterology. 2013;1(3):198–205.
11. Xu Y, Levy BT, Daly JM, Bergus GR, Dunkelberg JC. Comparison of patient preferences for fecal immunochemical test or colonoscopy using the analytic hierarchy process. BMC Health Serv Res. 2015;15(1):175.
12. Wilschut JA, Habbema JD, van Leerdam ME, et al. Fecal occult blood testing when colonoscopy capacity is limited. J Natl Cancer Inst. 2011;103(23):1741–51.
13. Hawley ST, McQueen A, Bartholomew LK, et al. Preferences for colorectal cancer screening tests and screening test use in a large multispecialty primary care practice. Cancer. 2012;118(10):2726–34.
14. Hol L, de Bekker-Grob EW, van Dam L, et al. Preferences for colorectal cancer screening strategies: a discrete choice experiment. Br J Cancer. 2010;102(6): 972–80.
15. Lv D, Hol L, Bekker-Grob EW. What determines individuals' preferences for colorectal cancer screening programmes? A discrete choice experiment. Eur J Cancer. 2010;46(1):150–9.
16. Marshall DA, Johnson FR, Phillips KA, Marshall JK, Thabane L, Kulin NA. Measuring patient preferences for colorectal cancer screening using a choice-format survey. Value Health. 2007;10(5):415–30.
17. Wolf RL, Basch CE, Brouse CH, Shmukler C, Shea S. Patient preferences and adherence to colorectal cancer screening in an urban population. Am J Public Health. 2006;96(5):809–11.
18. Bowyer HL, Vart G, Kralj-Hans I, et al. Patient attitudes towards faecal immunochemical testing for haemoglobin as an alternative to colonoscopic surveillance of groups at increased risk of colorectal cancer. J Med Screen. 2013;20(3):149–56.
19. Droste JS T s, van Turenhout ST, Oort FA, et al. Faecal immunochemical test accuracy in patients referred for surveillance colonoscopy: a multi-centre cohort study. BMC Gastroenterol. 2012;24:12–94.
20. de Wijkerslooth TR, Stoop EM, Bossuyt PM, et al. Immunochemical fecal occult blood testing is equally sensitive for proximal and distal advanced neoplasia. Am J Gastroenterol. 2012;107(10):1570–8.
21. Quintero E, Carrillo M, Gimeno-García AZ, et al. Equivalency of Fecal Immunochemical Tests and Colonoscopy in Familial Colorectal Cancer Screening. Gastroenterology. 2014;147(5):1021–30.e1.
22. Ghanouni A, Halligan S, Plumb A, Boone D, Wardle J, von Wagner C. Non- or full-laxative CT colonography vs. endoscopic tests for colorectal cancer screening: A randomised survey comparing public perceptions and intentions to undergo testing. Eur Radiol. 2014;24(7):1477–86.

23. Department for Communities and Local Government. The English indices of deprivation 2010. 2011. https://www.gov.uk/government/statistics/english-indices-of-deprivation-2010. Accessed 8 Apr 2015.
24. Segnan N, Senore C, Andreoni B, et al. Comparing attendance and detection rate of colonoscopy with sigmoidoscopy and FIT for colorectal cancer screening. Gastroenterology. 2007;132(7):2304–12.
25. Denberg TD, Melhado TV, Coombes JM, et al. Predictors of nonadherence to screening colonoscopy. J Gen Intern Med. 2005;20(11):989–95.
26. Wong RK, Wong ML, Chan YH, Feng Z, Wai CT, Yeoh KG. Gender differences in predictors of colorectal cancer screening uptake: a national cross sectional study based on the health belief model. BMC Public Health. 2013;13:677–77.
27. Ussui VS, Silva ALW, Borges LV, Silva JGN, Zeitune JMR, Hashimoti CL. What are the most important factors regarding acceptance to the colonoscopy?: Study of related tolerance parameters. Arq Gastroenterol. 2013;50:23–30.
28. Shah SG, Brooker JC, Thapar C, Williams CB, Saunders BP. Patient pain during colonoscopy: An analysis using real-time magnetic endoscope imaging. Endoscopy. 2002;34(06):435–40.
29. Park DI, Kim HJ, Park JH, et al. Factors affecting abdominal pain during colonoscopy. Eur J Gastroenterol Hepatol. 2007;19(8):695–9. doi:10.1097/01.meg.0000219097.32811.24.
30. Clarke N, Sharp L, Osborne A, Kearney PM. Comparison of Uptake of Colorectal Cancer Screening Based on Fecal Immunochemical Testing (FIT) in Males and Females: A Systematic Review and Meta-analysis. Cancer Epidemiol Biomarkers Prev. 2015;24(1):39–47.
31. de Wijkerslooth TR, de Haan MC, Stoop EM, et al. Burden of colonoscopy compared to non-cathartic CT-colonography in a colorectal cancer screening programme: randomised controlled trial. Gut. 2012;61(11):1552–9.
32. Stegeman I, van Doorn SC, Mundt MW, et al. Participation, yield, and interval carcinomas in three rounds of biennial FIT-based colorectal cancer screening. Cancer Epidemiol. 2015;39:388–93.

4

Role of vitamin D_3 combined to alginates in preventing acid and oxidative injury in cultured gastric epithelial cells

Francesca Uberti*, Claudio Bardelli, Vera Morsanuto, Sabrina Ghirlanda and Claudio Molinari

Abstract

Background: Gastric diseases are a worldwide problem in modern society, as reported in the USA, in the range of 0.5–2 episodes/year/person and an incidence of 5–100 episodes/1000/week according to seasons and age. There is convincing evidence that oxidative stress is involved in the pathogenesis of acute gastric injury. Acid secreted from gastric parietal cells determines mucosal injuries which in turn cause inflammation and oxidative stress. Consequent inflammation produces free radicals by mitochondria thus causing lipid peroxidation, oxidative and acidic stress, which can lead to cell apoptosis. Vitamin D_3, the active form of vitamin D, may counteract intracellular cell death and improve epithelial regeneration.

Methods: This study was planned to assess whether vitamin D_3 is a protective factor against acid injury and oxidative stress in gastric epithelial cells. Primary epithelial cells and GTL-16 cells have been used to test the effects of Grisù® alone or in combination with vitamin D_3 during oxidative stress or high acid exposition measuring cell viability, ROS production, cellular adhesion time along with apoptotic, autophagic and survival pathways. The combined effect of Grisù® and vitamin D_3 was found more effective in counteracting the negative consequences of oxidative stress and acidity conditions than some other gastroprotective agents, such as Maalox® or Gaviscon®.

Results: In case of oxidative stress or acidity condition the stimulation with Grisù® alone caused an improvement of cell viability and a reduction of ROS production on epithelial gastric cells. In addition, the adhesion time of the cells was improved. All these effects were increased by the presence of vitamin D_3. Similar data were also observed in primary gastric epithelial cells confirming the results obtained in GTL-16 cells.

Conclusions: These results suggest that Grisù® in combination with vitamin D_3 may exert a gastroprotective effect to maintain or restore the integrity of gastric epithelium through an antioxidant pathway, inhibiting apoptosis and activating survival kinases. Moreover, the combination of Grisù® and vitamin D_3 improves cell viability and decreases ROS production compared to other gastroprotective agents combined with vitamin D_3. All these data were validated using primary cells isolated from gastric tissue.

Keywords: Active vitamin D, Gastric acid, Oxidative stress, Gastroprotective drugs

Background

The impact of gastric diseases (for example chronic gastritis, duodenal and gastric ulceration, adenocarcinoma and gastric MALT lymphoma) on human health is a worldwide problem in modern society [1, 2]. For example in the USA, studies have reported gastrointestinal illness rates in the range of 0.5–2 episodes/year/person and incidence of 5–100 episodes/1000/week according to seasons and age. The number of episodes of gastrointestinal illnesses is similar in both 40-year-old studies and in recent ones [3]. Human stomach is extremely vulnerable to various attacks; trauma can cause erosion and mucosal epithelium damage which lead to gastrointestinal tract bleeding and/or ulcer perforation and finally worsen the original disease [4]. The gastrointestinal epithelium is a fundamental barrier protecting the gastrointestinal mucosa from damage against the outside

* Correspondence: francesca.uberti@med.uniupo.it
Laboratory of Physiology, Department of Translational Medicine, University of Piemonte Orientale, via Solaroli 17, Novara 28100, Italy

environment [4]. The cytoprotective functions against damage may be accomplished in the early phase of epithelial repair known as restitution [5–7], which is the ability of epithelial cells to spread and migrate across the basement membrane to repair the damage. This event is the basis of repair of mucosae after injury and is an important element to grant continuity over broad areas within hours [8, 9]. This reparative event occurs rapidly [10]. The damage to gastric mucosa deriving from stress ulcer has been shown in in vivo models to be possibly repaired within 24 h [11]. Gastric acid (HCl) secreted from gastric parietal cells has been reported to determine gastric mucosal injuries such as peptic ulcer and to induce gastropathy [12]. A prolonged exposition to strong acidic environment causes coagulation necrosis resulting from the desiccating action of the acid on proteins in exposed tissues. A mild gastritis condition is often associated with overindulgence in food and alcohol or stress and each episode causes more lasting damage, eventually resulting in cellular injury which in turn causes inflammation [13]. Consequent inflammation produces free radicals which in turn create even more tissue destruction [14, 15] eventually injuring DNA and potentially leading to stomach cancer, which is one of the most lethal malignancies known so far [16]. In addition, HCl enhances the process of lipid peroxidation in gastric mucosa [17]; the dissipation of mitochondrial transmembrane potential thus induces the production of reactive oxygen species (ROS) by mitochondria causing lipid peroxidation [18, 19]. ROS, including H_2O_2, are a major cause of cellular oxidative damage [20] and they play a critical role in the pathogenesis of gastric disorders [2, 21]. Under physiological conditions, gastric epithelium is exposed to high levels of ROS, derived from physical, chemical, or microbiological agents existing in gastric lumen, far higher than in other tissues or biological fluids [22, 23]. Accumulation of intracellular ROS is caused by incomplete reduction of oxygen [24] and this imbalance leads to oxidative stress [24]. H_2O_2 is a stable, small and uncharged molecule, that freely diffuses through cell membranes. An excessive level of H_2O_2 causes apoptosis, necrosis, and other oxidative damages [25]. When the lower esophageal sphincter is weak, the acid unnaturally moves up into the esophagus, causing gastroesophageal reflux disease (GERD), whose cardinal symptom is heartburn, mainly occurring postprandially.

Therapeutic strategies aim at treating both symptoms and epithelial damage with chemical or mechanical approaches. However, a new molecular approach can be hypothesized in order to counteract intracellular mechanisms leading to cell death and to improve epithelial regeneration.

Recently, a crucial role for vitamin D in digestive system health has been described. Low levels of active form of vitamin D ($vitD_3$) are related to poor stomach emptying as well as bloating and constipation or "irritable bowel". Vitamin D links to several target tissues in the digestive system, in the oral region, epithelial cells of the oral cavity, tongue and gingiva, teeth odontoblast and ameloblast precursor pulp and stratum intermedium cells; in the salivary glands: epithelial cells of striated ducts and granular convoluted tubules, intercalated ducts and acinar cells, as well as myoepithelial cells; in the stomach: neck mucous cells of gastric glands, endocrine cells of the antrum, and muscle cells of the pyloric sphincter; in the small and large intestine: absorptive and crypt epithelial cells; in the pancreas, predominantly islet B-cells [26]. In gastric mucosa, vitamin D appears to have high preventive and therapeutic potentials by stimulating cell proliferation and differentiation [27], and is able to regulate endocrine and paracrine secretion of gastrin with secondary effects, for instance on parietal cell HCl and pepsinogen secreting chief cells [26]. In isolated perfused stomach of vitamin D-deficient rats, gastrin and gastric somatostatin secretion is impaired [27]. Moreover, vitamin D_3 has been shown to act on smooth muscle cells in pyloric region and in large areas of small intestine [26]. The activity of vitamin D_3 is mediated by vitamin D receptor (VDR) [28], whose expression has been described in many different tissues including epithelial cells from stomach antrum to duodenum [26]. VDR is a member of the nuclear receptor superfamily which has been shown to be mostly localized in nuclear environment by radiolabeling studies [29], although there is also evidence of their existence in the cytoplasm [30], especially in the absence of ligands and serum in cell culture. Binding its receptor, vitamin D_3 causes a variety of downstream events, including a protective role against oxidative stress [31], regulation of autophagic pathways [32], and the interplay between apoptosis and survival pathways [31]. In this context vitamin D_3 may have beneficial effects on gastric health. For this reason, its use could be of greater efficacy in association with other gastroprotective agents like raft-forming alginates, buffers, polysaccharides and biophenols (Grisù®) when compared to other gastroprotectants (e.g. Maalox® or Gaviscon®).

Since VDR/vitD signaling plays a role in growth control of gastric cells, it can be expected that an adequate vitamin D status is required to achieve benefits not only in cancer prevention but also in many other pathologies. Our aim is to demonstrate whether the active form of vitamin D ($vitD_3$) can act as a protective factor against oxidative stress in cultured gastric epithelial cells in a mutually supportive manner with other gastroprotective agents.

Methods

Cell culture

GTL-16 cell line is a clonal line derived from a poorly differentiated gastric carcinoma cell line [33] and is widely used as a model of gastric epithelial cells. This cell line was donated by the Laboratory of Histology of the University of Eastern Piedmont. Cells were cultured in Dulbecco's Modified Eagle Medium (DMEM) supplemented with 10 % foetal bovine serum (FBS), 1 % penicillin-streptomycin in incubator at 37 °C, 5 % CO_2. The cells for the experiments were plated in a different ways; to study cell viability (MTT test) and cell proliferation (crystal violet staining) $1x10^4$ cells were plated on 96 well-plates; to analyze radical oxygen species (ROS) production $1x10^5$ cells were plated on 24 well-plates; to perform immunohistochemistry studies $0.5x10^4$ cells were placed in Culture Slide (BD, Bedford, MA, U.S.A.) with 4 chambers; to analyze the intracellular pathways through Western blot analysis the cells were plated on 60 mm dishes until confluence. Before stimulations the cells were maintained in DMEM without red phenol and FBS and supplemented with 1 % penicillin/streptomycin, 2 mM L-glutamine and 1 mM sodium pyruvate in an incubator at 37 °C, 5 % CO_2, and 95 % humidity for 18 h. Then the cells were treated with different agents in DMEM without red phenol and supplemented with 0.5 % FBS, 1 % penicillin/streptomycin, 2 mM L-glutamine and 1 mM sodium pyruvate.

Experimental protocol

The cells were used to study two different biological aspects. In the first set of experiments, the influence of a new alginate preparation (Grisù®) alone or in combination with 100 nM vitD_3 on cellular adhesion was analyzed by measuring adhesion time through crystal violet assay and vitronectin/fibronectin staining by Western Blot. In this case the agents were used to coat the plates or chamber-slides for 20 min in incubator at 37 °C before seeding the cells. The adhesion time of GTL-16 (a specific number of cells) was checked from 2 min to 720 min (2 min, 5 min, 15 min, 30 min, 60 min, 90 min, 240 min, 720 min) [34]. In the absence of coating, the cells were adherent until 3–5 h.

In the second set of experiments the same agents were added directly in the cells plated for the experimental protocol without coating. Maalox®, Gaviscon® and a proton pump inhibitor (PPI) were tested in the preliminary experiments alone or in combination with 100 nM vitD_3 to compare the efficacy to Grisù® alone or in combination with 100 nM vitD_3 on cell viability. In addition, all these agents were also tested in presence of 200 μM H_2O_2 or HCl to determine the effects during oxidative stress or gastric acidity. The time of stimulation was from 15 min to 24 h (15 min, 30 min, 60 min, 90 min, 3 h, 24 h). Since the maximum effect was observed after 1 h of treatment this condition was maintained for all successive experiments. Moreover, Maalox®, Gaviscon® and PPI had negative effects on cell viability which were more important in presence of H_2O_2 or HCl. In the successive experiments these agents were not tested.

Agents preparations

Grisù® is a dietary supplement that combines the properties of calcium alginate in a buffer solution, resulting from alkaline salts useful to counteract situations of high acidity, with a tyndalized probiotic (Pylopass®) and an extract of prickly pear and olive leaves (Mucosave®): the extract of prickly pear is useful for its emollient and soothing characteristics at the level of the digestive system.

Grisù®, composed by Mucosave® (0.83 mg/ml), calcium alginate (1.66 mg/ml), magnesium hydroxide (2.66 mg/ml), potassium citrate (4.66 mg/ml) and Pylopass™ (0.66 mg/ml), was dissolved according to solubility reported in manufacturer's instructions, directly in the DMEM without red phenol and FBS but supplemented with 1 % penicillin/streptomycin, 2 mM L-glutamine and 1 mM sodium pyruvate when used for the adhesion study. Instead for the second set of experiments Grisù®, Maalox®, Gaviscon® and PPI were dissolved directly in the medium used for stimulations respecting the solubility reported in manufacturer's instructions. In both sets of experiments, the solutions were used without dilutions. The active form of vitamin D (1,25-dihydroxyvitamin D_3, catalog number: D1530, Sigma-Aldirch, Milan, Italy) was prepared in absolute ethanol at 10^{-3} M and used at final concentration of 100 nM prepared directly in medium. The percentage of ethanol was less than 0.001 %. HCl was used to prepare an acidified medium (pH 4) and added to the cells without dilution.

MTT test

At the end of each stimulation, MTT-based In Vitro Toxicology Assay Kit (Sigma-Aldrich) was used to determine cell viability, as previously described [31]. Cells were incubated with 1 % MTT dye for 2 h at 37 °C in incubator, and then, the purple formazan crystals were dissolved in equal volume of MTT Solubilization Solution. Cell viability was determined by measuring the absorbance through a spectrometer (VICTORX3 Multilabel Plate Reader) at 570 nm with correction at 690 nm, and calculated by comparing results to control cells (100 % viable).

Crystal violet staining

The cells treated with Grisù® alone or in combination with vitD_3 were also analyzed by crystal violet staining

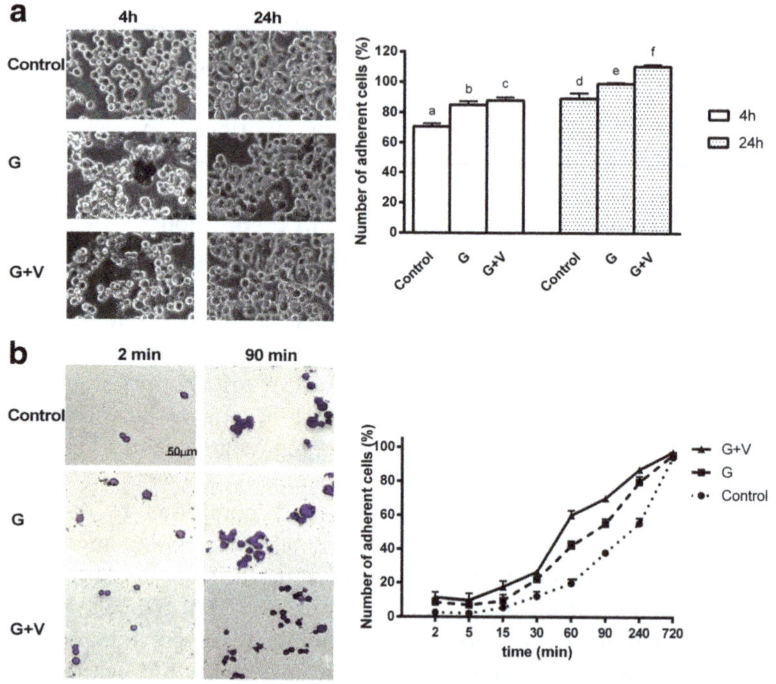

Fig. 1 Adhesion time analysis of GTL-16. In **a** on the left, optical microscopy images of adherent GTL-16 taken at original magnification 20X. On the right, the number of adherent cells for each treatment is reported. The ratio reports a mean ± (SD) (%) of adherent cells counted in 12 different areas. Data reported are means of 5 biological replicates. G = Grisù®; G + V = co-stimulation with Grisù® and vitD_3. b, c, d $p < 0.05$ *vs* a; a, f, e $p < 0.05$ *vs* d; e $p < 0.05$ *vs* b; f $p < 0.05$ *vs* c. In **b** on the left, optical microscopy images of the cells treated with Grisù® alone or in combination with vitD_3 after 2 min and 90 min are shown. The scale reported in the first picture is to be considered valid for all images. On the right, the cell counting of adherent cells during time (at 2 min, 5 min, 15 min, 30 min, 60 min, 90 min, 240 min, 720 min) is reported. The ratio reports a mean ± (SD) (%) of adherent cells counted in 12 different areas of 5 biological replicates. The abbreviations are the same reported in **a**. All samples are significant $p < 0.05$ *vs* control

to study adhesion. GTL-16 cells at the end of each time-point were fixed with 1 % glutaraldehyde for 15 min at RT, washed and stained with 100 μl of 0.1 % crystal violet for 20 min at RT. The multi-well plates were rinsed, dry and the images of adherent aqueous cells were taken and analyzed by ImageJ software. To obtain cell number estimation 100 μl of 10 % acetic acid were added and mixed before reading the absorbance at 595 nm through a spectrometer (VICTORX3 Multilabel Plate Reader). The number estimation was calculated by comparing results to the control cells (Control T0).

ROS production

The rate of superoxide anion release was measured using a standard protocol [31] and determined as a superoxide dismutase-inhibitable reduction of cytochrome C. In both treated and untreated cells, 100 μl of cytochrome C were added, and in another sample, 100 μL of superoxide dismutase were also added for 30 min in incubator (all substances from Sigma-Aldrich). The absorbance was measured at 550 nm in a spectrometer (VICTORX3 Multilabel Plate Reader) and the O_2 was expressed as means ± SD% of nanomoles per reduced cytochrome C per microgram of protein compared to control [35].

Western Blot

GTL-16 cells were lysed in iced Complete Tablet Buffer (Roche) supplemented with 2 mM sodium orthovanadate and 35 μg of proteins resolved on 15 or 5 % SDS-PAGE

Table 1 Cell counting of crystal violet staining

Time (min)	Control	G	G + V
2	2.67 ± 1.63	8.5 ± 2.12 [a]	11.33 ± 3.05 [a]
5	2.17 ± 0.98	7 ± 2.83	9.67 ± 4.04 [a]
15	5.5 ± 2.38	9.5 ± 3.54	17.5 ± 3.54 [a]
30	12 ± 2.83	22 ± 2.83 [a]	26.5 ± 0.71 [a]
60	19.67 ± 2.52	42 ± 2.84 [a]	60 ± 2.83 [a]
90	38 ± 2	55 ± 3 [a]	70 ± 2 [a]
240	55.33 ± 3.05	79.67 ± 3.215 [a]	87 ± 2 [a]
720	94.33 ± 2.082	95.68 ± 1.528	97.33 ± 1.15

Data are shown as a mean ± (SD) (%) of adherent cells counted in 12 different areas of 4 technical replicates. [a] $p < 0.05$ vs control. The abbreviations are the same described in figure legends

gels. Polyvinylidene fluoride membranes (PVDF, GE Healthcare Europe GmbH, Milan, Italy) were incubated overnight at 4 °C with specific primary antibody: anti-phospho-ERK$^{Thr202/Tyr204}$ (1:1000, Cell-SIgnaling), anti-VDR (1:250, Santa-Cruz), anti-Annexin V (1:1000, Sigma), anti-Beclin1 (1:250, Santa-Cruz), anti-Caspase 8 (1:400, Sigma), anti-Bax (1:200, Santa-Cruz), anti-Vitronectin (1:250, Santa-Cruz) and anti-Fibronectin

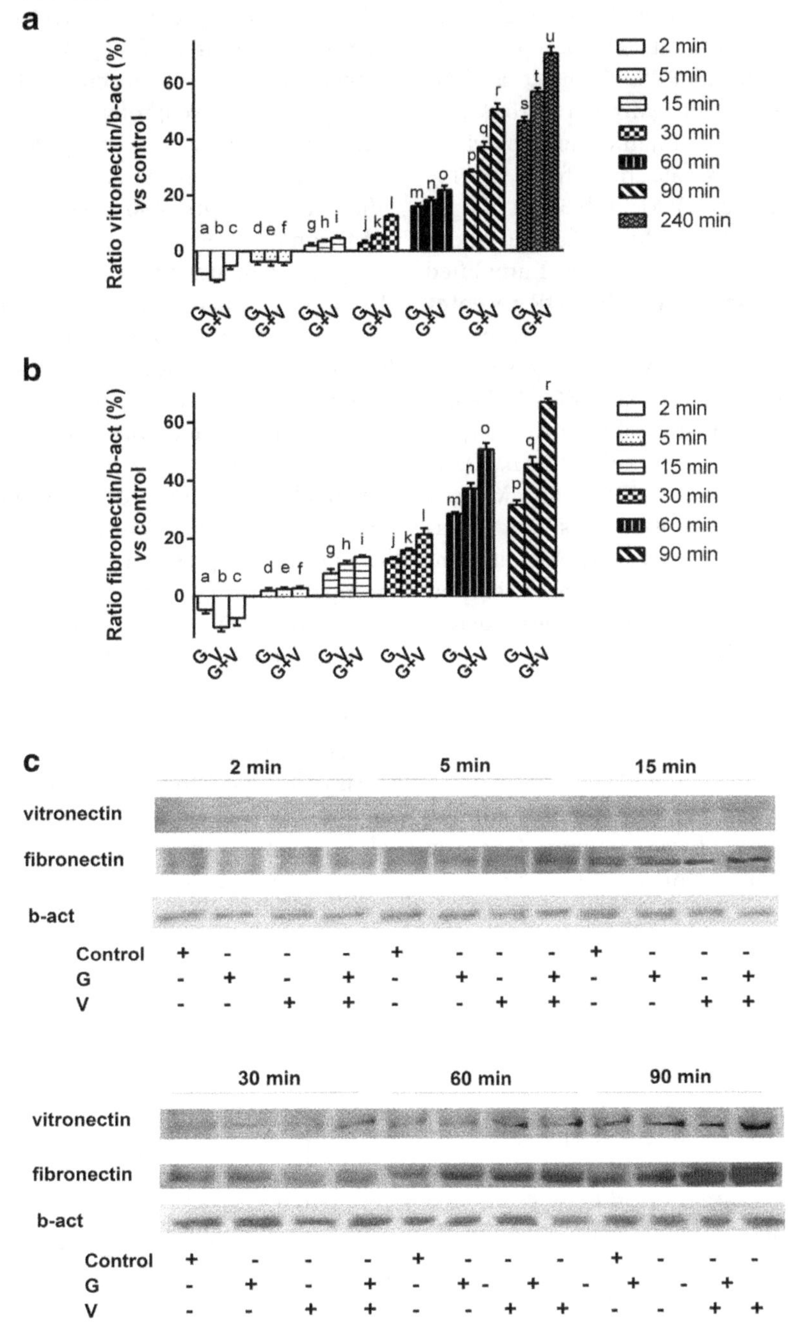

Fig. 2 Western blot and densitometric analysis of vitronectin and fibronectin. G = Grisù®; V = vitD$_3$; G + V = Grisù® combined with vitD$_3$. The ratio reports a mean ± (SD) (%) of 5 biological replicates normalized to control values (line 0 %). In **a** densitometric analysis of vitronectin normalized to control values during time (from 2 to 240 min). a, b, c, d, e, f, h, i, j, k, l, m, n, o, p, q, r, s, t, u $p < 0.05$ *vs* control; a, b $p < 0.05$ *vs* c; e $p < 0.05$ *vs* f; i $p < 0.05$ *vs* g; j, k $p < 0.05$ *vs* l; m, n, $p < 0.05$ *vs* o; p, q $p < 0.05$ vs r; s, t $p < 0.05$ *vs* u. In **b** densitometric analysis of fibronectin normalized to control values during time (from 2 to 90 min). d, e, f, g, h, i, j, k, l, m, n, o, p, q, r $p < 0.05$ *vs* control; g, h $p < 0.05$ *vs* i; j, k $p < 0.05$ *vs* l; m, n $p < 0.05$ *vs* o; p, q $p < 0.05$ *vs* r. In **c** an example of Western blot of protein extracts analyzed by immunoblotting with specific antibodies against the indicated proteins

(1:250, Abcam, UK). The protein expressions were normalized and verified through β-actin detection (1:5000; Sigma, Milan, Italy).

Immunocytochemistry

The cells cultured in chamber slides were fixed using an iced fixative solution (3.7 % formaldehyde, 3 % sucrose in PBS 1X) for 20 min at RT, permeabilized with ice 0.5 % Triton X-100 in PBS 1X in ice at 4 °C for 20 min, incubated with 3 % hydrogen peroxide in PBS 1X for 8 min and then maintained in a blocking solution (PBS 1X with 3 % albumin from bovine serum-BSA, Sigma, Milan, Italy) for 1 h in at RT, as previously described [36]. After this time the slides were incubated overnight at 4 °C in a humidified chamber with specific primary antibody VDR receptor (1:50). Then chamber slides were incubated before with diluted biotinylated secondary antibody solution (Dako Italia, Milan, Italy), then with VECTASTAIN® ABC Reagent (Dako Italia, Milan, Italy), and finally in peroxidase substrate solution (Peroxidase/DAB, Dako Italia, Milan, Italy), and counterstained with Mayer's hematoxylin. The number of positive cells was calculated as described elsewhere [37]; briefly, 12 different areas (1 mm^2) randomly selected from each section were taken, and the number of signals was determined using ImagePro 3 software (NIH, Bethesda, US). The results are expressed as means ± SD (%).

Statistical analysis

Results are expressed as means ± SD of at least 5 biological replicates for each experimental protocol and each replicate was reproduced 3 times. One-way ANOVA followed by Bonferroni post hoc test was used for statistical analysis. Mann-Whitney U test was used to compare percentages of responses. *P*-value <0.05 was considered statistically significant.

Results

Influence of Grisù® alone or in combination with vitD$_3$ on adhesion capacity

Grisù® acts as a physical barrier for gastric epithelial cells and protects against hyperacidity. The first set of experiments was performed because of a difference in cell adhesion after 4 h in the sample treated with Grisù® (85.17 ± 2.25 %) compared to control (70.63 ± 2.12 %, $p < 0.05$) (Fig. 1a). This augmented number of adherent cells was more evident after 24 h (99.2 ± 0.72 % compared to control 89.33 ± 3.51 %). The presence of vitD$_3$ improves this effect (at 4 h 88.07 ± 2.1 %; at 24 h 110.6 ± 1.25 %). Since this time is more suitable to explain the influence of Grisù®, the time-point was changed and Grisù® alone or in combination with vitD$_3$ was used to coat the plates. As reported in Fig. 1b and Table 1, in crystal violet staining, the number of adherent GTL-16 cells was time-dependent and in presence of Grisù® alone significantly increased ($p < 0.05$) starting from 2 min after seeding (8.5 ± 2.12 % compared to control 2.67 ± 1.63 %). This increase was enhanced in presence of vitD$_3$ (of about 33 % compared to Grisù® alone, $p < 0.05$). All these effects were more evident in the course of time ($p < 0.05$) and after 12 h almost all of the cells were attached ($p < 0.05$). Vitronectin and Fibronectin, two extracellular matrix glycoproteins well-known to be involved in adhesion, were analyzed by Western Blot, to explain the mechanism involved. As reported in Fig. 2a and c, Vitronectin expression assessed by Western blot and densitometric analysis, showed an increase in a time-dependent manner and the presence of Grisù® starting from 15 min was able to improve this expression (1.93 ± 0.9 %, $p < 0.05$) compared to control. The presence of co-stimulation with vitD$_3$ was able to amplify the effect of Grisù® alone starting from 15 min (4.69 ± 0.65 %) and this amplified effect was maintained for the entire test time, being evident at 90 min ($p < 0.05$) compared to Grisù® alone (of about 78 %). The effect of vitD$_3$ alone was also analyzed, but did not show a significant increase on vitronectin expression up to 60 min (18.06 ± 1 % compared to control), thus showing the significant ability of vitD$_3$ to improve the effect of Grisù®. The administration of Grisù® combined with vitD$_3$ after 4 h treatment was able to improve the Vitronectin expression according to the data observed in crystal violet staining ($p < 0.05$).

Similar time-dependent effects were also observed in Fibronectin expression, in GTL-16 treated with Grisù® alone or in combination with vitD$_3$, confirming the role of vitD$_3$ in modulating the capacity of Grisù®. These data obtained by Western Blot and densitometric analysis are shown in Fig. 2b and c.

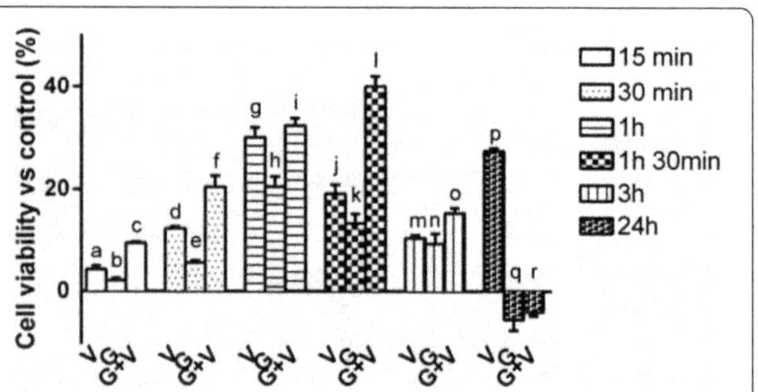

Fig. 3 Time course of cell viability in GTL-16. The effects of vitD$_3$ (V), Grisù® (G) and Grisù® combined with vitD$_3$ (G + V) *vs* control (line 0 %) from 15 min to 24 h are reported. Data represent as a mean ± (SD) (%) of 6 biological replicates. a, b, c, d, e, f, g, j, k, l, m, n, o, p; $p < 0.05$ *vs* control; a, b $p < 0.05$ *vs* c; c, d, e $p < 0.05$ *vs* f; c, f, h $p < 0.05$ *vs* i; i, j, k, o, r $p < 0.05$ *vs* l; n $p < 0.05$ *vs* o; o, p $p < 0.05$ *vs* r

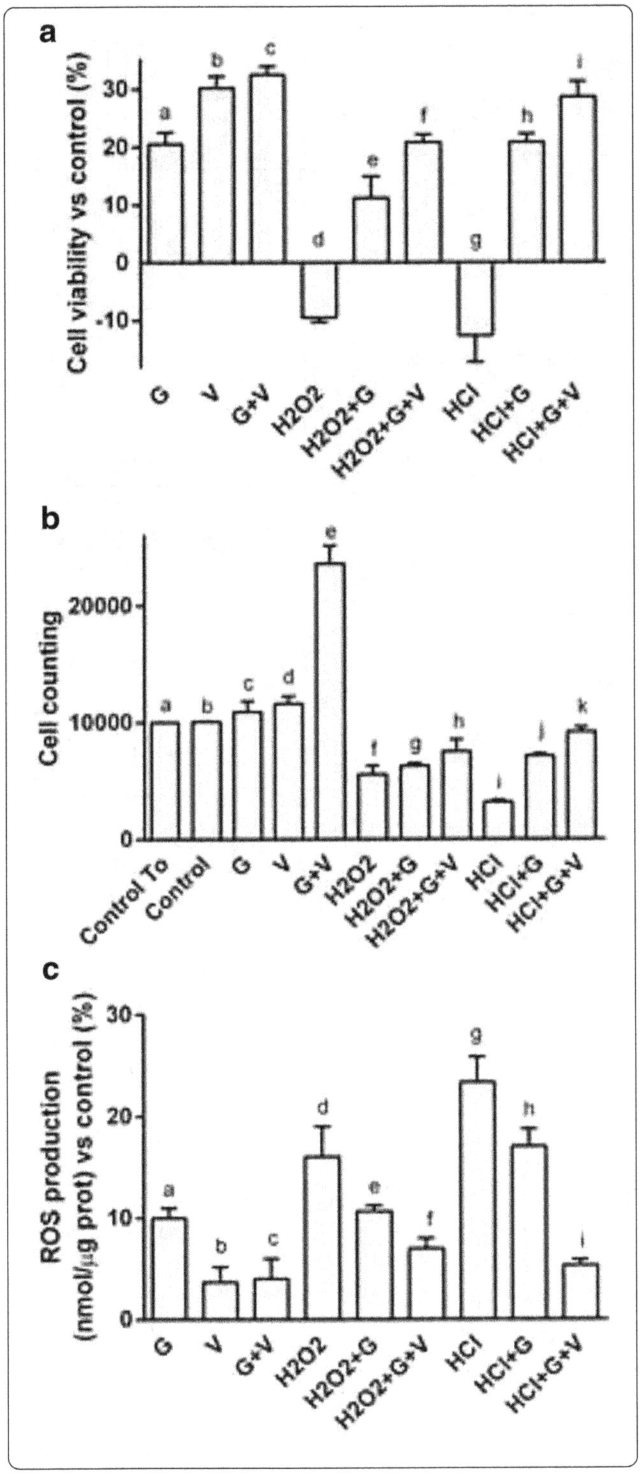

Fig. 4 Effects of Grisù® alone or in combination with vitD$_3$ during acidity and oxidative stress. G = Grisù®; V = vitD$_3$; G + V = Grisù® combined with vitD$_3$. Data represent a mean ± (SD) (%) of 6 biological replicates. In **a** cell viability: a, b, c, d, e, f, g, h, i $p < 0.05$ *vs* control (line 0 %); c $p < 0.05$ *vs* a; e, f $p < 0.05$ *vs* d; f $p < 0.05$ *vs* e; h, i $p < 0.05$ *vs* g; i $p < 0.05$ *vs* h; i $p < 0.05$ *vs* f. In **b** cell counting: c, d, e, f, g, h, i, j $p < 0.05$ *vs* control; e $p < 0.05$ *vs* c; e $p < 0.05$ *vs* d; h $p < 0.05$ *vs* g; h $p < 0.05$ *vs* f; k, j $p < 0.05$ *vs* i; k $p < 0.05$ *vs* j; k $p < 0.05$ *vs* h. In **c** ROS production: a, c, d, e, f, g, h, i, $p < 0.05$ *vs* control (line 0 %); c, b $p < 0.05$ *vs* a; f, e $p < 0.05$ *vs* d; f $p < 0.05$ *vs* e; i, k $p < 0.05$ *vs* g; i $p < 0.05$ *vs* h

Mechanisms induced on cultured GTL-16 cells by Grisù® alone or in combination with vitD$_3$

MTT test was performed on a time-course study to determine the best stimulation time for the influence of Grisù® alone or in presence of 100 nM vitD$_3$ on cell viability. As reported in Fig. 3, the maximum effect of Grisù® alone was observed after 1 h of stimulation (20.55 ± 1.99 %, $p < 0.05$) and in presence of vitD$_3$ this effect was amplified of about 58 %, ($p < 0.05$). For this reason, this time of stimulation was maintained for all successive experiments.

In order to clarify the efficacy of Grisù® alone and in combination with 100 nM vitD$_3$ on cell viability, on cell proliferation and on ROS production in gastroprotection, all the following experiments were performed in presence or absence of pretreatment for 30 min with 200 μM H_2O_2 or HCl. As reported in Fig. 4 the pretreatment for 30 min with 200 μM H_2O_2 or HCl caused a significant reduction ($p < 0.05$) of cell viability and cell proliferation and increased ROS production ($p < 0.05$) compared to control. Grisù® alone was able to counteract the negative effects exerted by H_2O_2 or HCl on cell viability, cell proliferation and ROS production ($p < 0.05$); in particular, the most evident beneficial effects were observed in reversing the influence exerted by HCl. In presence of the combination with 100 nM vitD$_3$ the beneficial effects were amplified ($p < 0.05$) maintaining the efficacy in counteracting the influence of HCl. The apoptotic (in particular Annexin V, Bax, Caspase 8), autophagic (Beclin 1) and survival (ERK/MAPK) pathways were investigated to explain the intracellular mechanisms involved in the protective actions induced by Grisù® alone or in combination with 100 nM vitD$_3$. In addition, the VDR receptor was analyzed to study the role of vitD$_3$ in all these effects. Western blot and densitometric analysis (Fig. 5 and Additional file 1) showed a significant increase of Annexin V, Bax and caspase-8 expressions ($p < 0.05$) compared to control in presence of pretreatment with 200 μM hH_2O_2 or HCl alone and the maximum effects were observed with HCl. On the contrary the markers of autophagy and survival pathways were maintained at a basal level. Either Grisù® or vitD$_3$

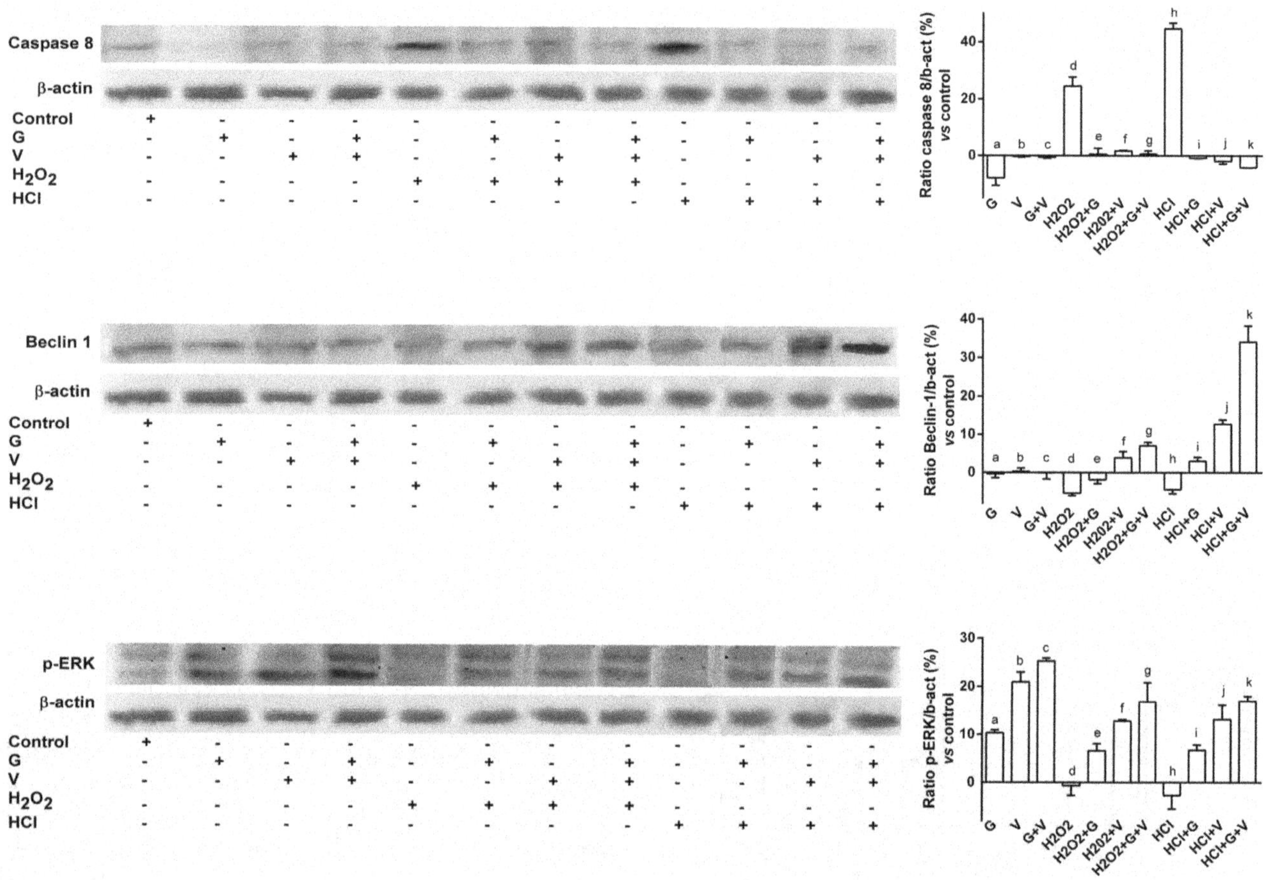

Fig. 5 Western blot and densitometric analysis of apoptotic, autophagic and survival pathways. The images and data reported are obtained from 5 biological replicates. G = Grisù®; V = vitD_3; G + V = Grisù® combined with vitD_3. Densitometric analysis are expressed as means ± (SD) (%) normalized to control values (defined as 0 %). Caspase 8 $p < 0.05$: a, d, h, k *vs* control; e, f, g *vs* d; g *vs* k; f, j *vs* b; a, k *vs* c; i, j, k *vs* h; c, i, j *vs* k; e, j *vs* a. Beclin $p < 0.05$: d, f, g, h, j, k *vs* control; g, k *vs* c; e, f, g *vs* d; e, k *vs* g; f, j *vs* b; i, j, k *vs* h; i, j *vs* k; i *vs* a. ERK: a, b, c, e, f, g, i. j, k *vs* control; e *vs* g; i *vs* k; a, g, k *vs* c; e, f, g *vs* d; i, j, k *vs* h; f, j *vs* b; e, i *vs* a

alone caused an increase in ERK1/2 and VDR expression compared to control ($p < 0.05$). The combination of Grisù® and vitD_3 amplified ($p < 0.05$) the effects on ERK1/2 and VDR expressions (25.26 ± 0.64 % and 39.12 ± 3.46 %, respectively) compared to Grisù® (10.31 ± 0.59 % and 0.33 ± 1.15 %, respectively) or vitD_3 alone (20.96 ± 2.05 % and 29.48 ± 1.34 %, respectively). The same stimulations performed after the treatments with 200 μM H_2O_2 or HCl, were able to reverse the negative effects acting on the expression of ERK1/2 and Beclin 1; in particular the combination of Grisù® and vitD_3 was able to amplify the activation of autophagic and survival pathways. In addition, this combination was able to improve the reduction of the apoptotic marker, such as Annexin V, Bax and caspase 8.

Finally, the involvement of VDR in the beneficial effects above described was also confirmed by immunocytochemical staining (Fig. 6) and by Western Blot analysis (Additional file 1).

The effects of combination of Grisù® and vitD_3 were compared to other gastroprotective agents on cell viability and ROS production, to confirm their ability to protect the epithelial gastric cells from oxidative stress or acidity injury. As reported in Fig. 7, the combination of Grisù® with vitD_3 was able to induce the maximal beneficial effects on cell viability and ROS production compared to other gastroprotective agents alone (Maalox®, Gaviscon® or PPI, $p < 0.05$). In addition, in presence of oxidative stress caused by H_2O_2 or HCl acidified medium, the combination of Grisù® with vitD_3 was able to positively modulate these negative conditions and significantly reduce ROS production. This effect was significantly better if compared to Maalox®, Gaviscon® and PPI.

In some additional tests, vitD_3 was added to other gastroprotective agents (Maalox®, Gaviscon® and PPI) and the effects have been compared to those induced by Grisù® combined with vitD_3. As shown in Fig. 7, Grisù®

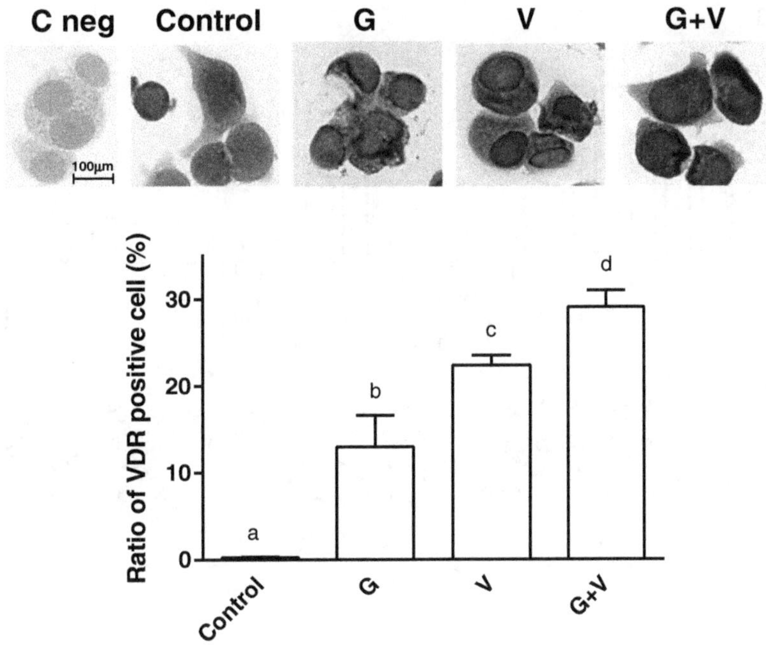

Fig. 6 Study of VDR by immunocytochemistry staining. G = Grisù®; V = vitD3; G + V = co-stimulation with Grisù® and vitD3. b, c, d $p < 0.05$ *vs* control; b, c $p < 0.05$ *vs* d. The images were taken by optical microscopy at original magnification 20X. Data reported are expressed as means ± (SD) (%) of 5 biological replicates

with vitD$_3$ showed greater effectiveness to counteract the negative effects of oxidative stress and acidity condition on cell viability and ROS release compared to other gastroprotectants.

Similar data were also observed in primary gastric cell cultures, where Grisù® with vitD$_3$ was able to counteract more effectively than other gastroprotectants, the negative effects of oxidative and acidic stress.

Validation in primary epithelial cells

Further experiments were carried out in primary gastric epithelial cells, in order to confirm previously obtained results about the protective effects exerted by Grisù® alone or combined with vitD$_3$ during oxidative and acidity injury. Method used to isolate the primary cell cultures is described in Additional file 2. Other methods were the same used in GTL-16 cells experiments. Some results on primary gastric cells were reported in Additional file 2. Particularly, the improvement of adhesion properties induced by Grisù® combined with vitD$_3$; the beneficial effects on cell viability and ROS production in counteracting H_2O_2 or HCl oxidative injury; the involvement of survival kinase in preventing apoptosis, are shown.

Here are reported two of most important effects of Grisù alone and combined with vitD$_3$ on cell viability and ROS production. As reported in Fig. 8a the time-course study confirms that Grisù® alone and Grisù® combined with vitD$_3$ are able to enhance cell viability in similar manner to what observed in GTL-16. The maximum effect was observed after 1 h 30 min ($p < 0.05$). So, time of stimulation was maintained for all subsequent experiments. Finally, in primary gastric cells have been also confirmed the efficacy of Grisù® alone and combined with vitD$_3$ compared to others gastroprotectants to prevent the damage induced by oxidative stress and acidity. As reported in Fig. 8b, vitD$_3$ can modulate the negative effects on ROS production only in presence of Grisù®. This effect was also observed in GTL-16 cells. Therefore, it can be hypothesized that Grisù® could act like a substrate capable of promoting the effects of vitD$_3$.

Discussion

The integrity of gastrointestinal epithelium and mucosa is known to be maintained by a number of secreted factors [38] and mediated by rapid proliferation and migration of mucosal epithelial cells [4] to resurface epithelial defects after various forms of mucosal epithelium injury [4] and to establish a barrier against the stress inducers. As reported in literature in several in vitro and in vivo studies, these factors protect gastric mucosal epithelium from a variety of noxious agents, including bacterial toxins, chemicals and drugs [4]. Epithelial migration, which is a fundamental phase in the healing process after gastric ulcer, is characterized by complex alterations

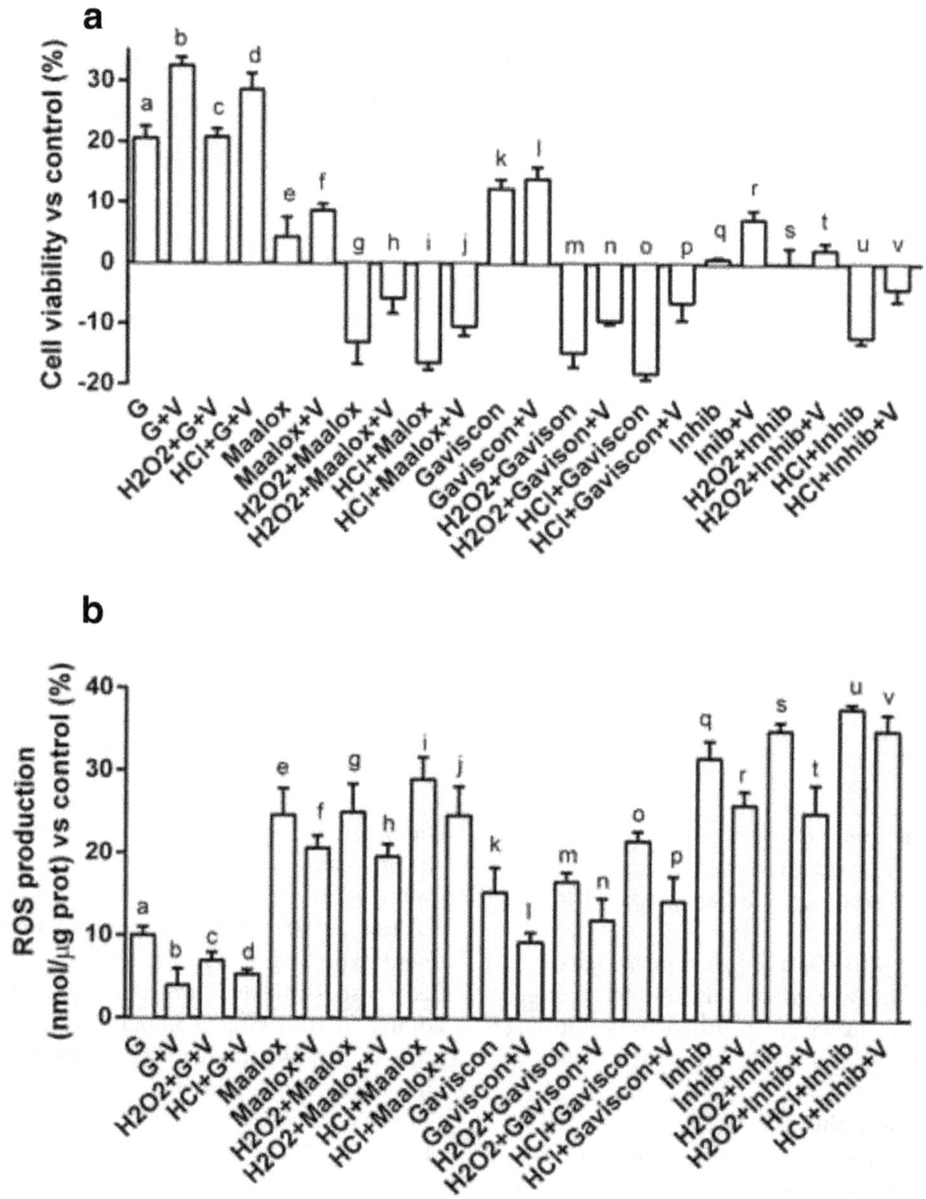

Fig. 7 Cell viability and ROS production in GTL-16 treated with other gastroprotectants with vitD_3. G = Grisù®; V = vitD_3; G + V = co-stimulation with Grisù® and vitD_3. Data reported are expressed as means ± (SD) (%) of 5 biological replicates. In **a**: a, b, c, d, f, g, h, i, j, k, l, m, n, o, p, r, u, v $p < 0.05$ *vs* control (line 0 %); b, d, e, f, g, h, i, j, k, l, m, n, o, p, q, r, s, t, u, v $p < 0.05$ *vs* a; a, c, e, f, g, h, i, j, k, l, m, n, o, p, q, r, s, t, u, v $p < 0.05$ *vs* b; g, h, m, n, s, t $p < 0.05$ *vs* c; i, j, o, p, u, v $p < 0.05$ *vs* d; g, h, i, j $p < 0.05$ *vs* e; h, j, $p < 0.05$ *vs* f; m, n, o, p $p < 0.05$ *vs* k; n, p $p < 0.05$ *vs* l; r, u, v $p < 0.05$ *vs* q. In **b**: a, c, e, f, g, h, i, j, k, l, m, n, o, p, q, r, s, t, u, v $p < 0.05$ *vs* control (line 0 %); b, e, f, g, h, i, j, m, o, q, r, s, t, u, v $p < 0.05$ *vs* a; e, f, g, h, i, j, k, m, n, o, p, q, r, s, t, u, v $p < 0.05$ *vs* b; g, h, m, s, t $p < 0.05$ *vs* c; i, j, o, p, u, v $p < 0.05$ *vs* d; o $p < 0.05$ *vs* k; t, u $p < 0.05$ *vs* q; v $p < 0.05$ *vs* r

in adhesion between cells and the extracellular matrix [39]. In this study the effects of vitD_3 on an in vitro experimental model of gastric cells have been observed. Findings of this work demonstrate that vitD_3 can exert beneficial effect on gastric cells in terms of improved viability and adhesivity or reduced ROS production. Moreover, this study permits to demonstrate that Grisù® alone is able to improve the adhesivity of cells, reducing the time of action (starting from 2 min from seeding, also measured by cell counting) but this effect is amplified by the presence of vitD_3. Moreover, we have found out that this effect is crucial on cells migration and that two important extracellular matrix glycoproteins, Vitronectin and Fibronectin, are involved in this effect mediated by Grisù® both alone and in presence of vitD_3. This consideration is even more important because it indicates

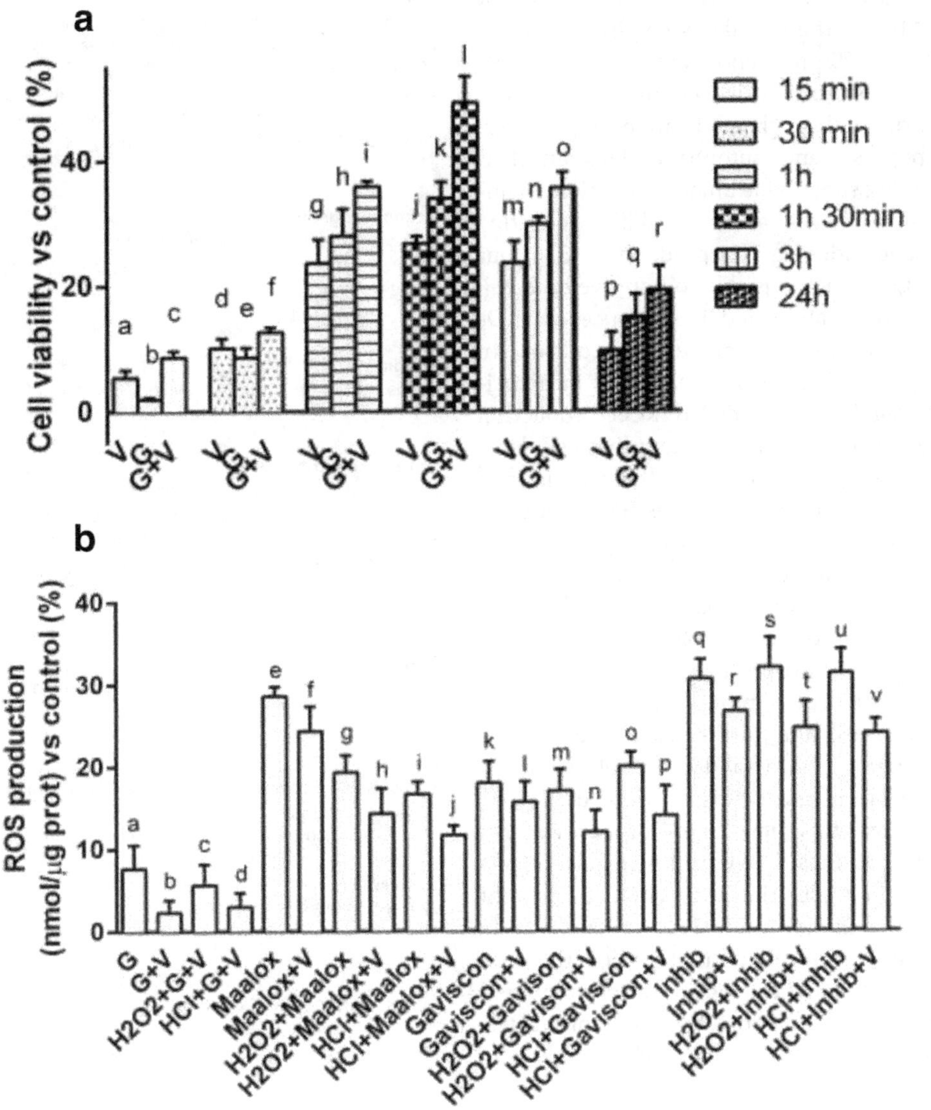

Fig. 8 Time-course of cell viability and ROS production in primary gastric cells. In **a** primary gastric cells treated with Grisù® alone or combined with vitD_3 analyzed at 15 min, 30 min, 1 h, 1 h 30 min, 3 h, and 24 h. V = vitD_3; G = Grisù®; G + V = Grisù® combined with vitD_3. Data are reported as means ± (SD) (%) of 3 biological replicates. a, c, d, e, f, g, h, i, j, k, l, m, n, o, p, q, r $p < 0.05$ *vs* control (line 0 %); c $p < 0.05$ *vs* b; g, h $p < 0.05$ *vs* i; j, k $p < 0.05$ *vs* l; m $p < 0.05$ *vs* o; p $p < 0.05$ *vs* r. In **b** the effect on ROS production of Grisù® combined with vitD_3 was compared to the effects of different gastroprotectants alone and with vitD_3. The results are expressed as means ± (SD) (%) of 3 biological replicates. G = Grisù®; V = vitD_3; G + V = Grisù® combined with vitD_3. a, e, f, g, h, i, j, k, l, m, n, o, p, q, r, s, t, u, v $p < 0.05$ *vs* control (line 0 %); e, f, g, h, i, k, l, m, o, p, q, r, s, t, u, v $p < 0.05$ *vs* a; e, f, g, h, i, j, k, l, m, n, o, p, q, r, s, t, u, v $p < 0.05$ *vs* b; g, h, m, n, t $p < 0.05$ *vs* c; i, j, o, p, u, v $p < 0.05$ *vs* d; g, h, i, j $p < 0.05$ *vs* e; h, j $p < 0.05$ *vs* f; v $p < 0.05$ *vs* q

that vitD_3 is able to improve the beneficial effects induced by alginates, thus supporting data about the mechanism of gastroprotection induced by alginates [40]. This hypothesis is also supported by other in vitro studies where VDR activation has been shown not only to enhance intracellular junctions but also to promote mucosal wound repair and to mediate the activity of vitD_3 thus inducing junction proteins expression [41]. As observed by Miyazaki et al., the reparative events following acute gastric injury occur rapidly [10]. There is evidence that oxidative stress plays an important role in the pathogenesis of acute gastric injury [42–44]. For example, the role of oxidative stress in gastrointestinal pathogenesis was first described in acute intestinal injury in ischemia/reperfusion models [42]. Following studies suggested that ROS are generally involved in acute injury of the gastrointestinal tract [43, 44]. It is noteworthy that experimental evidence shows how ROS production or superoxide (O_2^-) are induced both by cellular exposure to an alkaline environment and/or by acid injury [12, 44]. All these findings confirm the cytotoxic action both of ROS production and of acidic exposure leading to cells apoptosis. It is well known that $vitD_3$ may prevent cell death through modulation of the interplay between apoptosis and autophagy. This effect is obtained by inhibiting superoxide anion generation, maintaining mitochondria function and cell viability, activating survival kinases, and inducing NO production [31]. Our results show that Grisù® alone is able to improve both cell viability and cell proliferation and in presence of $vitD_3$ these effects are increased compared to control. In addition, after H_2O_2 or HCl exposure, Grisù® in association with $vitD_3$ significantly reduced ROS production and decreased cell viability loss, suggesting that cell damage and cytotoxicity can be prevented by the combination of Grisù® with $vitD_3$. These results suggest that Grisù® in combination with $vitD_3$ may exert a better gastroprotective effect through an antioxidant pathway, inhibiting apoptosis and activating survival kinases. Such effect was stronger in preventing epithelial damage than what observed using other gastroprotective agents such as Gaviscon®, Maalox® or proton pump inhibitors.

Since GTL-16 is a cell line, further experiments were carried out in primary cells to validate the observed results. Cells isolated from gastric tissue were used. The results obtained from this new series of experiments have allowed us to significantly confirm beneficial effects of Grisù®, alone or in association with $vitD_3$, to prevent the oxidative and acid injury.

In conclusion, this work demonstrates for the first time that $vitD_3$ has a beneficial effect when combined with an alginate-based gastroprotector agent on gastric epithelial cells, joining the effects of a mechanical barrier with the modulation of intracellular pathways in order to maintain or restore the integrity of gastric epithelium.

Conclusion

These in vitro results suggest that Grisù® in combination with $vitD_3$ may exert a gastroprotective effect to maintain or restore the integrity of gastric epithelium through an antioxidant pathway, inhibiting apoptosis and activating survival kinases better than other gastroprotective agents.

However, further in vivo or research will be necessary in order to assess, with histological and immunocytochemical methods, the efficacy of Grisù® and $vitD_3$ on gastric mucosa undergoing oxidative and/or acidic stress. The experimental data could thus provide a basis for the execution of clinical studies.

The combination of Grisù® with $vitD_3$ significantly decreased the reactive oxygen species production and decreased cell viability loss, suggesting that cell damage and cytotoxicity can be reduced.

Abbreviation

BSA: Albumin from bovine serum; DMEM: Dulbecco's Modified Eagle's medium; FBS: Fetal bovine serum; GERD: Gastroesophageal reflux disease; MALT: Mucose-associated lymphoid tissue; MTT: 3-(4,5-dimethylthiazol-2-yl)-2,5-diphenyltetrazolium bromide; NO: Nitric oxide; PBS: Phosphate-buffered saline; PPI: Proton Pump inhibitor; ROS: Reactive oxygen species; VDR: Vitamin D receptor; $vitD_3$: Vitamin D_3

Acknowledgements

Authors thank Dr. Mariangela Fortunato for her precious help with language. Laborest S.r.l (particularly Dr. Lorenzo Secondini) contributed to the study by donating Grisù®.

Funding

Funds derived from private donations to author's laboratory.

Authors' contributions

FU designed the study, performed the experiments, analyzed the data and wrote the manuscript; CB performed some experiments; VM performed some experiments and analyzed the data; SG analyzed the data and drew the figures; CM provided a major contribution in revising the manuscript. All authors read and approved the final manuscript.

Competing interests

The authors declare that they have no competing interests.

References

1. Boland CR, Luciani MG, Gasche C, Goel A. Infection, inflammation, and gastrointestinal cancer. Gut. 2005;54:1321–31.
2. Hu XT, Ding C, Zhou N, Xu C. Quercetin protects gastric epithelial cell from oxidative damage *in vitro* and *in vivo*. Eur J Pharmacol. 2015;754:115–24.
3. Payment P, Hunter PR. Endemic and epidemic infectious intestinal disease and its relationship to drinking water. Water Quality: Guidelines, Standards and Health. In: Lorna Fewtrell and Jamie Bartram. IWA Publishing, London: 2001. p. 61-88.
4. Sun Z, Liu H, Yang Z, Shao D, Zhang W, Ren Y, et al. Intestinal trefoil factor activates the PI3K/Akt signaling pathway to protect gastric mucosal epithelium from damage. Int J Oncol. 2014;45:1123–32.
5. Podolsky DK. Mucosal immunity and inflammation. V. Innate mechanisms of mucosal defense and repair: the best offense is a good defense. Am J Physiol. 1999;277:G495–9.
6. Wright NA. Aspects of the biology of regeneration and repair in the human gastrointestinal tract. Philos Trans R Soc Lond B Biol Sci. 1998;353:925–33.
7. Podolsky DK. Healing the epithelium: solving the problem from two sides. J Gastroenterol. 1997;32:122–6.
8. Santos MF, McCormack SA, Guo Z, Okolicany J, Zheng Y, Johnson LR, et al. Rho proteins play a critical role in cell migration during the early phase of mucosal restitution. J Clin Invest. 1997;100:216–25.
9. Dieckgraefe BK, Santoro SA, Alpers DH. Immunolocalization of alpha-integrin subunits and extracellular matrix components during human colonic organogenesis. Gastroenterology. 1996;110:58–71.
10. Miyazaki Y, Shinomura Y, Tsutsui S, Yasunaga Y, Zushi S, Higashiyama S, et al. Oxidative stress increases gene expression of heparin-binding EGF-like growth factor and amphiregulin in cultured rat gastric epithelial cells. Biochem Biophys Res Commun. 1996;226:542–6.
11. Wang JY, Johnson LR. Induction of gastric and duodenal mucosal ornithine decarboxylase during stress. Am J Physiol. 1989;257:G259–65.
12. Matsui H, Nagano Y, Shimokawa O, Kaneko T, Rai K, Udo J, et al. Gastric acid induces mitochondrial superoxide production and lipid peroxidation in gastric epithelial cells. J Gastroenterol. 2011;46:1167–76.
13. Davidson G, Kritas S, Butler R. Stressed mucosa. Nestle Nutr Workshop Ser Pediatr Program. 2007;59:133–42.
14. Boeckxstaens GE. Neuroimmune interaction in the gut: from bench to bedside. Verh K Acad Geneeskd Belg. 2006;68:329–35.
15. Iezzi A, Ferri C, Mezzetti A, Cipollone F. COX-2: friend or foe? Curr Pharm Des. 2007;13:1715–21.

16. Fox JG, Wang TC. Inflammation, atrophy, and gastric cancer. J Clin Invest. 2007;117:60–9.
17. Brzozowski T, Konturek PC, Konturek SJ, Drozdowicz D, Kwiecień S, Pajdo R, et al. Role of gastric acid secretion in progression of acute gastric erosions induced by ischemia–reperfusion into gastric ulcers. Eur J Pharmacol. 2000;398:147–58.
18. Murphy MP, Smith RA. Drug delivery to mitochondria: the key to mitochondrial medicine. Adv Drug Deliv Rev. 2000;41:235–50.
19. Nagano Y, Matsui H, Muramatsu M, Shimokawa O, Shibahara T, Yanaka A, et al. Rebamipide significantly inhibits indomethacin induced mitochondrial damage, lipid peroxidation, and apoptosis in gastric epithelial RGM-1 cells. Dig Dis Sci. 2005;50:S76–83.
20. Brand MD, Buckingham JA, Esteves TC, Green K, Lambert AJ, Miwa S, et al. Mitochondrial superoxide and aging: uncoupling protein activity and superoxide production. Biochem Soc Symp. 2004;71:203–13.
21. Bhattacharyya A, Chattopadhyay R, Mitra S, Crowe SE. Oxidative stress: an essential factor in the pathogenesis of gastrointestinal mucosal diseases. Physiol Rev. 2014;94:329–54.
22. Halliwell B, Clement MV, Ramalingam J, Long LH. Hydrogen peroxide. Ubiquitous in cell culture and *in vivo*? IUBMB Life. 2000;50:251–7.
23. Hiraishi H, Terano A, Sugimoto T, Harada T, Razandi M, Ivey KJ. Protective role of intracellular superoxide-dismutase against extracellular oxidants in cultured rat gastric cells. J Clin Investig. 1994;93:331–8.
24. Valko M, Leibfritz D, Moncol J, Cronin MTD, Mazur M, Telser J. Free radicals and antioxidants in normal physiological functions and human disease. Int J Biochem Cell Biol. 2007;39:44–84.
25. Veal EA, Day AM, Morgan BA. Hydrogen peroxide sensing and signaling. Mol Cell. 2007;26:1–14.
26. Wang Y, Zhu J, DeLuca HF. Where is the vitamin D receptor? Arch Biochem Biophys. 2012;523:123–33.
27. Kurose T, Seino Y, Ishida H, Tsuji K, Fukumoto H, Koh G, et al. Effect of vitamin D on gastrin and gastric somatostatin secretion from isolated perfused rat stomach. Life Sci. 1988;42:1995–2001.
28. Menezes RJ, Cheney RT, Husain A, Tretiakova M, Loewen G, Johnson CS, et al. Vitamin D receptor expression in normal, premalignant, and malignant human lung tissue. Cancer Epidemiol Biomarkers Prev. 2008;17:1104–10.
29. Stumpf WE, Sar M, Reid FA, Tanaka Y, DeLuca HF. Target cells for 1,25-dihydroxyvitamin D_3 in intestinal tract, stomach, kidney, skin, pituitary, and parathyroid. Science. 1979;206:1188–90.
30. Jones G, Strugnell SA, DeLuca HF. Current understanding of the molecular actions of vitamin D. Physiol Rev. 1998;78:1193–231.
31. Uberti F, Lattuada D, Morsanuto V, Nava U, Bolis G, Vacca G, et al. Vitamin D protects human endothelial cells from oxidative stress through the autophagic and survival pathways. J Clin Endocrinol Metab. 2014;99:1367–74.
32. Sun J. VDR/vitamin D receptor regulates autophagic activity through ATG16L1. Autophagy. 2016;12:1057–8.
33. Giordano S, Di Renzo MF, Ferracini R, Chiadò-Piat L, Comoglio PM. p145, a protein with associated tyrosine kinase activity in a human gastric carcinoma cell line. Mol Cell Biol. 1988;8:3510–7.
34. Humphries MJ. Cell adhesion assays. Mol Biotechnol. 2001;18(1):57–61.
35. Sun HY, Wang NP, Kerendi F, Halkos M, Kin H, Guyton RA, et al. Hypoxic postconditioning reduces cardiomyocyte loss by inhibiting ROS generation and intracellular Ca^{2+} overload. Am J Physiol Heart Circ Physiol. 2005;288:H1900–8.
36. Lattuada D, Uberti F, Colciaghi B, Morsanuto V, Maldi E, Squarzanti DF, et al. Fimbrial cells exposure to catalytic iron mimics carcinogenic changes. Int J Gynecol Cancer. 2015;25:389–98.
37. Lee SH, Lee SJ, Chung JY, Jung YS, Choi SY, Hwang SH, et al. p53, secreted by K-Ras-Snail pathway, is endocytosed by K-ras-mutated cells; implication of target-specific drug delivery and early diagnostic marker. Oncogene. 2009;28:2005–14.
38. Wright NA, Hoffmann W, Otto WR, Rio MC, Thim L. Rolling in the clover: trefoil factor family (TFF)-domain peptides, cell migration and cancer. FEBS Lett. 1997;408:121–3.
39. Pignatelli M. Modulation of cell adhesion during epithelial restitution in the gastrointestinal tract. Yale J Biol Med. 1996;69:131–5.
40. Thomas E, Wade A, Crawford G, Jenner B, Levinson N, Wilkinson J. Randomised clinical trial: relief of upper gastrointestinal symptoms by an acid pocket-targeting alginate-antacid (Gaviscon Double Action)- a double-blind, placebo-controlled, pilot study in gastro-oesophageal reflux disease. Aliment Pharmacol Ther. 2014;39(6):595–602.
41. Kong J, Zhang Z, Musch MW, Ning G, Sun J, Hart J, et al. Novel role of the vitamin D receptor in maintaining the integrity of the intestinal mucosal barrier. Am J Physiol Gastrointest Liver Physiol. 2008;294:G208–216.
42. Granger DN, Rutili G, McCord JM. Superoxide radicals in feline intestinal ischemia. Gastroenterology. 1981;81:22–9.
43. Itoh M, Guth PH. Role of oxygen-derived free radicals in hemorrhagic shock-induced gastric lesions in the rat. Gastroenterology. 1985;88:1162–7.
44. Hirota M, Inoue M, Ando Y, Hirayama K, Morino Y, Sakamoto K, et al. Inhibition of stress-induced gastric injury in the rat by glutathione. Gastroenterology. 1989;97:853–9.

5

Quality of life and impact of bile reflux after retro colic retro gastric gastrojejunostomy in Whipple surgery

Rohan Chaminda Siriwardana[1*], Rajapaksha Walimuni Mudiyanselage Anuradha Lokubandara[1], Shivanthi Janaki De Silva Hewavisenthi[2], Saumya Kumuduni Liyanage[2], Dona Subani Priyangika Jayatunge[1] and Chandika Anuradha Habarakada Liyanage[1]

Abstract

Background: Delayed gastric emptying and bile reflux are common concerns in long-term survivors after Whipple surgery. The study was designed to assess modified retro colic retro gastric gastrojejunostomy in reducing macro and microscopic bile reflux and impact on dyspepsia related quality of life in long-term survivors.

Methods: Out of 43 patients operated, 23 long-term survivors were included. All underwent gastroscopy and bile reflux was grouped as normal, yellowish bile lakes and presence of greenish bile lakes. Six standard gastric biopsies were taken. Microscopic bile reflux index (BRI) was calculated and a score more than 14 was considered significant. Validated Nepean dyspepsia index-short form (NDI-SF) was used to assess the severity of dyspepsia-related quality of life and compared with age and gender-matched control.

Results: The median age was 48 (21–70) years. Median survival of the group was 37 months (6–40). Endoscopically, 20/23 (87%) had macroscopic bile reflux (74% yellowish bile lakes, 13% greenish bile lakes). None had stomal ulcers or macroscopic inflammation. Mean bile reflux index score was 9.7 (range 1.77–34). Mean NDI–SF score of Whipple group was 23.1 (SD 8.88). In controls, mean score was 19.9 (SD 8.23), showing no significant difference ($p = 0.245$).

Conclusions: Though there was macroscopic bile reflux, clinical symptoms and microscopic changes were minimal. The modified technique had good long-term results.

Keywords: Whipple surgery, Bile reflux, Quality of life

Background

Whipple surgery was once a procedure associated with high morbidity and mortality rates. However over the years, perioperative outcome has improved. Currently it is a safe surgery with low morbidity and mortality [1, 2]. Now the focus has shifted from improving perioperative outcome to improving long-term survival and quality of life [3, 4] . Delayed gastric emptying and bile reflux gastritis are the main concerns of long-term survivors [3]. Many surgical techniques are being used by different centers to overcome this. Pylorus preservation, the use of separate loop to drain bile and use of retro colic loop are some of the adaptations used [5–7]. Khan et.al described a novel technique in performing the gastrojejunostomy and reported superior early results with the technique [8]. During this reconstruction, posterior gastrojejunostomy is pulled in to the infra colic compartment and anchored to the transverse mesocolon. This helps the anastomosis to retain in a dependent anatomical position. However long-term outcome is not reported. This study looks at intermediate results of patients who underwent retro colic retro gastric gastrojejunostomy with a mesocolic stich.

* Correspondence: rohansiriwardana@yahoo.com
[1]Department of Surgery, Faculty of Medicine, University of Kelaniya, Ragama, Sri Lanka
Full list of author information is available at the end of the article

Methods

Forty three patients who underwent Whipple surgery from January 2012 for malignant disease were included in the study. Patients with recurrence of primary malignancy, those who had immediate post-operative complications that needed relaporotomy, those who underwent chemotherapy within the last 6 months, and those who did not consent were excluded from the study. There were 23 patients who fulfilled the inclusion criteria (Fig. 1). There were no pancreatic leaks in the group. All surgeries were done by two hepatobiliary surgeons who worked in parallel. A standard technique was used for Whipple surgery in all cases. The common bile duct was divided at the level of the cystic duct. All the nodes to the right of the common hepatic artery were taken as specimen. Pancreatic division was done at the level of the neck. The uncinate process was completely removed clearing all the tissues to the right of the superior mesenteric artery. The stomach was divided at the level of the incisura. After the dissection, reconstruction was done using a single Roux loop taken through a window in the transverse mesocolon. The pancreas was anastomosed using ‘end to side two layer’ technique. This was followed by ‘end to side biliary reconstruction’. A 60 cm gap was left between hepaticojejunostomy and gastrojejunostomy. A separate mesenteric window was made in the left edge of the transverse mesocolon and the small bowel was taken to the supracolic compartment through this window. A two layer longitudinal 4 cm hand-sewn gastrojejunostomy was made in the posterior surface of the stomach close to the distal end of the gastric stump. The anastomosed distal stomach was then pulled down in to the infracolic compartment. The gastric stump was anchored to the mesenteric window to prevent retraction. All 23 patients were being followed up at the hepatobiliary clinic at regular intervals.

The patients were evaluated at 6 months after the surgery. The patients who fulfilled the inclusion criteria underwent upper gastric endoscopy. Two observers documented the macroscopic appearance of the gastric mucosa. Sample color photographs were used as a guide to categorize the macroscopic appearance. Macroscopic appearance was categorized as normal, presence of yellowish bile lakes, presence of greenish bile lakes, presence of gastric inflammation and presence of stromal ulcers. Six biopsies were taken from six standard sites to represent the stomach. Biopsy specimens were stained with Hematoxylin and Eosin. Giemsa stain was done to detect Helicobacter pylori. Two pathologists evaluated all specimens separately. Discrepancies in scores were resolved through discussion until both pathologists agreed on common scores. Bile reflux was reported using a previously published bile reflux index (BRI). The index was calculated using the formula: 7 x oedema of lamina propria + 3 x intestinal metaplasia + 4 x chronic

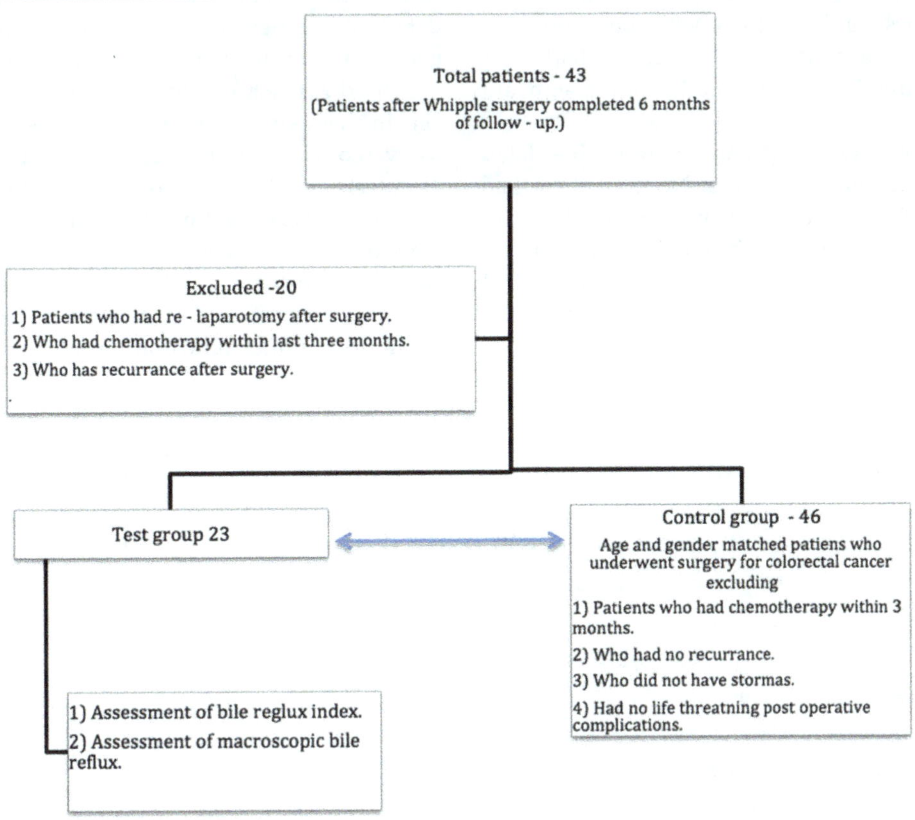

Fig. 1 Selection of patients and controls

inflammation—6 x *H.pylori*. An index over 14 was considered significant.

Patient's quality of life was assessed using Nepean dyspepsia short form quality of life (NDI-SF) questionnaire [9]. The questionnaire was translated to native language and was validated before using. Each patient was matched with two controls according to the age and gender. Controls were selected from a cohort of patients who had undergone lower abdominal surgeries for colorectal cancer. Patients who had recurrent disease, patients who had stomas, patients with bowel related complications or patients who were on chemotherapy within last 3 months were excluded. The NDI-SF score was compared between the two groups.

The study was approved by the Ethical Review Committee of the Faculty of Medicine, University of Kelaniya. All data were analyzed using SPSS 20. A p value of less than 0.05 was considered significant.

Results

The median survival of the group was 37 (6–40) months. 10 (45%) were males. The median age was 48 (21–70) years. Median body mass index was 20.32 kg/m^2 (15.03–30.07). 16 (69%) of them had diabetes. There were 10 (43%) patients with pancreatic cancers, 2 (8.6%) with bile duct cancers, 2 (8.6%) with neuro-endocrine tumours, and 9 (40%) with periampullary cancers. None of the patients in the group had early delayed gastric emptying. 6 (26%) Patients had adjuvant chemotherapy.

During endoscopy, 17 (74%) had yellowish bile lakes and 3 (13%) had greenish bile lakes. None of them had macroscopic gastric inflammation or stromal ulcers. In the microscopic assessment, the median BRI in the group was 9.7 (range 1.77–34). Only 5 patients had BRI over 14. *Helicobacor pylori* was not positive in any of the biopsies taken.

The quality of life was assessed in 10 areas. The overall score in the control was 19.9 (SD 8.23) while it was 23.1 (SD 8.88) in the test group indicating no significant difference ($p = 0.245$). The scores were comparable in the individual areas of NDI—SF (Table 1).

Discussion

In this cohort who had intermediate survival after Whipple surgery, bile was commonly noted in the distal part of the gastric stump. However biopsies did not show significant microscopic changes of bile reflux. Their quality of life was also comparable to the control. Maintaining the gastric stump in near-anatomical position, preventing stump retraction and angulation are considered important causes for good functional results after gastrectomy [6]. In the technique we use, the stomach is anchored to the root of the mesentery that helps to maintain its position. Furthermore there may be a mechanical advantage of keeping the gastric anastomosis in the infracolic compartment that facilitate the rapid emptying of the bile that enters in to the stomach.

Bile reflux gastritis is a well known histological entity characterized by foveolar hyperplacia, mucosal oedema, congestion and presence of acute and chronic inflammation [10]. Persistent bile reflux into the gastric remnant is known to cause significant clinical symptoms, structural changes and gastric carcinoma [10, 11]. However data looking specifically at bile reflux after Whipple surgery is limited in literature. Most data are from studies that used gastrectomy for distal gastric or duodenal cancer. In these studies, Roux en Y reconstruction was used to overcome bile reflux after distal gastrectomy [12, 13]. However, mobilizing a separate limb for biliary diversion adds more surgical time in addition to inherent problems of the Roux loop [14]. Another technique used is Braun enterostomy which has shown to reduce the incidence of bile reflux and delayed gastric emptying [15]. Additional jejunojejunostomy prolongs the surgical time

Table 1 Nepean dyspepsia index in the test and the control groups

	Study group mean (SD)	Control group mean (SD)	*P* value
General emotional well-being been disturbed by stomach problems	2.10 (1.07)	2.45 (1.39)	0.615
Irritable, tense or frustrated because of stomach problems	2.30 (1.13)	1.95 (1.10)	0.530
Ability to engage in things usually do for fun been disturbed by stomach problems	2.55 (1.47)	2.05 (1.32)	0.772
Enjoyment of things done usually for fun been disturbed by stomach problems	2.10 (1.33)	2.75 (1.48)	0.396
Ability to eat or drink been disturbed by stomach problems	2.15 (1.50)	2.10 (1.25)	0.726
Enjoyment of eating and/or drinking been disturbed by stomach problems	2.10 (1.25)	2.15 (1.18)	0.687
Feeling that they will always have stomach problems	2.45 (1.43)	2.00 (0.92)	0.353
Feeling of stomach problems might be due to a very serious illness.	2.05 (1.43)	1.75 (1.07)	0.289
Ability to work or study been disturbed by stomach problems	2.50 (1.70)	1.40 (1.23)	0.222
Enjoyment of work or study been disturbed by stomach problems	2.50 (1.70)	1.40 (1.14)	0.132
Total score	23.10 (8.88)	19.90 (8.23)	0.245

and can lead to other anastomosis related complications. In comparison to both these techniques, single loop reconstruction that we used is simple and is easy to perform.

Macroscopic bile reflux was noted in 87% of our cases. Bile pooled mainly in the distal stomach. Previous data from Fukuhara et.al [15] and others [16, 17] had shown a significant relationship between mucosal inflammation and presence of *Helicobacter pylori* infection. None of our patients had *Helicobacter pylori* present in the gastric mucosa. This could be an additional factor for not having significant mucosal inflammation. The median time for our evaluation since the surgery was 37 months. In a previous study, patients presenting with symptoms after gastrostomy showed bile reflux gastritis (BRG) in 60% of the cases after 14 years of surgery [18]. However other studies have shown mucosal changes much earlier [19]. Therefore median follow-up of 37 months in our cohort seems to be adequate to develop mucosal changes.

Delayed gastric emptying (DGE) is a well known complication after Whipple surgery. Incidence of early DGE is recorded to be around 20–30%. Its long-term impact and incidence of persistent symptoms is rarely discussed. Delayed gastric emptying is reported in around 10–20% of patients at 3 years after Whipple surgery [20]. In another study using standard reconstruction showed a similar incidence of DGE assessed with C13 acetate breath test at 24 months after surgery [21]. However gastric emptying studies need to be interpreted carefully in these patients who had lost a significant part of the stomach. In our study, gastric emptying time was not assessed. We feel that results of emptying studies have a little value in the absence of significant mucosal changes and symptoms.

One of the main drawbacks in the study is that it evaluates a smaller cohort of patients. Since this is the standard technique used in the center for reconstruction, we were not able to compare with a cohort reconstructed with an alternate technique. Since bile reflux index is a standard method in assessing bile reflux, we feel that having a lower BRI score without comparison is acceptable in arriving at our conclusion. However quality of life is best compared with a cohort having alternative reconstruction technique. To overcome this we selected a group of patients who had colonic surgeries unlikely to have upper gastric symptoms.

Conclutions

Patients with retro colic retro gastric gastrojejunostomy have good quality of life and minimal gastric mucosal changes. The technique seems to give good long-term results after Whipple surgery. This technique needs to be evaluated in a larger cohort.

Abbreviations

BRI: Bile reflux Index; NDI-SF: Nepean dyspepsia index-short form

Acknowledgements

We thank Mrs. Pathirana P. M. P. L Staff Technical Officer for performing laboratory analyses.

We thank Dr. Bandara L. M. P. M who assisted in statistical analysis and data collection of the study.

We thank Miss Vishaka Lakchani who assisted in statistical analysis and data collection of the study.

Funding

Self funded.

Authors' contributions

RCS is the corresponding author. He has coordinated the works done from the beginning to the end. Whipple surgery was performed under his supervision. Data collection, analysis and document works were organized by him. RWMAL assisted the surgeries. And he also contributed in the data collection. SJDSH has coordinated pathological analysis and pathological data collection data collections. SKL has contributed in pathological analysis and pathological data collections. DSPJ is the research assistant who was responsible in collecting and entering the data. She also analysed the data and helped in the process of writing the research works. CAH performed the surgeries and he has given his support in organizing the research to the primary researcher. All the authors have read understood and approved the manuscript and its contents.

Competing interests

There are no competing interest in our research.

Author details

[1]Department of Surgery, Faculty of Medicine, University of Kelaniya, Ragama, Sri Lanka. [2]Department of Pathology, Faculty of Medicine, University of Kelaniya, Ragama, Sri Lanka.

References

1. Grace PA, Pitt HA, Tompkins RK, Denbesten L, Longmire WP. Decreased morbidity and mortality after pancreatoduodenectomy. Am J Surg. 1986;151:141–9.
2. Trede M, Schwall G, Saeger HD. Survival after pancreatoduodenectomy. 118 consecutive resections without an operative mortality. Ann Surg. 1990;211:447–58.
3. Fitzmaurice C, Seiler CM, Büchler MW. Survival, mortality and quality of life after pylorus-preserving or classical Whipple operation. A systematic review with meta-analysis. Chirurg. 2010;81:454–71.
4. Ohtsuka T, Yamaguchi K, Ohuchida J, Inoue K, Nagai E, Chijiwa K, et al. Comparison of quality of life after pylorus-preserving pancreatoduodenectomy and Whipple resection. Hepatogastroenterology. 2003;50:846–50.
5. Eshuis WJ, Van Dalen JW, Busch ORC, van Gulik TM, Gouma DJ. Route of gastroenteric reconstruction in pancreatoduodenectomy and delayed gastric emptying. HPB. 2012;14:54–9.
6. Gangavatiker R, Pal S, Javed A, Dash NR, Sahni P, Chattopadhyay TK. Effect of antecolic or retrocolic reconstruction of the gastro/duodenojejunostomy on delayed gastric emptying after pancreaticoduodenectomy: a randomized controlled trial. J Gastrointest Surg. 2011;15:843–52.
7. Sobala GM, O'Connor HJ, Dewar EP, King RF, Axon AT, Dixon MF. Bile reflux and intestinal metaplasia in gastric mucosa. J Clin Pathol. 1993;46:235–40.
8. Khan AS, Hawkins WG, Linehan DC, Strasberg SM. A technique of gastrojejunostomy to reduce delayed gastric emptying after pancreatoduodenectomy. J Gastrointest Surg. 2011;15(8):1468–71.
9. Talley NJ, Haque M, Wyeth JW, Stace NH, Tytgat GN, Stanghellini V, et al. Development of a new dyspepsia impact scale: The Nepean Dyspepsia Index. Aliment Pharmacol Ther. 1999;13:225–35.
10. Dixon MF, O'Connor HJ, Axon AT, King RF, Johnston D. Reflux gastritis: distinct histopathological entity? J Clin Pathol. 1986;39:524–30.
11. Ritchie WP. Alkaline reflux gastritis. Can J Surg. 1982;25:248–9.
12. Osugi H, Fukuhara K, Takada N, Takemura M, Kinoshita H. Reconstructive procedure after distal gastrectomy to prevent remnant gastritis. Hepatogastroenterology. 2004;51:1215–8.

13. Cabrol J, Navarro X, Sancho J, Simo-Deu J, Segura R. Bile reflux in postoperative alkaline reflux gastritis. Ann Surg. 1990;211:239–43.
14. Hoya Y, Mitsumori N, Yanaga K. The advantages and disadvantages of a Roux-en-Y reconstruction after a distal gastrectomy for gastric cancer. Surg Today. 2009;39(8):647–51.
15. Watanabe Y, Ohtsuka T, Kimura H, Matsunaga T, Tamura K, Ideno N, et al. Braun enteroenterostomy reduces delayed gastric emptying after pylorus-preserving pancreatoduodenectomy: A retrospective review. Am J Surg. 2015;209:369–77.
16. Fukuhara K, Osugi H, Takada N, Takemura M, Lee S, Taguchi S, et al. Correlation between duodenogastric reflux and remnant gastritis after distal gastrectomy. Hepatogastroenterology. 2004;51:1241–4.
17. Fukuhara K, Osugi H, Takada N, Takemura M, Lee S, Taguchi S, et al. Duodenogastric reflux eradicates Helicobacter pylori after distal gastrectomy. Hepatogastroenterology. 2004;51:1548–50.
18. Vere CC, Cazacu S, Comănescu V, Mogoantă L, Rogoveanu I, Ciurea T. Endoscopical and histological features in bile reflux gastritis. Rom J Morphol Embryol. 2005;46:269–74.
19. Li XB, Lu H, Chen HM, Chen XY, Ge ZZ. Role of bile reflux and Helicobacter pylori infection on inflammation of gastric remnant after distal gastrectomy. J Dig Dis. 2008;9:208–12.
20. Matsumoto I, Shinzeki M, Asari S, Goto T, Shirakawa S, Ajiki T, et al. A prospective randomized comparison between pylorus- and subtotal stomach-preserving pancreatoduodenectomy on postoperative delayed gastric emptying occurrence and long-term nutritional status. J Surg Oncol. 2014;109(7):690–6.
21. Kawai M, Tani M, Hirono S, Okada K, Miyazawa M, Yamaue H. Pylorus-resecting pancreaticoduodenectomy offers long-term outcomes similar to those of pylorus-preserving pancreaticoduodenectomy: Results of a prospective Study. World J Surg. 2014;38:1476–83.

6

Rebamipide does not protect against naproxen-induced gastric damage

Thiago Gagliano-Jucá[1*], Ronilson A. Moreno[2], Tiago Zaminelli[3], Mauro Napolitano[4], Antônio Frederico N. Magalhães[5], Aloísio Carvalhaes[6], Miriam S. Trevisan[5], John L. Wallace[7] and Gilberto De Nucci[3,7,8]

Abstract

Background: Rebamipide is a gastroprotective agent with promising results against gastric damage induced by non-steroidal anti-inflammatory drugs. The present study evaluated if rebamipide protects against naproxen-induced gastric damage in healthy volunteers. Changes in gastric PGE2 tissue concentration were also evaluated.

Methods: After a preliminary endoscopy to rule out previous gastric macroscopic damage, twenty-four healthy volunteers of both sexes were divided into 2 groups. One group received sodium naproxen 550 mg b.i.d. plus placebo for 7 days, while the other group received sodium naproxen 550 mg b.i.d. plus rebamipide 100 mg b.i.d. At the end of treatment, a new endoscopy was performed. Gastric macroscopic damage was evaluated by the Cryer score and by the modified Lanza score. The primary outcome measure of the trial was the macroscopic damage observed in each treatment group at the end of treatment. Biopsies were collected at both endoscopies for PGE2 quantification and histopathological analysis (secondary outcomes). Tissue PGE2 was quantified by ELISA. The randomization sequence was generated using 3 blocks of 8 subjects each. Volunteers and endoscopists were blind to whether they were receiving rebamipide or placebo.

Results: All recruited volunteers completed the trial. Sodium naproxen induced gastric damage in both groups. At the end of the study, median Cryer score was 4 in both groups (Difference = 0; 95%CI = −1 to 0; $p = 0.728$). In the placebo group, the mean tissue PGE2 concentration was 1005 ± 129 pg/mL before treatment and 241 ± 41 pg/mL after treatment ($p < 0.001$). In the rebamipide group, the mean tissue PGE2 concentration was 999 ± 109 pg/mL before treatment, and 168 ± 13 pg/mL after treatment ($p < 0.001$). There was no difference in mean tissue PGE2 between the two groups (difference = 5; 95%CI from −334.870 to 345.650; $p = 0.975$). No significant change was observed at the histopathological evaluation, despite the evident macroscopic damage induced by naproxen.

Conclusion: Rebamipide does not protect against naproxen-induced gastric damage in healthy volunteers.

Keywords: NSAID, Histopathology, Human, ELISA, Endoscopy, Cryer score, Modified Lanza score

* Correspondence: thiagogagliano@gmail.com
[1]Institute of Biophysics Carlos Chagas Filho, Federal University of Rio de Janeiro (UFRJ), 21941-902 Rio de Janeiro, Brazil
Full list of author information is available at the end of the article

Background

Naproxen and other non-selective non-steroidal anti-inflammatory drugs (NSAIDs) induce gastrointestinal (GI) adverse events ranging from dyspepsia to upper and lower GI tract ulcers [1–3]. Naproxen 660 – 1000 mg per day administered for 2 to 14 days is used as a model for NSAID-induced gastroduodenal damage in healthy volunteers [4–8].

Rebamipide has been described as a GI mucosal protector agent with promising results in prophylaxis and treatment of GI ulcers caused by NSAIDs, *H. pylori* or endoscopic submucosal dissection [9–15]. Results from animal studies have suggested that the protective effects of rebamipide are attributable to stimulation of prostaglandin (PG) synthesis [16, 17]. In healthy volunteers, concomitant administration of rebamipide 100 mg with ibuprofen 600 mg t.i.d. for 7 consecutive days resulted in a mean gastric damage score of 1.3 ± 1.0, which was significantly lower than that of the control group (mean score of 2.9 ± 1.7), as assessed by the modified Lanza score ($p = 0.032$) [10]. In patients with rheumatic disease rebamipide 100 mg b.i.d. also showed a protective effect against NSAID-induced gastric damage [18].

The present study evaluated whether rebamipide could provide a protective effect against naproxen-induced gastric damage in healthy volunteers.

Methods

Volunteers

Volunteers of both sexes aged 18 years old or older without any significant cardiac, hepatic, renal, pulmonary, neurological, gastrointestinal or hematological diseases, as determined by their medical history, physical examination, and routine laboratory tests (hematology, blood biochemistry, urine analysis and fecal occult blood test), were invited to participate in this double-blind, randomized, parallel placebo-controlled phase II single-center trial. All subjects tested negative for hepatitis B and C (except for serologic scar), as well as HIV I and II, and were instructed to abstain from taking any medication including over-the-counter medication for 2 weeks prior to and during the study period. Pregnancy was an exclusion criterion. All women enrolled had negative β-HCG. All volunteers were informed about the aim and risks of the study by the clinical investigator and they all signed a written informed consent statement before entering the study. The study was performed according to the 2008 revised Declaration of Helsinki for bio-medical research involving human subjects and the 1996 rules of Good Clinical Practices. The study protocol was approved by the Committee of Research Ethics of the University of Sao Paulo, Sao Paulo, Brazil, on 26 November 2014 (before the initiation of the study procedures), and the study is registered at ClinicalTrials.gov, ID NCT02632812.

After performing a preliminary gastroduodenal endoscopy at the Vera Cruz Hospital (Campinas, Brazil) to rule-out prior macroscopic upper GI damage in the subjects, twenty-four healthy volunteers (12 men) were enrolled in the study. Other exclusion criteria were: achlorhydria (pH > 6.5); positive fecal occult blood test; drug abuse, including alcohol or tobacco.

Treatment

Volunteers were randomly divided into 2 groups: group A received 550 mg of sodium naproxen (Flanax® - Bayer) plus an effervescent placebo (Biolab Indústria Farmacêutica Ltda.) diluted in 200 mL of water b.i.d. for 7 consecutive days; group B received 550 mg of sodium naproxen (Flanax® - Bayer) plus 100 mg of effervescent rebamipide (Biolab Indústria Farmacêutica Ltda.) diluted in 200 mL of water b.i.d. for 7 consecutive days. The randomization sequence was determined using the randomization generator available at www.randomization.com, using 3 blocks of 8 subjects each. Volunteers were blind to whether they were receiving rebamipide or placebo. To assure adherence, the drugs were administered by a member of the research team (also blind to treatment allocation) early in the morning and late in the evening for the whole duration of the study. A pharmacist was responsible for labeling treatments as A or B, and for breaking the code at the end of the study. Volunteers were required to be fasted in the morning and were only allowed to eat at least 2 h after administration of medications. In the evening, volunteers were required to be at least for 2 h without ingestion of food, and were also asked to avoid eating for the following 2 h after the dose.

Adverse reactions were individually evaluated. Causality relationship to the treatment was assessed with the aid of the Karch & Lasagna algorithm [19]. The necessity of interruption of treatment or specific therapy was individually assessed by the Principal Investigator depending on the severity of the reaction and the causality relationship to the treatment.

Gastrointestinal damage evaluation

Gastroduodenal endoscopy was performed before the start of the study and in the morning of the 8th day of treatment in all volunteers. Exams were performed by a single endoscopist. The primary outcome measure of the trial was the macroscopic damage observed in each treatment group at the end of treatment. The number of mucosal erosions after treatment was counted and macroscopic mucosal injury scored according to Cryer [20] and to the modified Lanza score (MLS; Table 1) [9, 21]. Gastroduodenal ulcers were classified according to the Sakita-Miwa classification. Additionally, a second endoscopist retrospectively evaluated the exams, blind to

Table 1 Cryer and modified Lanza scores according to gastroduodenal mucosal injury

Score	Cryer score	Modified Lanza score
0	Normal or erythema	No hemorrhage or erosion observed
1	Any amount of submucosal hemorrhage or edema without erosions.	One or two hemorrhages or erosions observed in one gastric area.
2	1 erosion ± submucosal hemorrhage or edema.	Three to five hemorrhages or erosions observed in one gastric area.
3	2–4 erosions ± submucosal hemorrhage or edema.	Hemorrhages or erosions observed in two gastric areas; six or more hemorrhages or erosions observed in one gastric area, with the total number not exceeding ten in the entire stomach.
4	5 or more erosions and/or a single ulcer ± submucosal hemorrhage or edema.	Hemorrhages or erosions observed in three or more gastric areas; eleven or more hemorrhages or erosions observed widely in the entire stomach.
5	Multiple ulcers ± submucosal hemorrhage or edema.	Ulcer.

the scores given by the first endoscopist. If there was any difference between the score given by the two endoscopists, the final score would be the mean value of the two numbers. Both endoscopists were blind to treatment group allocation of volunteers. In each exam 3 biopsies were collected from the gastric antrum and 3 from the gastric corpus for PGE2 quantification. Samples were immediately washed in phosphate buffer saline at pH 7.4 and stored individually in a dry Eppendorf tube and kept at −20 °C until analysis. Another 2 biopsies from each stomach region (4 total) were collected at each endoscopic procedure for histological analysis. Volunteers were questioned about GI symptoms at every dose. Changes in gastric PGE2 concentration, histopathological characteristics and GI symptoms at the end of the study compared to baseline were evaluated as secondary outcome measures. A more detailed questionnaire about GI symptoms such as heartburn, abdominal pain, fullness, nausea, vomiting, blood in stools or others was completed before receiving the first dose and at the last day of treatment. In the questionnaires, when any symptom was reported, the volunteer was asked to describe the intensity and frequency of the symptom over the previous 7 days. Routine laboratory tests were repeated at the end of treatment, including fecal occult blood test.

PGE2 quantification

Tissue PGE2 concentration was quantified by enzyme-linked immunosorbent assay (ELISA) using Cayman Chemical Monoclonal Prostaglandin E_2 EIA Kit (item number 514010). Briefly, biopsies from the gastric antrum and corpus collected in both endoscopic procedures were weighted and homogenized individually for 20 s by a Polytron in 1 mL of Na_3PO_4 buffer solution (pH = 7.4). Aliquots of 200 μL of the homogenate were placed in a dry bath at 37 °C for 20 min and then centrifuged at 20,800 *g* for 30 s. Supernatant (150 μL) was collected and diluted 1:100 (v/v) to be used in the ELISA. Each aliquot was assayed in duplicate and final PGE2 concentrations were adjusted for initial sample mass. Data are displayed as mean ± SEM. The person responsible for the quantification of PGE2 was blind to treatment group allocation of volunteers.

Histopathological evaluation

Biopsies from gastric antrum and corpus were immediately put in formaldehyde after collection. Samples were stained in hematoxylin and eosin for characterization and graded according to a score described in Table **2**. Giemsa stain was used to diagnose *H. pylori* infection. The pathologist was also blind to treatments.

Statistical analysis

For evaluation of statistical difference of tissue PGE2 between treatments, a *t*-test was performed. A paired *t* test was used to compare tissue PGE2 before and after treatments within each group. Endoscopic and histopathological scores between treatment groups were compared using the Mann–Whitney *U*-test. Gastrointestinal symptoms after treatments were compared by Fisher's exact test. A p value <0.05 was considered significant. The sample size planned for the study was 24 volunteers of both sexes. This number was chosen based on the gastroprotective effects of rebamipide previously reported [9]. The calculation considered the Mann–Whitney *U* test analysis of the reported data on gastroduodenal damage scoring by MLS. The effect size observed (difference between treatments) was 67 % (median score after treatment of 3 and 1, in the placebo and rebamipide groups, respectively). Given a power of 80 % and a 0.05 chance of type 1 error, the original sample size estimation was 10 volunteers per group. The final number of 12 volunteers per group was chosen considering a 20 % rate of drop-out. Other studies with rebamipide in healthy volunteers also used similar sample sizes [10, 15].

Results

All 24 volunteers enrolled completed all procedures of the study. The median age of men was 24 years (range 18 – 49 years), mean weight was 75.7 kg (61.0 – 97.0 kg), mean height was 175 cm (152 – 186 cm), and mean body mass index was 24.8 kg/m^2 (20.2 – 28.7 kg/m^2). Women had a

Table 2 Histhopathologic grade score developed for microscopic injury evaluation

Score	Findings
0	Normal gastric mucosa or mild chronic inflammation
1	Chronic gastritis without activity
2	Chronic gastritis with activity on antrum
3	Chronic gastritis with activity on the body
4	Chronic gastritis with activity on antrum and on the body

median age of 24.5 years (range 20 – 42 years), mean weight was 69.5 kg (54.0 – 83.0 kg), mean height was 164 cm (153 – 170 cm), and mean body mass index was 25.9 kg/m^2 (20.7 – 28.7 kg/m^2). Three volunteers (two men) were not allowed to enroll in the study because of gastric damage observation in the preliminary endoscopy.

There was agreement between the endoscopists on the scores of all exams. Endoscopic findings and scores for each volunteer using the macroscopic scoring systems are summarized in Table 3. The median Cryer score was 4 in both placebo and rebamipide groups (Difference = 0; 95%CI = −1 to 0; $p = 0.728$). The median MLS was 4 in the placebo group and 3.5 in the rebamipide group (Difference = 0.5; 95%CI = −2 to 1; $p = 0.822$). In the placebo group 2 volunteers (16 %) presented GI ulcers (1 ulcer each), while 4 volunteers (32 %) in the rebamipide group had ulcers ($p = 0.320$). Figure 1a and b illustrate the macroscopic aspect of the gastric mucosa of volunteer 24 in the rebamipide group before treatment and at the end of the study.

The incidence of GI symptoms in each treatment group is displayed in Table 4. Individual data regarding

Table 3 Summary of findings in the endoscopic procedure at the end of treatments

Volunteer #	Treatment	Scores before treatment	Cryer Score	Lanza Score	Antrum	Duodenum	Other
2	Placebo	0	3	2	4 erosions		
5	Placebo	0	2	1	1 erosion + submucousal hemorrage		
7	Placebo	0	4	4	>20 erosions		
8	Placebo	0	4	5	2 erosions + 1 ulcer (Sakita A2)		
10	Placebo	0	4	4	>10 erosions		
12	Placebo	0	4	5	10 erosions + 1 ulcer (Sakita A2)		
14	Placebo	0	4	2	5 erosions		
16	Placebo	0	4	4	20 erosions		
17	Placebo	0	4	4	10 erosions	3 erosions	
18	Placebo	0	4	4	10 erosions		
19	Placebo	0	4	4	10 erosions		
23	Placebo	0	4	4	10 erosions		
1	Rebamipide	0	4	4	20–25 erosions		
3	Rebamipide	0	4	4	10 erosions		
4	Rebamipide	0	4	5	10 erosions	1 ulcer (Sakita A2)	
6	Rebamipide	0	3	1	2 erosions + erythema		
9	Rebamipide	0	3	2	3 erosions		
11	Rebamipide	0	3	3	2 erosions		Submucousal hemorrhage in gastric fundus
13	Rebamipide	0	5	5	Small erosions + 2 ulcers (Sakita A2)		
15	Rebamipide	0	4	2	5 erosions + erythema		
20	Rebamipide	0	3	2	4 erosions		
21	Rebamipide	0	4	5			Pylorus with edema and 1 ulcer (Sakita A2)
22	Rebamipide	0	3	2	3 erosions		
24	Rebamipide	0	5	5	10 erosions + 4 ulcers (Sakita A2)		

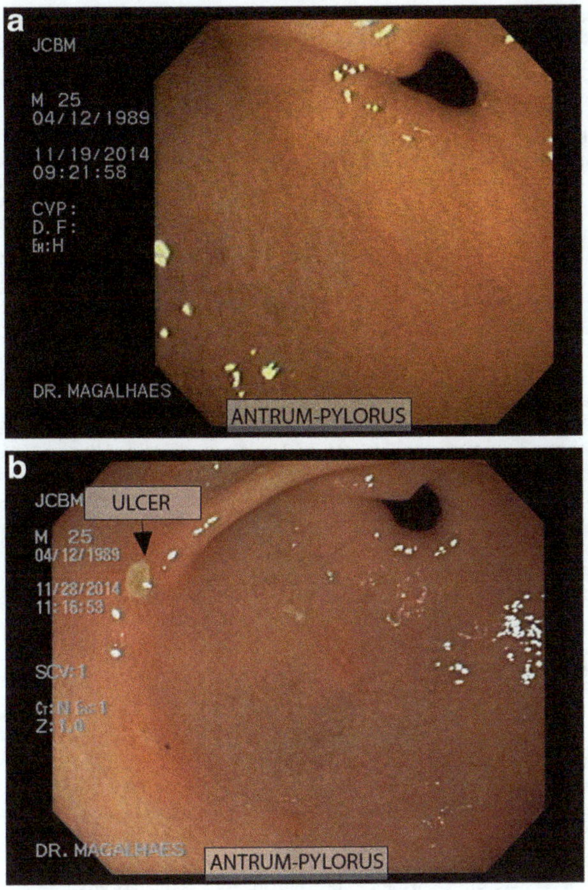

Fig. 1 Photographic documentation of the endoscopic procedure in a volunteer in the rebamipide group (**a**) before and (**b**) after treatment

GI symptoms is available in Additional file 1: Table S1. There were no statistical differences between treatment groups at the end of the study. All fecal occult blood tests were negative at the end of treatment.

PGE2 quantification

In the placebo group, the mean tissue PGE2 concentration was 1005 ± 129 pg/mL before treatment, and 241 ± 41 pg/mL after treatment (difference = 764; 95%CI from 477 to 1051), which corresponded to a mean inhibition of PGE2 synthesis of 76.0 % ($p < 0.001$). In the rebamipide group, the mean tissue PGE2 concentration was 999 ± 109 pg/mL before treatment, and 168 ± 13 pg/mL after treatment (difference = 831.5; 95%CI from 612 to 1051), a mean inhibition of 83.2 % ($p < 0.001$). There was no difference between the two groups in PGE2 tissue concentration before treatments (difference = 5; 95%CI from −334.870 to 345.650; $p = 0.975$). The individual PGE2 concentration found for each volunteer before and after treatment is available in Additional file 2: Table S2.

Table 4 Incidence of gastrointestinal symptoms

Gastrointestinal symptom	Placebo ($n = 12$)		Rebamipide ($n = 12$)		P value	
	Before	After	Before	After	Before	After
Any	3	5	5	3	0.67	0.33
Abdominal pain	2	3	3	2	0.50	0.50
Heartburn	2	2	3	1	0.50	0.50
Nausea	1	2	1	1	0.76	0.50
Intestinal cramps	0	1	1	0	0.50	0.50
Fullness	1	0	0	0	0.50	1.00

Incidence of gastrointestinal symptoms in each treatment group before the beginning and at the end of the study. *P* value was calculated comparing incidence of symptoms between placebo and rebamipide groups before and after treatments by Fisher's exact test

Histopathological evaluation

At the initial endoscopic procedure, median histopathological scores were 1 in both groups (Difference = 0; 95%CI = −3 to 1; $p = 0.582$). At the end of the study, median histopathological scores were also 1 in both groups (Difference = 0; 95%CI = −1 to 1; $p = 0.997$). At the initial endoscopy, 5 volunteers in each group were *H. pylori* positive. At the end of treatments, 6 subjects in each group were *H. pylori* positive. The individual histopathological score for each patient as well as *H. pylori* status before and after treatment is available in Additional file 3: Table S3.

Discussion

The present study did not find any evidence of a gastroprotective effect of rebamipide on naproxen-induced gastroduodenal damage as assessed by endoscopic macroscopic evaluation. This result differs from previous findings, in which rebamipide treatment resulted in less severe gastric damage induced by NSAIDs [9, 10, 15]. One possible explanation for the different results found in the present work is that naproxen was more aggressive than others models of NSAID-induced gastric damage. To evaluate this possibility, previously published data was further analyzed. Treatment with indomethacin at 75 mg/day without rebamipide for 7 consecutive days resulted in a median MLS of 3. When treatment was associated with rebamipide 100 mg t.i.d., median MLS was 1 [9]. Treatment with ibuprofen 1800 mg/day for 7 consecutive days without rebamipide resulted in a median MLS of 3. When volunteers received rebamipide concomitantly with ibuprofen, median MLS was 2 [10]. By performing the Mann–Whitney *U*-test to compare MLS scores from the placebo group in the present study to those found in the placebo groups of the previously mentioned studies, no difference in gastric lesion scores among these 3 models of NSAID-induced gastric damage was observed (indomethacin vs. naproxen, $p = 0.475$; ibuprofen vs. naproxen, $p = 0.343$; indomethacin vs. ibuprofen, $p = 1.0$). However, since the characteristics of volunteers enrolled in the aforementioned studies are very different from those of the present study and trials designs are not the same, final conclusions cannot be drawn from these statistical analyses.

Since all the aforementioned studies evaluated Japanese or Korean subjects [9, 10, 13, 15, 18], population characteristics may have influenced the results. Higher gastric pH is known to be a protective factor in NSAID-induced gastric damage. The incidence of hypochlorhydria in the Japanese population is higher than in western countries, affecting more than 40 % of individuals over 50 year olds in Japan [22], while in the Unites States the incidence varies from 8 % in young adults to 11 % in the elderly [23, 24]. The higher gastric pH might facilitate the observation of the protective effect of rebamipide reported in Asian individuals. Another possibility for differences in rebamipide effects in NSAID-induced gastric damage is the genetic and dietary characteristics of the populations evaluated in each study.

One difference of the present study is that the daily dose of rebamipide was 200 mg, while most previous reports treated volunteers with 300 mg of rebamipide per day [9–15, 25, 26]. However, rebamipide at 200 mg/day in patients with rheumatic disease showed a protective effect in NSAID-induced gastroduodenal mucosal injury [18]. It is unlikely that a reduction in 33 % of the dose would abolish the supposed effect of rebamipide. A lower dosage of rebamipide was chosen due to safety concerns. Most of the safety data about rebamipide comes from studies in Asian populations. This is the first time a study evaluated effects of rebamipide in a Brazilian population.

Increased PG synthesis was previously suggested as a possible mechanism for mucosal protection of rebamipide [16, 17]. If so, rebamipide should not have a protective effect in NSAID-induced gastric damage through modulation of PG synthesis, since NSAIDs block the activity of cyclooxygenases.

In the present study, no significant histopathological change of the gastric mucosa was seen at the end of treatment in neither groups, despite the clear aggressiveness of naproxen observed on macroscopy. These results confirm previous reports that identified the histological features characteristic of NSAID users only in a subset of patients, and that microscopic findings do not correlate with macroscopical damage [27, 28]. This may reflect that the histological parameters used lack sufficient sensitivity or else, the mechanism responsible for the appearance of erosions and ulcers is independent of the degree of inflammation.

Conclusion

Rebamipide 200 mg/day does not protect against naproxen-induced gastroduodenal damage in healthy volunteers.

Abbreviations

ELISA, Enzyme-linked immunosorbent assay; GI, Gastrointestinal; MLS, Modifies Lanza score; NSAIDs, Non-steroidal anti-inflammatory drugs; PG, Prostaglandin.

Acknowledgements

Not applicable.

Funding

The study was funded by Biolab Indústria Farmacêutica Ltda. The funding body approved the study design and the methods that were used for data acquisition and analysis, but had no involvement with the interpretation of data or with the composition of the manuscript.

Authors' contributions

TGJ and GDN designed the research; TGJ, RAM, TZ, MN, AFNM, AC and MST performed the research; TGJ, RAM, TZ, MN, AFNM, AC, MST, JLW and GDN analyzed the data; TGJ, JLW and GDN wrote the paper. All authors read and approved the final manuscript.

Authors' information

Not applicable.

Competing interests

The authors declare that they have no competing interests.

Author details

[1]Institute of Biophysics Carlos Chagas Filho, Federal University of Rio de Janeiro (UFRJ), 21941-902 Rio de Janeiro, Brazil. [2]Galeno Research Unit, Campinas, Brazil; Faculty of Medical Sciences, Metropolitan University of Santos, Santos, Brazil. [3]Department of Pharmacology, Faculty of Medical Sciences, State University of Campinas (UNICAMP), Campinas, Brazil. [4]Department of Pharmacology, ICB – University of Sao Paulo (USP), 05508-900 Sao Paulo, Brazil. [5]Department of Gastroenterology, Faculty of Medical Sciences, State University of Campinas (UNICAMP), Campinas, Brazil. [6]Brazilian Society for Digestive Endoscopy (SOBED), Sao Paulo, Brazil. [7]Unicastelo Medical School, University Camilo Castelo Branco (UNICASTELO), Fernandopolis, Brazil. [8]Department of Pharmacology, ICB – University of Sao Paulo (USP), Sao Paulo, Brazil.

References

1. Wolfe MM, Lichtenstein DR, Singh G. Gastrointestinal toxicity of nonsteroidal antiinflammatory drugs. N Engl J Med. 1999;340(24):1888–99. doi:10.1056/NEJM199906173402407.
2. Maiden L, Thjodleifsson B, Theodors A, Gonzalez J, Bjarnason I. A quantitative analysis of NSAID-induced small bowel pathology by capsule enteroscopy. Gastroenterology. 2005;128(5):1172–8.
3. Sostres C, Gargallo CJ, Arroyo MT, Lanas A. Adverse effects of non-steroidal anti-inflammatory drugs (NSAIDs, aspirin and coxibs) on upper gastrointestinal tract. Best Pract Res Clin Gastroenterol. 2010;24(2):121–32. doi:10.1016/j.bpg.2009.11.005.
4. Aadland E, Fausa O, Vatn M, Cohen H, Quinlan D. Protection by misoprostol against naproxen-induced gastric mucosal damage. Am J Med. 1987;83(1A):37–40.
5. Aabakken L, Osnes M. Gastroduodenal lesions induced by naproxen. An endoscopic evaluation of regional differences and natural course. Scand J Gastroenterol. 1990;25(12):1215–22.
6. Oddsson E, Gudjonsson H, Thjodleifsson B. Comparison between ranitidine and omeprazole for protection against gastroduodenal damage caused by naproxen. Scand J Gastroenterol. 1992;27(12):1045–8.
7. Sarosiek J, Marcinkiewicz M, Parolisi S, Peura DA. Prostaglandin E2 content in residual gastric juice reflects endoscopic damage to the gastric mucosa after naproxen sodium administration. Am J Gastroenterol. 1996;91(5):873–8.
8. Bianchi Porro G, Lazzaroni M, Petrillo M. Double-blind, double-dummy endoscopic comparison of the mucosal protective effects of misoprostol

versus ranitidine on naproxen-induced mucosal injury to the stomach and duodenum in rheumatic patients. Am J Gastroenterol. 1997;92(4):663–7.
9. Naito Y, Yoshikawa T, Iinuma S, Yagi N, Matsuyama K, Boku Y, et al. Rebamipide protects against indomethacin-induced gastric mucosal injury in healthy volunteers in a double-blind, placebo-controlled study. Dig Dis Sci. 1998;43(9 Suppl):83S–9S.
10. Kim HK, Kim JI, Kim JK, Han JY, Park SH, Choi KY, et al. Preventive effects of rebamipide on NSAID-induced gastric mucosal injury and reduction of gastric mucosal blood flow in healthy volunteers. Dig Dis Sci. 2007;52(8): 1776–82. doi:10.1007/s10620-006-9367-y.
11. Terano A, Arakawa T, Sugiyama T, Suzuki H, Joh T, Yoshikawa T, et al. Rebamipide, a gastro-protective and anti-inflammatory drug, promotes gastric ulcer healing following eradication therapy for Helicobacter pylori in a Japanese population: a randomized, double-blind, placebo-controlled trial. J Gastroenterol. 2007;42(8):690–3. doi:10.1007/s00535-007-2076-2.
12. Kobayashi M, Takeuchi M, Hashimoto S, Mizuno K, Sato Y, Narisawa R, et al. Contributing factors to gastric ulcer healing after endoscopic submucosal dissection including the promoting effect of rebamipide. Dig Dis Sci. 2012; 57(1):119–26. doi:10.1007/s10620-011-1850-4.
13. Kim JH, Park SH, Cho CS, Lee ST, Yoo WH, Kim SK, et al. Preventive efficacy and safety of rebamipide in nonsteroidal anti-inflammatory drug-induced mucosal toxicity. Gut Liver. 2014;8(4):371–9. doi:10.5009/gnl.2014.8.4.371.
14. Kurokawa S, Katsuki S, Fujita T, Saitoh Y, Ohta H, Nishikawa K, et al. A randomized, double-blinded, placebo-controlled, multicenter trial, healing effect of rebamipide in patients with low-dose aspirin and/or non-steroidal anti-inflammatory drug induced small bowel injury. J Gastroenterol. 2014; 49(2):239–44. doi:10.1007/s00535-013-0805-2.
15. Tozawa K, Oshima T, Okugawa T, Ogawa T, Ohda Y, Tomita T, et al. A randomized, double-blind, placebo-controlled study of rebamipide for gastric mucosal injury taking aspirin with or without clopidogrel. Dig Dis Sci. 2014;59(8):1885–90. doi:10.1007/s10620-014-3108-4.
16. Kleine A, Kluge S, Peskar BM. Stimulation of prostaglandin biosynthesis mediates gastroprotective effect of rebamipide in rats. Dig Dis Sci. 1993; 38(8):1441–9.
17. Qi Z, Jie L, Haixia C, Xiaoying Z. Effect of rebamipide on quality of peptic ulcer healing in rat. Dig Dis Sci. 2009;54(9):1876–83. doi:10.1007/s10620-008-0577-3.
18. Seo YI, Park SH, Min DJ, Kim WU, Min JK, Lee SH, et al. Effects of rebamipide against nonsteroidal anti-inflammatory drugs (NSAIDs)induced gastroduodenal mucosal injury. J Korean Rheum Assoc. 2001;8(2):73–80.
19. Karch FE, Lasagna L. Toward the operational identification of adverse drug reactions. Clin Pharmacol Ther. 1977;21(3):247–54.
20. Cryer B, Feldman M. Effects of very low dose daily, long-term aspirin therapy on gastric, duodenal, and rectal prostaglandin levels and on mucosal injury in healthy humans. Gastroenterology. 1999;117(1):17–25.
21. Lanza FL, Royer Jr GL, Nelson RS, Chen TT, Seckman CE, Rack MF. A comparative endoscopic evaluation of the damaging effects of nonsteroidal anti-inflammatory agents on the gastric and duodenal mucosa. Am J Gastroenterol. 1981;75(1):17–21.
22. Morihara M, Aoyagi N, Kaniwa N, Kojima S, Ogata H. Assessment of gastric acidity of Japanese subjects over the last 15 years. Biol Pharm Bull. 2001; 24(3):313–5.
23. Dressman JB, Berardi RR, Dermentzoglou LC, Russell TL, Schmaltz SP, Barnett JL, et al. Upper gastrointestinal (GI) pH in young, healthy men and women. Pharm Res. 1990;7(7):756–61.
24. Russell TL, Berardi RR, Barnett JL, Dermentzoglou LC, Jarvenpaa KM, Schmaltz SP, et al. Upper gastrointestinal pH in seventy-nine healthy, elderly, North American men and women. Pharm Res. 1993;10(2):187–96.
25. Talley NJ, Riff DS, Schwartz H, Marcuard SP. Double-blind placebo-controlled multicentre studies of rebamipide, a gastroprotective drug, in the treatment of functional dyspepsia with or without Helicobacter pylori infection. Aliment Pharmacol Ther. 2001;15(10):1603–11.
26. Mizukami K, Murakami K, Hirashita Y, Hisamatsu A, Ogawa R, Uchida M, et al. Efficacy of rebamipide for low-dose aspirin-related gastrointestinal symptoms. J Clin Biochem Nutr. 2012;51(3):216–20. doi:10.3164/jcbn.12-27.
27. El-Zimaity HM, Genta RM, Graham DY. Histological features do not define NSAID-induced gastritis. Hum Pathol. 1996;27(12):1348–54.
28. Frezza M, Gorji N, Melato M. The histopathology of non-steroidal anti-inflammatory drug induced gastroduodenal damage: correlation with Helicobacter pylori, ulcers, and haemorrhagic events. J Clin Pathol. 2001; 54(7):521–5.

Findings in young adults at colonoscopy from a hospital service database audit

Stephanie Wong[1], Ilmars Lidums[1], Christophe Rosty[2,3,4], Andrew Ruszkiewicz[5,6], Susan Parry[7], Aung Ko Win[8], Yoko Tomita[9], Sina Vatandoust[10], Amanda Townsend[9], Dainik Patel[10], Jennifer E. Hardingham[9,11], David Roder[12], Eric Smith[9,11], Paul Drew[13,14], Julie Marker[15], Wendy Uylaki[1,9], Peter Hewett[16], Daniel L. Worthley[11,17], Erin Symonds[18,19], Graeme P. Young[18], Timothy J. Price[9,11] and Joanne P. Young[9,11,20*]

Abstract

Background: Colorectal cancer (CRC) diagnosed at <50 years is predominantly located in the distal colon and rectum. Little is known about which lesion subtypes may serve as CRC precursors in young adults. The aim of this work was to document the prevalence and histological subtype of lesions seen in patients aged <50 years, and any associated clinical features.

Methods: An audit of the colonoscopy database at The Queen Elizabeth Hospital in Adelaide, South Australia over a 12-month period was undertaken. Findings were recorded from both colonoscopy reports and corresponding histological examination of excised lesions.

Results: Data were extracted from colonoscopies in 2064 patients. Those aged <50 comprised 485 (24%) of the total. CRC precursor lesions (including sessile serrated adenoma/polyps (SSA/P), traditional serrated adenomas, tubular adenomas ≥10 mm or with high-grade dysplasia, and conventional adenomas with villous histology) were seen in 4.3% of patients aged <50 and 12.9% of patients aged ≥50 (P <0.001). Among colonoscopies yielding CRC precursor lesions in patients under 50 years, SSA/P occurred in 52% of procedures (11/21), compared with 27% (55/204) of procedures in patients aged 50 and older ($P = 0.02$). SSA/P were proximally located in (10/11) 90% of patients aged under 50, and 80% (43/54) of those aged 50 and older ($P = 0.46$).

Conclusions: SSA/P were the most frequently observed CRC precursor lesions in patients aged <50. Most CRCs in this age group are known to arise in the distal colon and rectum suggesting that lesions other than SSA/P may serve as the precursor for the majority of early-onset CRC.

Keywords: Adenoma, Sessile serrated adenoma, Early-onset colorectal cancer

Background

Colorectal cancer (CRC) in young adults (diagnosed before age 50 years) accounts for 7.5% of the total CRC burden in the Australian population [1], and its incidence has been increasing during the last two decades in both Australia and the USA [2–4]. Though the early age of onset for CRC is thought to reflect an increased genetic predisposition, the majority appear to be sporadic [5, 6]. CRC in young adults associated with known hereditary conditions such as Lynch syndrome comprises a minor component (15–17%) [7–10], whilst a further subset of cases have a clear familial basis with no attributable genetic aetiology [11]. Some authors have raised the possibility that sporadic early-onset CRC may result from the inheritance of multiple predisposing genetic variants, both rare and common [12], rather than the slow accumulation of somatic changes seen in sporadic CRC from older patients. Attempts to identify rare predisposing variants outside the known genetic syndromes have been undertaken on CRC patients under 40 years of age, and have encountered considerable heterogeneity, with few rare loss-of-function variants being recurrent [13]. Hence the origin of most early-onset CRC remains unexplained.

* Correspondence: joanne.young@adelaide.edu.au
[9]Department of Haematology and Oncology, The Queen Elizabeth Hospital, Woodville South 5011, Adelaide, South Australia, Australia
[11]School of Medicine, University of Adelaide, Adelaide 5000, South Australia, Australia
Full list of author information is available at the end of the article

A number of authors have suggested that early-onset CRC is a distinct entity based on clinico-molecular analyses [14, 15]. Early-onset CRC occurs more frequently in the distal colorectum compared with CRC in older adults [3]. In addition, the CRC are more likely to display mucinous and signet ring cell differentiation, and high histologic grade. Early-onset CRC has also been reported to have a different molecular profile than that occurring in older adults [11]. In particular, early-onset CRC demonstrates less frequent *BRAF* mutation (7% vs 19%) and more frequent isolated *PIK3CA/PTEN* mutation (16% vs 1%) than tumours from patients aged over 70 at CRC diagnosis [16]. CRC develop from two *major* subclasses of precursor lesions; conventional adenomas and serrated polyps. The molecular pathogenesis of CRC frequently reflects the lesion from which the CRC arises; however, studies of precursor lesion histological subtypes in the young are limited, as this age group is not undergoing population screening. Lesion subtypes are associated with a number of lifestyle risk factors [17, 18], and therefore may be studied to provide clues to the triggers for early-onset colorectal neoplasia. The aim of this study was to document the prevalence, location and histological subtype of CRC precursor lesions in patients undergoing colonoscopy before age 50 years in a hospital colonoscopy service and compare the findings with those from patients aged 50 years and older, with a view to increasing the current understanding of bowel neoplasia in young adults and seeking clues to its potential risk factors.

Methods

This is a cross-sectional study using an audit of 2613 procedures recorded within the colonoscopy database at The Queen Elizabeth Hospital (a tertiary teaching hospital) in Adelaide, South Australia over a 12-month period from March 2013. Data from each procedure were extracted in sequence by a gastroenterology registrar (SW) and recorded in a purpose-dedicated database. Findings were obtained from both the colonoscopy report within a ProVation endoscopy procedure documentation system (Wolters Klewer) [19], and the corresponding pathology report concerning histological examination of excised lesions. Lesion sizes were derived from colonoscopy reports. Indications for colonoscopy were derived from admission notes in ProVation including self-reported family history of CRC (any non-specified relative with CRC), personal medical history of colonic neoplasia, bowel symptoms (pain, change of habit, diarrhoea, constipation), occult or overt bleeding, confirmed iron-deficiency anaemia, and confirmed or suspected inflammatory bowel disease. The study was approved by the Human Research Ethics Committee of the Central Adelaide Local Health Network under protocol number HREC/14/TQEHLMH/194.

Definitions

Lesion subtypes were reported on a *per colonoscopy* basis. *Any serrated lesion* included hyperplastic polyps, sessile serrated adenoma/polyps (SSA/P) and traditional serrated adenomas (TSA) [20]. *Any conventional adenoma* comprised conventional adenomas with tubular and/or villous histology and low- or high-grade dysplasia. *CRC precursor lesions* (CPL), comprised SSA/P with or without dysplasia, TSA, tubular adenomas ≥10 mm in size or with high-grade dysplasia (ATA) and any conventional adenoma with villous histology (TVA or VA). *Proximal colon* refers to caecum, ascending colon, and transverse colon. *Distal colon* refers to splenic flexure, descending colon, sigmoid colon and rectum.

Statistical analysis

Prevalence of characteristics of patients, indications for colonoscopy and findings were compared between two groups (<50 vs ≥50 years) using Pearson's chi-squared test. Continuous variables were compared using a *t*-test. All statistical association tests were performed using SPSS Version 23 for Mac (IBM). Two-tailed statistics were used throughout with a significance level of *P*-value <0.05.

Results

Of the total 2613 available reports, 398 (15%) were excluded due to incomplete data, and a further 77 procedures (3%) were not completed due to poor bowel preparation, looping or patient discomfort, leaving 2138 complete procedures (82%). Within this group, sixty-six patients underwent multiple colonoscopies during the study period. In instances of multiple procedures, data were drawn from the initial procedure only, leaving a total of 2064 individual patients whose data contributed to the study. Characteristics of patients and colonoscopy findings are given in Table 1.

Indications

Patients aged <50 were more likely to be having a procedure for *family history* of CRC (*P* = 0.001), whereas those aged ≥ 50 years were more likely to have a *personal history* of CRC or polyps (*P* <0.001). Five patients were known to have a DNA mismatch repair gene mutation (Lynch syndrome) prior to the procedure, and all were females and aged under 50 years. Confirmed or suspected inflammatory bowel disease, abdominal pain and change in bowel habit were more frequently reported as an indication for colonoscopy in young patients (*P* <0.001 in all instances). Young patients had a higher prevalence of overt bleeding as an indication for their procedure (*P* <0.001), whereas older patients demonstrated a higher prevalence of occult bleeding (*P* <0.001).

Table 1 Characteristics of patients, and polyp findings in each age group

		All	%	Age <50	%	Age ≥50	%	*P*-value <50 vs ≥50
Totals		*n* = 2064		*n* = 485		*n* = 1579		
Mean age		59.7		39.2		66.0		
Median age		60		42		65		
Age range		18–96		18–49		50–96		
Sex	Males	984	47.6	220	45.4	764	48.4	0.13
	Females	1080	52.4	265	54.6	815	51.6	
Indications								
	IBD	90	4.4	49	10.1	41	2.6	*<0.001*
	Overt bleeding	348	16.8	108	22.2	240	15.2	*<0.001*
	Occult bleeding	350	16.9	29	5.9	321	20.3	*<0.001*
	Pain	227	11	77	15.9	150	9.5	*<0.001*
	Bowel habit	194	9.4	74	15.3	120	7.6	*<0.001*
	FH CRC	117	5.7	42	8.7	75	4.8	*0.001*
	PH CRC	83	4	4	0.8	79	5	*<0.001*
	PH polyps	303	14.9	34	7	274	17.4	*<0.001*
Findings								
	Any polyps	714	34.6	80	16.5	584	37	*<0.001*
	Serrated polyps	205	9.9	41	8.5	164	10.4	0.21
	Conventional adenomas	523	25.3	46	9.5	477	30.2	*<0.001*
	Multiple polyps	406	19.7	35	7.2	371	23.5	*<0.001*
	CPL	225	10.9	21	4.3	204	12.9	*<0.001*
Polyp sub-types								
	SSA/P	65	3.1	11	2.3	54	3.4	0.20
	TSA	1	0.01	0	0	1	0.06	
	TVA	95	4.6	8	1.6	87	5.5	*<0.001*
	ATA	76	3.7	3	0.6	73	4.6	*<0.001*
	VA	2	0.01	0	0	2	0.13	
Cancers								
	CRC	55	2.7	5	1	50	3.2	*0.01*
	Distal CRC Site	28	49.1	4	80	24	48.1	0.35

IBD Inflammatory bowel disease (Crohns disease, ulcerative colitis, NOS), *FH CRC* Family history of CRC, *PH CRC* Personal history of CRC, *PH* Polyps Personal history of polyps, *CPL* known CRC precursor lesions, *SSA/P* Sessile serrated adenoma/polyps, *TVA* Tubulovillous adenoma, *ATA* Advanced tubular adenoma (≥10 mm, and/or high-grade dysplasia), *TSA* Traditional serrated adenoma, *VA* Villous adenoma
Significant *p*-values are shown in italics

Precursor polyps and cancers

Histologically confirmed neoplastic lesions were observed in 16.5% (80/485) of patients aged <50 and 37% (584/1579) of patients aged ≥50 (P <0.001) (Table 1). Polyps known to serve as CRC precursor lesions (CPL) were seen in 4.3% (21/485) of patients aged <50 and 12.9% (204/1579) of patients aged ≥50 (P <0.001). When all polyps were assessed according to subtype, there was no evidence for a difference in serrated polyp prevalence (any serrated subtypes including hyperplastic polyps) when data were partitioned at age 50 ($P = 0.21$). In contrast, conventional adenomas were more prevalent in the older age group (P <0.001). The distribution of CPL subtypes also differed between age groups (Table 1 and Fig. 1). The prevalence in the study population of SSA/P did not differ between the two age groups ($P = 0.20$) but both TVA (P <0.001) and ATA (P <0.001) were more prevalent in the older age group (Fig. 1a,b). SSA/P were removed from 11/21 (52%) colonoscopies bearing known precursor lesions in patients <50 year, compared with 55/204 (27%) colonoscopies in patients aged 50 and older ($P = 0.02$) (Fig. 1c). SSA/P were located in the proximal colon in 90% of cases within the patient group aged <50 years, and in 80% in those aged ≥50 ($P = 0.45$). Average size of SSA/P in the <50 age group was 6.8 mm (range 2–15 mm) and in those aged ≥50 was 8.7 mm

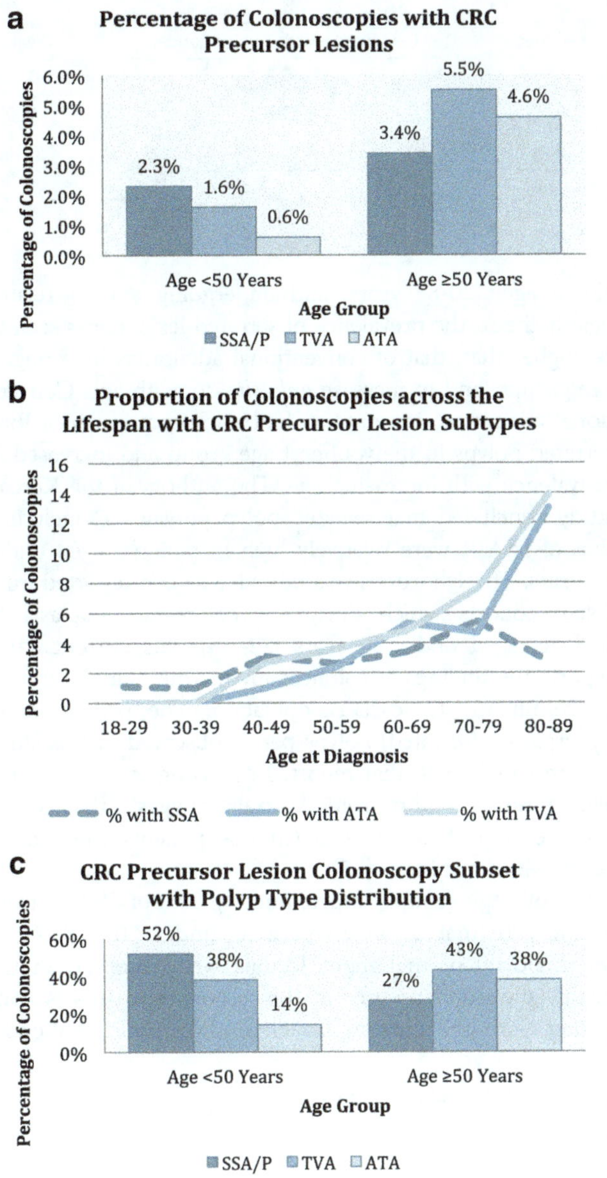

Fig. 1 Distribution of Polyp Subtypes. Graphs showing the distribution of polyp subtypes **a** across all colonoscopies partitioned by age group, **b** within the colonoscopies which yielded known CRC precursor lesions (CPL) partitioned by age group and **c** the percentage of colonoscopies which yielded the three major subtypes of CRC precursor lesions, SSA/P, TVA and ATA across the lifespan. *SSA/P* sessile serrated polyp, *TVA* tubulovillous adenoma, *ATA* advanced tubular adenoma (≥10 mm or high-grade dysplasia)

(range 2–25 mm) ($P = 0.36$). There was no difference between the prevalence of SSA/P in each sex overall ($P = 0.35$) or within the younger patient age group ($P = 0.59$). The prevalence of CPL or CRC did not differ between the sexes in patients aged <50, however males were more likely than females to develop CPL or CRC in patients aged ≥50 years ($P = 0.007$) (Table 2). The service-based adenoma detection rate was 297/984 (30%) for males and 226/1080 (21%) for females.

CRC was detected in 1.0% (5/485) of patients aged <50 vs 3.2% (50/1579) of patients aged ≥50 ($P = 0.01$). Colonoscopy-detected CRC in patients aged <50 was found in the distal colon in 4/5 (80%) compared with 24/50 (48%)($P = 0.35$). Of the five patients known to have Lynch syndrome, only one was found to have CRC in the setting of long-standing ulcerative colitis, and the remaining four patients showed no pathology. All high-grade dysplasia in the audit was observed in the older age group in 16 polyps from 15 patients (12 females; average age 74). The polyps comprised 4 tubular adenomas and 11 tubulovillous adenomas. In addition, several rare polyp types were observed during the audit including a single, proximally located SSA/P with dysplasia in a 67 year old female, a villous adenoma in a 79 year old female, and a traditional serrated adenoma in a 51 year old female.

Synchronously occurring lesion types

The co-occurrence of CPL subtypes in patients in each age group is shown in Table 3. Having at least one SSA/P was associated with any conventional adenoma across all patients ($P = 0.002$), with any conventional tubular adenoma ($P = 0.001$), whilst there was no evidence for an association with advanced tubular adenomas ($P = 0.09$) or tubulovillous adenomas ($P = 0.99$). The association between SSA/P and any conventional adenoma or any tubular adenoma remained significant when patients ≥50 years were considered ($P = 0.02$ and $P = 0.008$ respectively) but failed to attain statistical significance when patients aged under 50 years were analysed ($P = 0.08$ and $P = 0.05$ respectively). Co-occurrence between conventional adenomas, or tubular adenomas, and SSA/P was present regardless of family history of CRC.

Bleeding and polyp types

Patients who were having a colonoscopy for occult or active bleeding were more likely to have been diagnosed with CPL or CRC ($P = 0.005$) compared with patients not reporting any bleeding. This finding was seen in the older age group ($P = 0.03$), though not in younger patients ($P = 0.18$). When bleeding was stratified into overt and occult forms, occult bleeding was associated with CPL or CRC ($P = 0.03$), or with advanced conventional adenoma specifically ($P = 0.009$), in patients diagnosed at ≥50 years, but there was no evidence for this association in patients under 50 years. No associations emerged between bleeding and SSA/P in either age group ($P = 0.99$)(Table 4).

Table 2 Medium to high-risk polyps or cancer grouped by sex and age

Group	Males	Percentage with CPL or cancer	Females	Percentage with CPL or cancer	*P*-value*
<50 years	11	5	15	5.7	0.75
≥50 years	140	18.3	109	13.4	*0.007*
All	151	15.3	124	11.5	*0.01*

*Comparison of proportion of each feature between males and females
CPL known CRC precursor lesions
Significant *p*-values are shown in italics

Family history of CRC

There was no evidence for association between family history of CRC and CPL, or CRC specifically, in those aged under 50 at colonoscopy. There was some evidence for patients aged 50 and older to have an association between a family history of CRC and a diagnosis of CRC specifically ($P = 0.08$). SSA/P showed an association with family history of CRC ($P = 0.04$) in those aged 50 and older. No evidence for an association between family history of CRC and conventional adenomas was observed in either age group.

Discussion

The results of this study suggest that, in contrast to older patients, SSA/P comprise a significantly higher *proportion* of the known CRC precursors [21] removed from patients aged under 50 in a routine colonoscopy service. Overall, SSA/P prevalence did not differ between the two age groups in the study, whereas advanced adenoma prevalence increased steadily with age, in parallel to some degree with the higher prevalence of cancer in the older age group, and consistent with what would be expected in the general population. A similar pattern to these observations has been reported previously among all polyp subtypes [22]. In a retrospective cohort of 28,544 asymptomatic patients from Korea aged 20-88 years, and undergoing a work-related health check, the prevalence of serrated lesions was seen to be higher than that of conventional adenomas in youngest age groups, and to increase *only slightly* with age. Conventional adenomas, in contrast, had a lower prevalence than serrated polyps in the youngest age group and increased in prevalence with increasing age. The authors of the Korean study concluded that serrated polyp prevalence, including that of SSA/P, were relatively high in patients aged under 50 years. Though extensive studies have been reported from Asian cohorts which document colorectal neoplasia in patients aged under 50 years [22–24], this current study reports the findings at colonoscopy in young adults from a predominantly Caucasian population. The prevalence of hyperplastic (serrated) polyps per se observed in this study is comparable with that reported by Wong et al [23], however a recent report from Australia suggests that SSA/P subtype is relatively rare in Chinese patients when compared with Caucasians [25].

In both age groups, approximately 80% of SSA/P arose in the proximal colon. In patients under 50 with CRC, the majority of malignant lesions was observed in the distal colon and rectum in this report, and this is consistent with the current understanding that early-onset

Table 3 Co-occurrence of adenoma subtypes with SSA/P in patients with conventional adenomas

SSA/P co-occurring with...		SSA/P present (n)	(%)	SSA/P absent (n)	(%)	*P*-value*
Any AD	<50 years	3/11	27.3	43/474	9.1	0.08
	≥50 years	25/55	46.3	452/1523	29.7	*0.02*
	All	28/66	43.1	495/1997	24.8	*0.002*
Any TA	<50 years	3/11	27.3	37/474	7.8	0.05
	≥50 years	24/55	44.4	403/1524	26.4	*0.008*
	All	27/66	41.5	440/1998	22.0	*0.001*
ATA	<50 years	1/11	9.1	2/474	0.4	0.07
	≥50 years	4/55	7.4	69/1524	4.5	0.32
	All	5/66	7.7	71/1998	3.6	0.09
TVA	<50 years	0/11	0.0	8/485	1.7	0.99
	≥50 years	3/55	5.6	84/1524	5.5	0.99
	All	3/66	4.6	92/1998	4.6	0.99

*Comparison of proportions of specified condition present (i.e. SSA/P present among those with any adenoma, any tubular adenoma, an advanced tubular adenoma, or a tubulovillous adenoma) between young adults (<50 years) and older adults (≥50 years) compared to patients with the specified adenoma only
SSA/P sessile serrated adenoma/polyp, *Any AD* any conventional adenoma, *Any TA* any tubular adenoma, *ATA* advanced tubular adenoma (≥10 mm and/or high-grade dysplasia), *TVA* tubulovillous adenoma
Significant *p*-values are shown in italics

Table 4 Associations between significant neoplasia and bleeding observations in patients with bleeding

		Age <50 *n*=	%	P-value	Age ≥50 *n*=	%	*P*-value	All *n*=	%	*P*-value
Totals	Patients with bleeding	137			561			698		
Any bleeding	With CPL/CRC	10	7.3	0.18	101	18.0	*0.03*	111	15.9	*0.005*
	With SSA/P	5	3.6	0.2	17	3.0	0.53	22	3.2	0.99
	With AA	4	2.9	0.54	65	11.6	*0.03*	69	9.9	*0.008*
Totals	Patients with overt bleeding	*n* = 108			*n* = 240			*n* = 348		
Overt bleeding	With CPL/CRC	8	7.4	0.17	40	16.7	0.31	48	13.8	0.34
	With SSA/P	4	3.7	0.21	8	3.3	0.56	12	3.4	0.42
	With AA	4	3.7	0.21	23	9.6	0.49	27	7.8	0.52
Totals	Patients with occult bleeding	*n* = 29			*n* = 321			*n* = 350		
Occult bleeding	With CPL/CRC	2	6.9	0.45	61	19.0	*0.03*	63	18.0	*0.002*
	With SSA/P	1	3.4	0.5	9	2.8	0.31	10	2.9	0.44
	With AA	0	0.0	0.5	42	13.1	*0.009*	42	12.0	*0.001*

CPL/CRC CRC precursor lesions and/or CRC, *SSA/P* sessile serrated polyp, *AA* advanced conventional adenoma (≥10 mm or high-grade dysplasia or villous histology)
Significant *p*-values are shown in italics

CRC is predominantly a malignancy of the distal large bowel [3, 12, 26, 27]. SSA/P, being located in the proximal colon in young adults, are therefore unlikely to be the precursor lesion for most early-onset CRC. In support of this premise, somatic *BRAF* mutation, the molecular genetic hallmark of SSA/P, is relatively rare in CRC from young adults, being present at (3/45) 7% in a Norwegian study [16], 1/68 (2%) in a Spanish report [8], and in 0/39 (0%) from France [14]. Activating mutations in *BRAF* are present in 14–16% of all population-based CRC [28, 29].

It is not known for certain whether SSA/P have always been present in young patients undergoing colonoscopy. Indeed, growing awareness of SSA/P has occurred only in recent decades, and may have contributed to this observation. Alternatively, the presence of SSA/P in young patients may be a surrogate marker for mucosal abnormalities and future risk of advanced neoplasia, related to an emerging population risk factor among young adults. Smoking has been consistently associated with SSA/P, and, though it is thought by some authors that the induction time in young adults is insufficient to produce neoplasia [3, 30, 31], a recent report has presented evidence that it may be a contributory factor [32]. Associations between obesity and diabetes and a diagnosis of SSA/P have been reported inconsistently [33, 34]. However, metabolic risk scores for prediction of advanced colorectal neoplasia demonstrate their greatest effects in patients aged under 60 years [35]. More recently, diabetes has been identified as an independent risk factor for colorectal neoplasia in patients aged 40–49 years [23] and diabetes has been identified elsewhere as a risk factor for early-onset CRC [36].

The study also incidentally highlights a number of features of SSA/P. It presents indirect evidence for a prolonged dwell time for these lesions, and suggests that SSA/P may arise early and be present in the colon for decades without a significant increase in size [37]. Bleeding as an indication for colonoscopy was not associated with SSA/P in our data [38], in contrast to this symptom showing a significant association with advanced conventional adenomas. In addition, the study confirms a previous observation of an association between SSA/P and a family history of CRC [39], though this was not apparent in patients under 50. In patients under 50, the lower overall age of first-degree relatives may be a contributing factor to this observation.

The study observed a significant likelihood for SSA/P to co-occur with *non-villous* conventional adenomas specifically, though association between SSA/P and conventional adenomas generally has long been recognised [38, 40–44]. A recent report provided indirect evidence for our finding in that conventional adenomas which occur synchronously with SSA/P lack *KRAS* mutation [45] which is a known feature of villous histology [46]. A further report has shown that proximal serrated polyps have been associated with multiple non-advanced conventional adenomas in Chinese patients [43]. These findings may be related to a predisposed mucosa [47], and as such may serve as a *marker* for increased risk of advanced neoplasia, rather than as precursors per se. The presence of small SSA/P in association with a small tubular adenoma has recently been associated with a significantly increased rate of metachronous advanced neoplasia during surveillance when compared to small tubular adenomas alone (18.2% vs 7.8%, $P = 0.02$). In addition, the presence of small SSA/P had a risk of metachonous advanced neoplasia comparable with an index high-risk conventional adenoma (17.9% for a small isolated SSA/P vs 15.9% for a high-risk conventional adenoma) [48]. It has been suggested that isolated small SSA/P therefore be considered for new surveillance interval recommendations [48]. These observations highlight the clinical relevance of findings in our current study, as there may be potential benefit of increased longitudinal follow-up in young adults with SSA/P, *regardless of size*. That there was no association between SSA/P and adenomas with villous histology may reflect genetic background in patients who develop SSA/P [49].

A previous report has suggested that rectal bleeding is less useful for prediction of advanced neoplasia in patients under 50 years [50], and this observation has also emerged in our study. The differences in occult versus active bleeding may have some implications when we look at mechanisms to reduce the impact from an increasing rate of CRC in patients aged under 50 years. Only 6% of those <50 years had occult bleeding compared to 20.3% for those aged over 50 years ($p = <0.001$). The low rate may reflect a lower uptake of the testing, as expected, because young patients are not undergoing screening. It also highlights a difference in timing of presentation with younger patients more likely to await symptoms and there is evidence of more advanced disease potentially supportive of this [51]. Although education around testing for occult bleeding will still be relevant, more general education approaches around screening, symptoms and early presentation to a health care provider may be just as important, both targeting patients and the health care profession, and may involve other markers of increased risk such as family history of malignancy and personal history of diabetes.

The study has a number of limitations. Patients under 50 are undergoing procedures for a different range of indications, although this does reflect real world practice. The number of young adults with neoplastic findings was relatively low and may have affected the power of a subset of comparisons. However, the presence of SSA/P in young adults is an important observation which has the potential to identify those aged under 50 who are at higher than population risk. In addition, the population did not include cases of advanced neoplasia diagnosed by sigmoidoscopy or imaging, and it is difficult to know whether this has influenced the ability to generalise to all young adults undergoing investigations. Colonoscopies were performed at a single tertiary centre involving multiple colonoscopists, and individual adenoma detection rates were not available. However, our service-based adenoma detection rate is within the updated limits suggested for a quality colonoscopy service of at least 30% for males and 20% for females [52]. Family history was self-reported and not systematically verified, and indications for colonoscopy were extracted from admission notes. Allowing for these limitations, results showed that adenoma prevalence rises with age, and this is in keeping with what would be expected in the general population [53]. This report also confirms a recent publication demonstrating that advanced polyps in patients under 45 are more likely to be sporadic than associated with family history, as family history of CRC was reported in 7.1% of those with any advanced neoplasia [54].

Conclusions

In summary, proximal SSA/P comprised a greater proportion of lesions with malignant potential in patients under age 50, compared with older patients. However most CRC in this age group occurs in the distal colon and rectum, both in this study, and consistently in the literature [3, 12, 26, 27], suggesting that SSA/P are unlikely to serve as the premalignant lesion for the majority of early-onset CRC, but may have a potential role as *markers* of future increased risk for advanced neoplasia. Further, SSA/P in both age groups co-occurred significantly with conventional non-villous adenomas, a combination with increased risk for subsequent advanced neoplasia [48].

Abbreviations

AA: Advanced conventional adenoma; ATA: Advanced tubular adenoma (≥10 mm, and/or high-grade dysplasia); CPL: Known CRC precursor lesions; FH CRC: Family history of CRC; IBD: Inflammatory bowel disease (Crohns disease, ulcerative colitis, NOS); PH CRC: Personal history of CRC; PH Polyps: Personal history of polyps; SSA/P: Sessile serrated adenoma/polyp; TSA: Traditional serrated adenoma; TVA: Tubulovillous adenoma; VA: Villous adenoma

Acknowledgement

The authors thank Sheona Page for assistance with ethics applications.

Funding

AKW is an NHMRC Early Career Fellow.

Authors' contributions

SW performed the audit, interpreted results, contributed to and approved the final manuscript, IL Contributed to the audit, interpreted results, contributed to and approved the final manuscript, CR interpreted results, contributed to and approved the manuscript, AR interpreted results, contributed to and approved the final manuscript, SP interpreted results, contributed to and approved the final manuscript, AKW contributed to data analysis, interpreted results, contributed to and approved the final manuscript, YT interpreted results, contributed to and approved the final manuscript, SV interpreted results, contributed to and approved the final manuscript, AT interpreted results, contributed to and approved the final manuscript, DP interpreted results, contributed to and approved the final manuscript, JEH interpreted results, contributed to and approved the final manuscript, DR contributed to analysis of data, interpreted results, contributed to and approved the final manuscript, ES interpreted results, contributed to and approved the final manuscript, PD interpreted results, contributed to and approved the final manuscript, JM contributed to results, contributed to and approved the final manuscript, WU assisted with the audit, formatted results, contributed to and approved the final manuscript, PH interpreted results, contributed to and approved the final manuscript, DW interpreted results, contributed to and approved the final manuscript, ES interpreted results, contributed to and approved the final manuscript, GPY interpreted results, provided critical input to and approved the final manuscript, TJP interpreted results, provided critical input to and approved the final manuscript, JPY conceived the design, analysed the results, wrote the manuscript. All authors read and approved the final manuscript.

Competing interests
The authors declare they hold no conflict of interest with respect to this work.

Author details
[1]Department of Gastroenterology, The Queen Elizabeth Hospital, Woodville South 5011, Adelaide, South Australia, Australia. [2]Envoi Specialist Pathologists, Kelvin Grove 4059, Brisbane, QLD, Australia. [3]School of Medicine, University of Queensland, Herston 4006, Brisbane, QLD, Australia. [4]Department of Pathology, Colorectal Oncogenomics Group, Genetic Epidemiology Laboratory, The University of Melbourne, Parkville 3010, Melbourne, VIC, Australia. [5]Division of Anatomical Pathology, SA Pathology, Adelaide 5000, South Australia, Australia. [6]Centre for Cancer Biology, University of South Australia, Adelaide 5000, South Australia, Australia. [7]Familial GI Cancer Service and Ministry of Health Bowel Cancer Programme, Auckland City Hospital, Auckland, New Zealand. [8]Centre for Epidemiology and Biostatistics, Melbourne School of Population and Global Health, The University of Melbourne, Parkville 3010, Melbourne, VIC, Australia. [9]Department of Haematology and Oncology, The Queen Elizabeth Hospital, Woodville South 5011, Adelaide, South Australia, Australia. [10]Flinders Medical Centre, Bedford Park 5042, Adelaide, South Australia, Australia. [11]School of Medicine, University of Adelaide, Adelaide 5000, South Australia, Australia. [12]Cancer Epidemiology and Population Health, University of South Australia, Adelaide 5000, South Australia, Australia. [13]School of Nursing and Midwifery, Flinders University, Bedford Park 5042, Adelaide, South Australia, Australia. [14]Basil Hetzel Institute, The Queen Elizabeth Hospital, Woodville South 5011, Adelaide, South Australia, Australia. [15]Cancer Voices SA, Kensington Park 5068, Adelaide, South Australia, Australia. [16]University of Adelaide Department of Surgery, The Queen Elizabeth Hospital, Woodville South 5011, Adelaide, South Australia, Australia. [17]Cancer Theme, South Australian Health and Medical Research Institute, Adelaide 5000, South Australia, Australia. [18]Flinders Centre for Innovation in Cancer, Flinders University, Bedford Park 5042, Adelaide, South Australia, Australia. [19]Bowel Health Service, Repatriation General Hospital, Daw Park 5041, Adelaide, South Australia, Australia. [20]SAHMRI Colorectal Node, Basil Hetzel Institute, Woodville South, Adelaide, South Australia 5011, Australia.

References
1. AIHW. Cancer in Australia: an overview 2014. Cancer series No 90. Cat. no. CAN 88. Canberra: AIHW. Cancer series Canberra, 2014.
2. O'Connell JB, Maggard MA, Liu JH, et al. Rates of colon and rectal cancers are increasing in young adults. Am Surg. 2003;69:866–72.
3. Siegel RL, Jemal A, Ward EM. Increase in incidence of colorectal cancer among young men and women in the United States. Cancer Epidemiol Biomarkers Prev. 2009;18:1695–8.
4. Young JP, Win AK, Rosty C, et al. Rising Incidence of Early-Onset Colorectal Cancer in Australia over Two Decades: Report and Review. J Gastroenterol Hepatol. 2015;30:6–13.
5. Chubb D, Broderick P, Dobbins SE, et al. Rare disruptive mutations and their contribution to the heritable risk of colorectal cancer. Nat Commun. 2016;7:11883.
6. Liang J, Kalady MF, Church J. Young age of onset colorectal cancers. Int J Colorectal Dis. 2015;30:1653–7.
7. Perea J, Rodriguez Y, Rueda D, et al. Early-Onset Colorectal Cancer is an Easy and Effective Tool to Identify Retrospectively Lynch Syndrome. Ann Surg Oncol. 2011;18:3285–91.
8. Pearlman R, Frankel WL, Swanson B, et al. Prevalence and Spectrum of Germline Cancer Susceptibility Gene Mutations Among Patients With Early-Onset Colorectal Cancer. JAMA Oncol. 2016. doi:10.1001/jamaoncol.2016.5194.
9. Plunkett M, Murray M, Frizelle F, Teague L, Hinder V, Findlay M. Colorectal adenocarcinoma cancer in New Zealand in those under 25 years of age (1997-2007). ANZ J Surg. 2014;84(5):371–5.
10. Southey MC, Jenkins MA, Mead L, et al. Use of molecular tumor characteristics to prioritize mismatch repair gene testing in early-onset colorectal cancer. J Clin Oncol. 2005;23:6524–32.
11. Silla IO, Rueda D, Rodriguez Y, et al. Early-onset colorectal cancer: a separate subset of colorectal cancer. World J Gastroenterol. 2014;20:17288–96.
12. Stigliano V, Sanchez-Mete L, Martayan A, et al. Early-onset colorectal cancer: a sporadic or inherited disease? World J Gastroenterol. 2014;20:12420–30.
13. Tanskanen T, Gylfe AE, Katainen R, et al. Exome sequencing in diagnostic evaluation of colorectal cancer predisposition in young patients. Scand J Gastroenterol. 2013;48:672–8.
14. Kirzin S, Marisa L, Guimbaud R, et al. Sporadic early-onset colorectal cancer is a specific sub-type of cancer: a morphological, molecular and genetics study. PLoS One. 2014;9:e103159.
15. Perea J, Rueda D, Canal A, et al. Age at Onset Should Be a Major Criterion for Subclassification of Colorectal Cancer. J Mol Diagn. 2014;16:116–26.
16. Berg M, Danielsen SA, Ahlquist T, et al. DNA sequence profiles of the colorectal cancer critical gene set KRAS-BRAF-PIK3CA-PTEN-TP53 related to age at disease onset. PLoS One. 2010;5:e13978.
17. Burnett-Hartman AN, Passarelli MN, Adams SV, et al. Differences in epidemiologic risk factors for colorectal adenomas and serrated polyps by lesion severity and anatomical site. Am J Epidemiol. 2013;177:625–37.
18. Wallace K, Grau MV, Ahnen D, et al. The association of lifestyle and dietary factors with the risk for serrated polyps of the colorectum. Cancer Epidemiol Biomarkers Prev. 2009;18:2310–7.
19. Tran Cao HS, Cosman BC, Devaraj B, et al. Performance measures of surgeon-performed colonoscopy in a Veterans Affairs medical center. Surg Endosc. 2009;23:2364–8.
20. Snover D, Ahnen DJ, Burt RW, et al. Serrated polyps of the colon and rectum and serrated polyposis. In: WHO Classification of Tumours of the Digestive System. Fourth edth ed. Lyon: IARC; 2010.
21. Tinmouth J, Henry P, Hsieh E, et al. Sessile serrated polyps at screening colonoscopy: have they been under diagnosed? Am J Gastroenterol. 2014; 109:1698–704.
22. Kim HY, Kim SM, Seo JH, et al. Age-specific prevalence of serrated lesions and their subtypes by screening colonoscopy: a retrospective study. BMC Gastroenterol. 2014;14:82.
23. Wong JC, Lau JY, Suen BY, Ng SC, Wong MC, Tang RS, Wong SH, Wu JC, Chan FK, Sung JJ. Prevalence, distribution, and risk factor for colonic neoplasia in 1133 subjects aged 40-49 undergoing screening colonoscopy. J Gastroenterol Hepatol. 2017;32(1):92–7.
24. Wong MC, Ching JY, Chiu HM, et al. Risk of Colorectal Neoplasia in Individuals With Self-Reported Family History: A Prospective Colonoscopy Study from 16 Asia-Pacific Regions. Am J Gastroenterol. 2016;111:1621–9.
25. Kumbhari V, Behary J, Hui JM. Prevalence of adenomas and sessile serrated adenomas in Chinese compared with Caucasians. J Gastroenterol Hepatol. 2013; 28:608–12.
26. Myers EA, Feingold DL, Forde KA, et al. Colorectal cancer in patients under 50 years of age: A retrospective analysis of two institutions' experience. World J Gastroenterol. 2013;19:5651–7.
27. Perea J, Alvaro E, Rodriguez Y, et al. Approach to early-onset colorectal cancer: Clinicopathological, familial, molecular and immunohistochemical characteristics. World J Gastroenterol. 2010;16:3697–703.
28. English DR, Young JP, Simpson JA, et al. Ethnicity and risk for colorectal cancers showing somatic BRAF V600E mutation or CpG island methylator phenotype. Cancer Epidemiol Biomarkers Prev. 2008;17:1774–80.
29. Weisenberger DJ, Siegmund KD, Campan M, et al. CpG island methylator phenotype underlies sporadic microsatellite instability and is tightly associated with BRAF mutation in colorectal cancer. Nat Genet. 2006;38:787–93.
30. Botteri E, Iodice S, Bagnardi V, et al. Smoking and colorectal cancer: a meta-analysis. JAMA. 2008;300:2765–78.
31. Giovannucci E. An updated review of the epidemiological evidence that cigarette smoking increases risk of colorectal cancer. Cancer Epidemiol Biomarkers Prev. 2001;10:725–31.
32. Shankar A, Shankar U, Dignan M. Effect of genetic and epigenetic characteristics on higher incidence of early-onset colorectal cancer in southeastern Appalachian Kentucky. J Clin Oncol. 2016;34:e13101.
33. Anderson JC, Rangasamy P, Rustagi T, et al. Risk factors for sessile serrated adenomas. J Clin Gastroenterol. 2011;45:694–9.
34. Haque TR, Bradshaw PT, Crockett SD. Risk factors for serrated polyps of the colorectum. Dig Dis Sci. 2014;59:2874–89.
35. Orannapalai N, Attawettayanon W, Kanngern S, et al. Predicting the occurrence of cancer-associated colorectal polyp using a metabolic risk score. Mol Clin Oncol. 2014;2:124–8.

36. Win AK, Taunde SA, Jayasekara H, et al. Role of lifestyle factors on risk of early-onset colorectal cancer. Asia Pac. J Clin Oncol. 2014;10:245.
37. Bettington M, Walker N, Rosty C, Brown I, Clouston A, McKeone D, Pearson SA, Leggett B, Whitehall V. Clinicopathological and molecular features of sessile serrated adenomas with dysplasia or carcinoma. Gut. 2017;66(1):97–106.
38. Zorzi M, Senore C, Da Re F, Barca A, Bonelli LA, Cannizzaro R, de Pretis G, DiFuria L, Di Giulio E, Mantellini P, Naldoni C, Sassatelli R, Rex DK, Zappa M, Hassan C, Equipe Working Group. Detection rate and predictive factors of sessileserrated polyps in an organised colorectal cancer screening programme with immunochemical faecal occult blood test: the EQuIPE study (Evaluating Quality Indicators of the Performance of Endoscopy). Gut. 2016. [Epub ahead of print].
39. Rustagi T, Rangasamy P, Myers M, et al. Sessile serrated adenomas in the proximal colon are likely to be flat, large and occur in smokers. World J Gastroenterol. 2013;19:5271–7.
40. Alvarez C, Andreu M, Castells A, et al. Relationship of colonoscopy-detected serrated polyps with synchronous advanced neoplasia in average-risk individuals. Gastrointest Endosc. 2013;78:333–41. e1.
41. Hazewinkel Y, de Wijkerslooth TR, Stoop EM, et al. Prevalence of serrated polyps and association with synchronous advanced neoplasia in screening colonoscopy. Endoscopy. 2014;46:219–24.
42. Li D, Jin C, McCulloch C, et al. Association of large serrated polyps with synchronous advanced colorectal neoplasia. Am J Gastroenterol. 2009;104: 695–702.
43. Ng SC, Ching JY, Chan VC, et al. Association between serrated polyps and the risk of synchronous advanced colorectal neoplasia in average-risk individuals. Aliment Pharmacol Ther. 2015;41:108–15.
44. Schreiner MA, Weiss DG, Lieberman DA. Proximal and large hyperplastic and nondysplastic serrated polyps detected by colonoscopy are associated with neoplasia. Gastroenterology. 2010;139:1497–502.
45. Pai RK, Mackinnon AC, Joseph L, et al. Identification of histologically distinct conventional adenomas that arise predominately in patients with sessile serrated adenomas. Am J Surg Pathol. 2010;34:355–63.
46. Vogelstein B, Fearon ER, Hamilton SR, et al. Genetic alterations during colorectal-tumor development. N Engl J Med. 1988;319:525–32.
47. Rosty C, Parry S, Young JP. Serrated polyposis: an enigmatic model of colorectal cancer predisposition. Pathol Res Int. 2011;2011:157073.
48. Melson J, Ma K, Arshad S, Greenspan M, Kaminsky T, Melvani V, Bishehsari F, Mahon B, Jakate S. Presence of small sessile serrated polyps increases rate of advanced neoplasia upon surveillance compared with isolated low-risk tubular adenomas. Gastrointest Endosc. 2016;84(2):307–14.
49. Wynter CV, Walsh MD, Higuchi T, et al. Methylation patterns define two types of hyperplastic polyp associated with colorectal cancer. Gut. 2004;53:573–80.
50. Lee JS, Rieger NA, Stephens JH, et al. Six-year prospective analysis of the rectal bleeding clinic at the Queen Elizabeth Hospital, Adelaide, South Australia. ANZ J Surg. 2007;77:553–6.
51. Vatandoust S, Price TJ, Ullah S, Roy AC, Beeke C, Young JP, Townsend A, Padbury R, Roder D, Karapetis CS. Metastatic Colorectal Cancer in Young Adults: A Study From the South Australian Population-Based Registry. Clin Colorectal Cancer. 2016;15(1):32–6.
52. Rex DK, Schoenfeld PS, Cohen J, et al. Quality indicators for colonoscopy. Gastrointest Endosc. 2015;81:31–53.
53. Adelstein BA, Macaskill P, Turner RM, et al. The value of age and medical history for predicting colorectal cancer and adenomas in people referred for colonoscopy. BMC Gastroenterol. 2011;11:97.
54. Kushnir VM, Nalbantoglu I, Watson R, et al. Advanced colorectal adenomas in patients under 45 years of age are mostly sporadic. Dig Dis Sci. 2014;59:2757–64.

8

Relationship of body weight with gastrointestinal motor and sensory function: studies in anorexia nervosa and obesity

Sena Bluemel[1], Dieter Menne[3], Gabriella Milos[4], Oliver Goetze[1], Michael Fried[1,5], Werner Schwizer[1,5], Mark Fox[1,5] and Andreas Steingoetter[1,2*]

Abstract

Background: Whether gastrointestinal motor and sensory function is primary cause or secondary effect of abnormal body weight is uncertain. Moreover, studies relating continuous postprandial sensations of satiation to measurable pathology are scarce. This work assessed postprandial gastrointestinal function and concurrent sensations of satiation across a wide range of body weight and after weight change.

Methods: Patients with anorexia nervosa (AN) and obesity (OB) were investigated in reference to normal weight controls (HC). AN were additionally investigated longitudinally. Gastric emptying, antral contractions and oro-cecal transit after ingestion of a solid meal were investigated by MRI and ^{13}C-lactose-ureide breath test. The dependency of self-reported sensations of satiation on the varying degree of stomach filling during gastric emptying was compared between groups.

Results: 24 AN (BMI 14.4 (11.9–16.0) kg/m^2), 16 OB (34.9 (29.6–41.5) kg/m^2) and 20 HC (21.9 (18.9–24.9) kg/m^2) were studied. Gastric half-emptying time (t_{50}) was slower in AN than HC ($p = 0.016$) and OB ($p = 0.007$), and a negative association between t_{50} and BMI was observed between BMI 12 and 25 kg/m^2 ($p = 0.007$). Antral contractions and oro-cecal transit were not different. For any given gastric content volume, self-reported postprandial fullness was greater in AN than in HC or OB ($p < 0.001$). After weight rehabilitation, t_{50} in AN tended to become shorter ($p = 0.09$) and postprandial fullness was less marked ($p < 0.01$).

Conclusions: A relationship between body weight and gastric emptying as well as self-reported feelings of satiation is present. AN have slower gastric emptying and heightened visceral perception compared to HC and OB. Longitudinal follow-up after weight rehabilitation in AN suggests these abnormalities are not a primary feature, but secondary to other factors that determine abnormal body weight.

Keywords: Gastric emptying, Gastrointestinal transit, Visceral sensations, Anorexia Nervosa, Obesity

* Correspondence: steingoetter@biomed.ee.ethz.ch
[1]Division of Gastroenterology and Hepatology, University Hospital Zurich, Raemistrasse 100, CH-8091 Zurich, Switzerland
[2]Institute for Biomedical Engineering, University and ETH Zurich, Zurich, Switzerland
Full list of author information is available at the end of the article

Background

Clinically relevant over- and underweight states have been attributed to genetic, psychological and environmental factors that influence food intake [1–4]. The central perception of satiation and satiety regulates food intake and is modulated by biophysical and neurohormonal feedback mechanisms originating from the gastrointestinal (GI) tract [5–8]. By regulating digestive function, these signals link central perceptions with GI motility [9]. However, observational and interventional trials studying the interrelation between GI motor and postprandial sensory function with body weight have not provided definitive findings. Previous studies have focused on either under- or overweight patients. In addition, the interpretation of published data is difficult because the technologies applied to assess GI function (e.g., γ-scintigraphy, ^{13}C-breath test) varied greatly between studies. Moreover, the relation of self-reported postprandial sensations of satiation and stomach volumes with body weight has not been demonstrated without invasive methods.

Individuals with morbid obesity have a delayed postprandial onset of satiation and less fullness [10]. Some authors suggest that this is related to relatively rapid gastric emptying compared to normal weight controls, but continuous assessments of sensations in the postprandial period are missing [11–15]. Moreover, observations varied between studies [16–21], so the role of altered gastric emptying and postprandial sensations in obesity remains controversial.

At the other extreme, many morbidly underweight patients with anorexia nervosa complain of prolonged fullness, bloating and nausea after meals [22]. These sensations have been linked to abnormal stomach function [23–26] – in particular, prolonged gastric emptying [25, 27–32]. However, the association between slow solid gastric emptying and clinically relevant postprandial symptoms is weak [33, 34] and it is not known whether this abnormality restricts meal consumption in this patient group.

This study aimed to clarify the relationship of postprandial GI motor and sensory function with body weight. The specific hypothesis tested was that the "GI response to feeding varies inversely with body weight" such that gastric emptying and oro-cecal transit increase and postprandial sensations of satiation decrease from under- to overweight. If present, then these findings would support the idea that the neurohormonal response to feeding is heightened in underweight and weakened in overweight patients and provide a physiological basis for the peripheral GI control of body weight (mediated by food intake). To this end, GI motor and sensory function in participants across a wide range of body weight including anorexic, normal weight and obese participants were investigated. In order to further test whether GI motor and sensory function are a primary cause or a secondary effect of abnormal body weight the participants with abnormal body weight were intended to be tested before and after weight rehabilitation.

Methods

Participants

Anorexia nervosa (AN) patients met DSM-IV criteria [35] and had a BMI <15.5 kg/m^2 at inclusion. AN were recruited from an inpatient psychotherapy unit for patients with severe eating disorders of the Psychiatric Department of the University Hospital. After a somatic and psychiatric stabilization period at the Eating Disorders Centre of the Clinic for Psychiatry and Psychotherapy within the first 4 weeks following admission, the participants should regularly gain approximately 1 kg of weight per week. This was attained by interdisciplinary multimodal inpatients therapy, consisting of assisted meals, group and individual psychotherapy, body-perception therapy, creativity therapy, nutritional counselling and other therapies. Recruitment and visit 1 occurred within the first 2 to 4 weeks of the program (orientation phase), before patients start to gain weight. Visit 2 (group AN2) occurred after AN patients attained BMI >17.5 kg/m^2. Normal weight, healthy controls (HC) with BMI 18.5–24.9 kg/m^2 were recruited via public announcements. Obese participants (OB) with BMI >30 kg/m^2 were recruited via the outpatient clinic of the Endocrinology Department of the University Hospital. Visit 2 was planned after patients lost >5% of body weight. Exclusion criteria were age <18 years and >60 years; history of gastrointestinal, cardiorespiratory (including hypertension), hematologic, renal or atopic disorders, diabetes, drug or alcohol abuse; abdominal surgery; regular intake of medication altering gut function (e.g. anticholinergics, laxatives, proton-pump inhibitors); presence of metallic foreign bodies interacting with magnetic resonance imaging (MRI); claustrophobia; body dimensions too large to fit into MRI scanner; pregnancy and lactation.

Study design

At the screening visits for the cross-sectional and longitudinal comparison, participants meeting the inclusion criteria completed the short-form Leeds Dyspepsia Questionnaire (LDQ), Gastroparesis Cardinal Symptom Index (GCSI), Beck Depression Inventory II (BDI) and the State-Trait-Anxiety Inventory (STAI). Participants fasted for minimum eight hours and refrained from smoking prior to study days. On study days, women were tested for pregnancy by urine analysis, normogylcaemia was confirmed. Participants were not allowed to eat or drink apart from the offered food and beverages.

As outlined in Fig. 1, following baseline measurements the muffin test meal (430 kcal, 21% fat, 63% carbohydrate, 16% protein) and the ^{13}C-breath test marker were eaten together with 200 ml of tap water while seated on the MRI scanner table. After ingestion (time t = 0 min), participants were placed in supine position inside the scanner and postprandial gastric volumes, antral motility, breath samples and sensation scores were acquired at regular time intervals (ref. Fig. 1). After 240 min, participants had to eat another unlabelled muffin meal. After 360 min, an *ad libitum* buffet was provided consisting of water, tomato soup, cheese, apples, chocolate, crackers and butter.

Magnetic resonance imaging

MRI was performed in a 1.5 T whole-body system (1.5 T Achieva; Philips Healthcare, The Netherlands). Gastric volume was derived from 30 axial MRI image planes covering the gastric region, performed during a single breath hold. Gastric content volume (GCV) was semi-automatically segmented at each time point using a custom designed image analysis software developed for MATLAB 7.4 (MathWorks Inc., Natick, MA, USA) [36]. Gastric motility scans consisted of 70 consecutive dynamic scans covering the gastric antrum and pylorus and recorded over 100 s during free-breathing [37].

^{13}C-Lactose-ureide breath test

Oro-cecal transit time (OCTT) was assessed by ^{13}C-lactose-ureide (^{13}C-LU) (Euriso-Top, Saint-Aubin Cedex, France) breath test after priming of the colonic bacterial flora with five 100 milligram doses of unlabelled lactose-ureide the day prior to the study (validated by authors). On the study day 500 mg ^{13}C-lactose-ureide blended into 2 grams of butter on 1x1 cm white bread was ingested immediately before the muffin meal [38]. Breath samples were collected into aluminized bags and analysed by non-dispersive isotope selective infrared spectroscopy (NDIRS, IRIS, Wagner Analysen Technik, Bremen, Germany). The increase of $^{13}CO_2$ concentration in the exhaled air referenced to the baseline value (delta over baseline, DOB) was used for data analyses.

Sensation scores

Participants were asked to rate their sensations of *hunger, fullness, nausea, bloating, abdominal pain, desire to eat* and *amount desired to eat* on a scale from 0 (*zero*, no sensation) to 10 (*ten*, maximal possible sensation) as described previously [39, 40].

Data analyses and statistics

Group size and power calculations were based on the primary study outcome measurement: half-time of gastric emptying (t_{50}). Published MRI data reported a mean difference of 29 min in t_{50} between a solid and a liquid test meal in 8 healthy participants, which was used as a clinically relevant effect size [41]. To detect the same difference with $\alpha = 0.05$ and power 90%, the required group size was estimated to be 16. Data plots and statistical analyses were performed with the software R, version 2.13.1 (R Foundation for Statistical Computing, Vienna, Austria).

MRI gastric content emptying curves were fitted by a power-exponential function to derive t_{50} [42]. To compensate for heteroscedasticity (reduction of the number of outliers and homogenization of variances), values of t_{50} were log-transformed for linear model analysis. Differences in $\log(t_{50})$ between groups are given as ratios (with confidence intervals). Gastric motility data were analyzed by a linear mixed-effect model.

OCTT was determined from the DOB-versus-time plots by a web-based consensus application (mean from four separate raters). Results were censored at OCTT >480 min. Analysis was based on Kaplan-Meier estimates and log-rank (Mantel-Haenszel) tests.

LDQ and GCSI were analyzed as previously described [43, 44]. The LDQ asks for the frequency and severity of indigestion, heartburn, regurgitation and nausea within

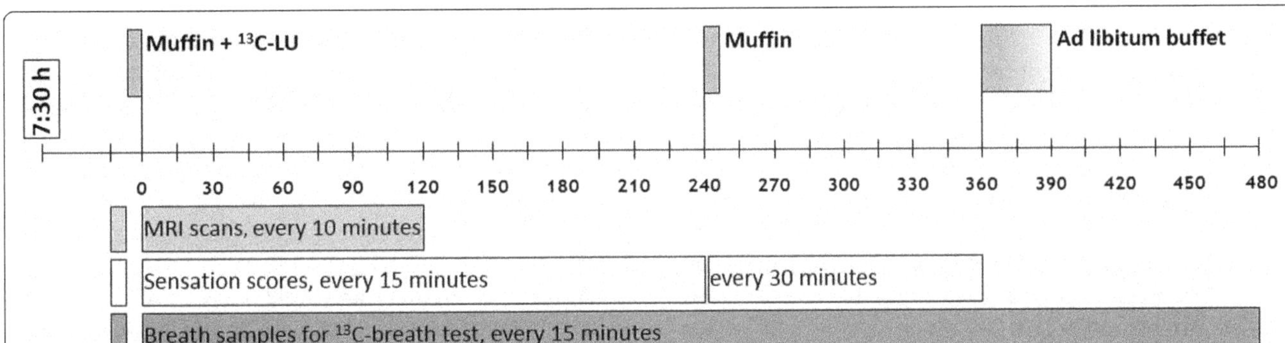

Fig. 1 Overview of study day. Baseline measurements were acquired before ingestion of the ^{13}C-labelled test meal. MRI scans of gastric content volume and motility, breath samples and sensation scores were acquired as indicated. ^{13}C-LU = ^{13}C-lactose-ureide breath test marker

the preceding 2 months. Each item scores 0 to 4, and the sum (0 to 32) indicates severity of dyspeptic symptoms. The GCSI scores 0 to 5 for nausea, retching, vomiting, stomach and excessive fullness, inability to finish a meal, loss of appetite, bloating, and abdominal distention. A mean score of <3 indicates mild, a score of 3.0 to 3.9 moderate and a score of ≥4.0 severe gastroparesis symptoms [45]. BDI and STAI were analyzed according to the German manuals [46, 47]. The BDI evaluates self-reported depression symptoms using 21 questions. Each answer scores between 0 and 3, and the sum of scores indicates depressive symptoms (≤12: no depression symptoms, 13–19: mild symptoms, 20–29 moderate symptoms, ≥30 severe symptoms). The STAI uses 20 questions to evaluate "state" anxiety (temporary emotion) and 20 questions to evaluate "trait" anxiety (anxious personality). Both parts are interpreted separately, and each answer scores between 1 and 4. The higher the score, the higher the anxiety. Differences in distributions of questionnaire scores and demographic data between the groups were analyzed by Kruskal-Wallis test. Healthy controls were expected to have the lowest scores.

Differences in initial group-wise sensation scores were tested with a bootstrapped median test because of the highly skewed distribution (package *pairwiseCI* for program R) [48]. To analyze the dependency of sensations of satiation on gastric content volume, the cumulative link mixed model package *ordinal* and function *clmm2* for the program R were applied. Linear fits were computed to the cumulative logits (ordinal logistic regression) of *hunger* and *fullness* scores with group as fixed effect [49]. This was followed by a logistic transformation in order to obtain the cumulative probability that a participant chooses a defined satiation score.

All tests based on linear models were corrected for 3-fold multiple testing using the Tukey method. Computed data are given as mean and 95% confidence interval (CI) unless otherwise stated.

Results

Demographics and descriptive statistics

The study was conducted between October 2010 and July 2012. Demographic data of the study population included in the cross-sectional comparison are given in Table 1. The majority of patients in all groups were female. The age in the obese participant group was wider spread ($p < 0.001$). The distributions of dyspepsia, anxiety and depression scores (ref. Table 1) were different between groups (all $p < 0.01$).

12 of 24 AN patients included in the cross-sectional study were re-investigated after 112 (69 to 161) days of weight rehabilitation. These AN2 patients achieved a mean BMI increase of 3.4 (2.7 to 4.1) kg/m^2 to a mean BMI of 18.1 kg/m^2. The individual changes between visits for dyspepsia, anxiety and depression are displayed in Additional file 1: Figure S1. No participant with OB lost sufficient weight to meet the criteria for re-investigation during the study period.

Table 1 Demographic and descriptive data of study population for the cross-sectional comparison

	AN	HC	OB
# participants (men)	24 (0)	20 (3)	16 (5)
Age [years]	23 (18–41)	24 (18–38)	32 (19–56)[a]
BMI [kg/m^2][b]	14.4 (11.9–16.0)	21.9 (18.9–24.9)	34.9 (29.6–41.5)
LDQ[b]	7 ± 2.6	1.3 ± 1.1	4.1 ± 2.0
GCSI[b]	2.1 ± 1.4	0.4 ± 0.6	0.7 ± 0.8
BDI[b]	26.0 ± 9.6	3.5 ± 2.0	7.6 ± 7.5
STAI (state)[b]	62.6 ± 8.6	45.1 ± 7.6	54.2 ± 6.2
STAI (trait)[b]	66.4 ± 10.1	45.0 ± 7.2	51.9 ± 10.6

Demographic data are given as mean (range); descriptive data are given as mean ± standard deviation

[a] indicates a significant different distribution of values in the labelled group compared to unlabelled groups

[b] indicates a significant different distribution between all groups (Kruskal-Wallis test, all $p < 0.01$)

Gastrointestinal motor function

GI motor function was determined by MRI (assessment of gastric emptying and antral contraction frequency) and ^{13}C-lactose-ureide breath test (oro-cecal transit). Respective t_{50} values were: AN 138.7 (121.3 to 158.5) minutes, HC 110 (94.9 to 127.4) minutes and OB 105.5 (89.4 to 124.5) minutes. The ratio of log-transformed t_{50} data showed slower gastric emptying in AN patients compared to HC and OB participants (HC:AN = 0.8 (0.7 to 1), $p = 0.016$; OB:AN = 0.8 (0.6 to 0.9), $p = 0.007$ and OB:HC = 1.0 (0.8 to 1.2), $p = 0.89$). A correlation between body weight and gastric emptying was observed up to a BMI of 25 kg/m^2 ($p = 0.0068$), but not at higher values (Fig. 2). All groups had similar mean antral contraction frequencies (~3/min; $p > 0.3$).

Oro-cecal transit time showed a tendency to decrease with increasing body weight, but median values were statistically not different: AN = 346 (294 to NA) minutes, HC = 308 (277 to 430) minutes and OB = 280 (266 to 401) minutes (log-rank test over all groups, $p = 0.564$).

In the longitudinal study, after weight rehabilitation in AN, gastric emptying time slightly decreased. The average t_{50} was 134.3 (109.9 to 148.4) and 121.5 (99.5 to 134.3) minutes for AN1 and AN2, respectively. The ratio of log-transformed values of t_{50} was 0.90 (0.82 to 1.00), $p = 0.087$. Mean antral contraction frequency did not change. For AN1 it was 2.7 (2.5 to 3)/min and for AN2 2.8 (2.6 to 3)/min, $p = 0.45$.

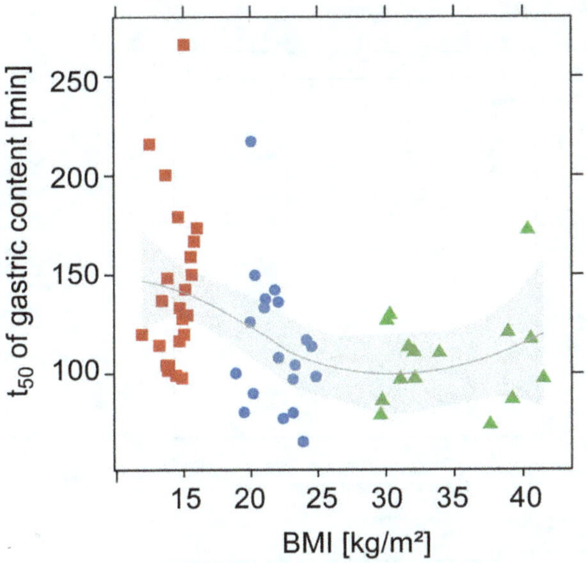

Fig. 2 Gastric emptying (t_{50}) over the full range of body weight (BMI). Participant groups are indicated by squares (participants with anorexia nervosa), dots (healthy controls) and triangles (participants with obesity). The solid line and shaded band show a smooth fit and the 95%-confidence range

Gastrointestinal sensory function

GI sensory function was determined by self-reported sensation scores and food intake at an *ad libitum* buffet. Postprandial sensations of *nausea*, *bloating* and *abdominal pain* were rarely reported after the test meal and were not different between groups. The dependency of self-reported sensations of *fullness* and *hunger* on the varying postprandial gastric content volume is displayed in Fig. 3. *Fullness* was maximal immediately after food intake (Fig. 3a and c). Postprandial *fullness* was greater in AN patients than in HC and OB participants at any given volume ($p < 0.001$). For example, all AN patients still rated *fullness* > *zero* when gastric content volume was 200 ml, whereas median *fullness* in HC dropped to *zero* between gastric content volume 300 to 250 ml. In contrast, OB participants occasionally rated *fullness* as *zero* even at maximal gastric volume after the meal.

The sensation of *hunger* was reported by all groups when postprandial gastric content volume decreased below 300 to 250 ml (ref. Fig. 3b and d). In AN patients, *hunger* increased more slowly as gastric emptying proceeded than in HC and OB participants ($p < 0.04$).

After weight gain, sensation scores in AN2 for both *fullness* and *hunger* were shifted towards larger gastric content volumes ($p < 0.001$), i.e. less abnormal values (ref. Fig. 3e and f).

Satiety was measured by *ad libitum* food intake, with higher satiety corresponding to lower food intake. AN ate less than HC and OB; however, there was no difference between OB and HC (HC-AN: 376 (178 to 574) kcal, $p < 0.001$; OB-AN: 511 (292 to 731) kcal, $p < 0.001$; OB-HC: 135 (-90 to 361) kcal, $p = 0.33$). AN preferred to eat carbohydrates, while HC and OB ate comparable amounts of fat and carbohydrates (detailed data on file). After weight rehabilitation, AN2 patients increased food intake by 6.1% ($p = 0.034$). The composition of food ingested remained unchanged.

Discussion

Postprandial gastrointestinal (GI) motor and sensory function was investigated across a wide spectrum of body weight. A relationship was detected between body weight and gastric emptying such that anorexic patients (AN) had slower gastric emptying than healthy controls (HC) or obese participants (OB). The dependency of postprandial sensations of satiation on the changing gastric content volume during emptying was extracted and displayed using an ordinal logistic regression approach based on the concurrent and continuous MRI volume data and sensation ratings. For any postprandial gastric content volume, AN reported markedly more *fullness* and less *hunger* compared to HC and OB participants. Taken together, these findings confirmed the hypothesis that GI response to feeding varies inversely with body weight. The additional longitudinal follow-up in anorexic patients demonstrated that both gastric emptying and sensations can become less abnormal following weight rehabilitation.

Gastrointestinal motor function and body weight

A relationship between gastric emptying and body weight was present in the BMI range from 12 to 25 kg/m^2, corresponding to AN patients and HCs. These findings are consistent with previous studies that often reported delayed gastric emptying for AN, but similar emptying in OB compared to HC [16–19, 25, 27–31, 50–52]. Interestingly, no difference in antral contraction frequency was present between groups. In this regard, it can be inferred that relatively slow gastric emptying in AN patients is not due to impaired breakdown (grinding) of the solid test meal by antral contraction waves, but due to other factors such as enhanced nutrient feedback from the small intestine. The oro-cecal transit time (OCTT) documented by ^{13}C-lactose-ureide breath test followed the same pattern as gastric emptying, i.e., it decreased with increasing BMI from AN to HC and OB. However, no statistical difference between groups was detected, due to high variability of OCTT. The latter might result from an undiagnosed small intestinal bacterial overgrowth (not tested during screening) that would result in a premature rise of $^{13}CO_2$ in the exhaled air. Previous studies have also reported normal or prolonged OCTT in AN [53, 54] with no consistent abnormality in OB patients [16, 55, 56]. The rate of gastric

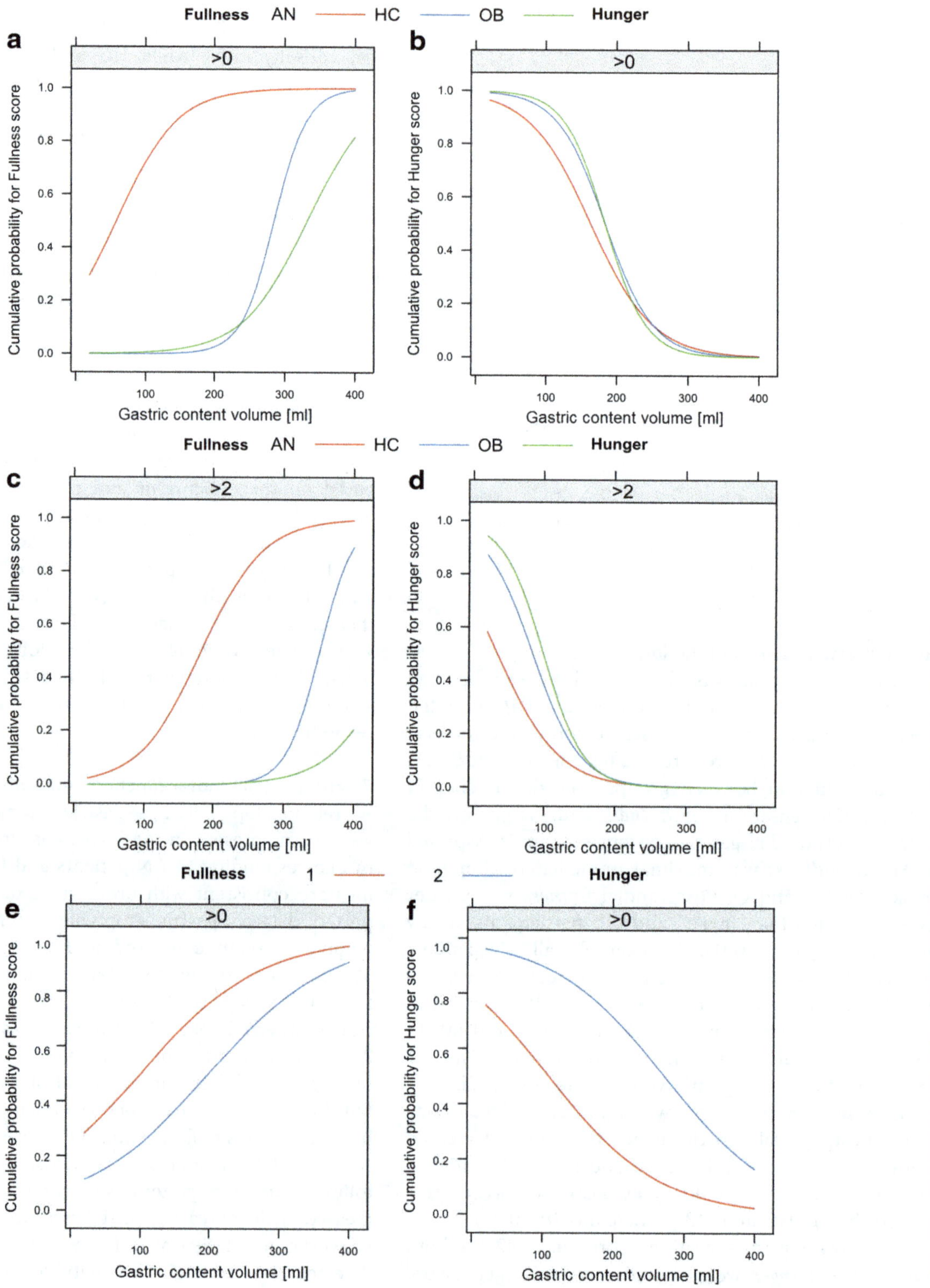

Fig. 3 (See legend on next page.)

(See figure on previous page.)

Fig. 3 Sensation scores for *hunger* and *fullness* in relation to gastric content volume. The plots display the probability (y-axis) that participants report *fullness* or *hunger* higher than a stated threshold (indicated above each panel) at a given gastric content volume (x-axis). The maximal postprandial content volume after the meal is plotted at the right of the x-axis. Compared to HC, the sensation of *fullness* reported by AN patients was significantly shifted to the left (i.e., increased visceral sensation) and for OB the relationship was shifted to the right (i.e., decreased visceral sensation). This is illustrated for *fullness* scores > *zero* (**a**) and > *two* (**c**). Conversely, at any given volume, the sensation of *hunger* reported by HC and OB was significantly greater than that reported by AN patients. This is illustrated for *hunger* scores > *zero* (**b**) and > *two* (**d**). The 12 AN patients included in the longitudinal analysis sensed less *fullness* (**e**) and more *hunger* (**f**) after the weight rehabilitation program. 1 = AN at visit 1, 2 = AN at visit 2

emptying and OCTT is thought to be modulated by secretion of GI peptide hormones (e.g. CCK, GLP-1, PYY) in response to nutrient sensing in the small bowel (termed "the ileal brake") [16, 29, 57–59]. The relevance of the major GI peptide hormones for gastric emptying and satiation in the diseased state, i.e., AN and OB compared to HC, will be evaluated by state-of-the-art multivariate modelling. Since this adds sizeable complexity to the data analyses, it was considered beyond the focus of this work. Besides any direct effects of GI peptide hormones, the differences in GI motor function for AN may also be explained by different dietary habits at study entry. As AN patients notoriously avoid fatty food (also observed during *ad libitum* buffet), it can be assumed that the muffin represents a high-fat meal for this group [60, 61]. Acute fat consumption following a fat-restricted diet has been shown to prolong gastric emptying in lean and obese humans [62–64]. Conversely, with chronic high-fat diet the gastric emptying rate increases over time [65, 66]. These effects are thought to be due to up- and down-regulation of intraluminal fat digestion and mucosal fat sensing, respectively, impacting on the neurohormonal GI response ("ileal brake") [66–68]. However, here the relationship of GI motility and nutritional habits remains speculative, as this study did not control for long-term food intake. The influence of female sex steroid hormones on gastric emptying might add to the observed differences in gastric emptying between the groups. While some studies could not find differences between the follicular and luteal phase of the menstrual cycle in women, other studies showed slower gastric emptying in premenopausal women investigated in the follicular phase and postmenopausal women taking hormone replacement [69–71]. This was accompanied by reduced contractility in the gastric antrum [71]. Here, the study days were not timed with the menstrual cycle of the female participants. However, a difference in antral contractions was not observed between groups. Furthermore, AN participants were amenorrheal and the majority took oral contraceptives. If this has the same effect on gastric emptying as hormone replacement in postmenopausal women has not yet been investigated.

In the longitudinal investigation of anorexic patients, a trend to faster gastric emptying after successful weight rehabilitation was observed. It should be noted that AN2 patients were still underweight (average BMI of 18.1 kg/m^2) and that this effect might have been more distinct with more pronounced increase in BMI. This finding is consistent with previous studies in AN with comparable follow-up time and BMI at follow-up [25, 27, 29, 50, 72]. These investigations found accelerated gastric emptying particularly in the restrictive type of anorexia nervosa, while gastric emptying in the purging type remained unchanged (here 9 of 12 patients that gained weight were classified as restrictive type AN at study entry). While AN patients at visit 1 had a restrictive eating behaviour, all AN2 patients were close to discharge and ate regularly a balanced, ca. 2400 kcal diet. Thus, at re-investigation the test meal was more similar to the habitual diet than at study entry, thereby contributing to a more normal gastric emptying. Psychological comorbidities, like anxiety or major depression, can additionally influence gastrointestinal motility [73]. This was addressed in a covariable analysis with data from 8 AN patients with complete data sets for t_{50}, BDI and STAI for both study visits (Additional file 1: Figure S1). None of the tests with this small data set showed evidence for an effect of STAI and BDI on the estimated differences in t_{50}. Recruitment of constitutionally thin and overweight individuals with comparable dietary habits and without psychiatric comorbidities could possibly overcome such confounders [74].

Whereas 50% of the AN patients attained the predefined weight change required for re-investigation, this was not achieved by any of the OB patients. This could have several reasons. First, the out-patient consultations of OB did not include behavioural and psychotherapy. As OB are less persistent and self-directive than AN patients [75, 76], this could have contributed to the failure of the weight rehabilitation program. Second, during the study period bariatric surgery became a health insurance paid treatment for BMI ≥35 kg/m^2, which might have reduced the motivation in some OB participants to lose weight conventionally [77].

Taken together, the results of the longitudinal study suggest that abnormal gastric emptying is not a primary feature of underweight, but more likely secondary to other factors (e.g. eating habits, diet, psychiatric comorbidities).

However, the lack of control for these factors does not allow for discrimination between these possibilities.

Gastrointestinal sensory function and body weight

Important differences in self-reported postprandial sensations of satiation were present between the three study groups. By combining continuous MRI volume data with postprandial sensation ratings and using an ordinal logistic regression approach, *fullness* and *hunger* ratings could directly be related to the degree of gastric filling after intake of the ~400 ml muffin test meal (Fig. 3a-d). Previous MRI studies described a linear relationship between fullness and gastric distention in healthy participants and patients with functional dyspepsia [78, 79]. The presented approach allows for a more detailed observation of this relationship without using invasive techniques such as barostat. This allowed the following conclusions: (i) Most HC sensed an "empty" stomach (i.e., *fullness* ratings ~ *zero*) while the stomach still contained 200 ml and started to report *hunger* (i.e., *hunger* ratings > *zero*) at a gastric content volume of <100 ml. (ii). Interestingly, a number of OB patients did not feel any *fullness* even at maximal stomach filling; however, overall, the sensation of *fullness* and *hunger* was comparable to HCs. (iii) In contrast, AN patients report heightened sensitivity to gastric filling compared to HC and OB patients with approximately 1 in 3 AN patients still reporting *fullness* and no *hunger* at all when the stomach was completely empty. Consistent with this experimental data, questionnaires also demonstrated more dyspeptic and gastroparesis symptoms in AN patients (Table 1). Additionally, satiety, as assessed by the *ad libitum* buffet, was also more marked in AN patients than in HC and, in particular, OB patients. These findings complement a previous study in obese individuals that reported reduced *fullness* at one single postprandial time point compared to normal weight controls [10]. In AN, a previous epidemiological study found severe postprandial dyspeptic symptoms, i.e., fullness and early satiety [22].

The relationship between sensations of satiation and gastric distention is mediated by gastric mechanosensitive receptors with the former being modulated by the macronutrient composition (especially fat content) of the ingested meal [79–81]. Chemo-sensitive nutrient sensors in the small intestine trigger the release of GI peptides (e.g. CCK, GLP-1, PYY). These act as neuro-hormones that modulate vagal afferent activity and central perception [5, 82, 83]. For example, CCK enhances the satiating effect of gastric filling (i.e., reduces hunger) and high postprandial CCK levels may explain the altered sensation of *fullness* and *hunger* in AN patients [83–85]. However, a meta-analysis of studies in AN patients revealed only slightly increased CCK levels at baseline compared to HC, but equivalent levels after meals [86]. Thus, analogous to the effects on gastric emptying, altered perception of *fullness* in AN and OB might not be related to direct effects of GI peptide hormones on gastric function, but rather to the habitual diet at study entry. It has been shown that chronic, high-fat diet leads to a decrease in postprandial *fullness* and *satiety* respectively [80, 87]. Therefore, it may be the composition of the test meal relative to the habitual diet of participants that explains the observed differences. Psychiatric comorbidity provides several other, possible explanations for differences in *fullness* and *hunger* sensations between the study groups. First, anxiety among AN patients (Table 1) could reduce gastric accommodation which would be expected to increase postprandial *fullness* [88]. Second, reduced reporting of *hunger* and higher *satiety* ratings may represent a "secondary gain" in AN patients undergoing weight rehabilitation [27]. Third, interoceptive awareness and visceral sensitivity are decreased in AN patients, resulting in diminished ability to discriminate *hunger* and *satiety* sensations [89, 90]. In summary, abnormal reports of sensations in this group could be exaggerated by abnormal GI physiology, attempts by patients to excuse eating less, or the psychiatric disease and related comorbidities.

Longitudinal investigation of AN1 vs. AN2 revealed that *fullness* and *hunger* ratings shifted towards more normal levels (Fig. 3e and f). There was also less *satiety*, as indicated by increased intake at the *ad libitum* buffet. As discussed above, such improvements could be the result of physiological adaptation to increased oral intake or behavioural change. Previous studies found an improvement of interoceptive awareness in AN patients with weight gain [91]. However, it is not possible to assess from study results whether this is a consequence of weight rehabilitation, adaption to regular food intake or improved psychological state. Of note, food intake increased by only 6%, thus, the trend to more normal postprandial sensations is more likely related to regular food intake and weight gain, than to psychological rehabilitation. The latter is also mirrored by unchanged anxiety, i.e., values of the STAI (state). Indeed, if the latter occurred, then one would expect AN patients to choose chocolate or cheese rather than apples and soup at the *ad libitum* buffet, which was never observed.

Conclusions

By investigating participants across a wide range of BMI, this study provides detailed insight into the relationship of GI motor and sensory function with body weight. Results indicate that gastric emptying rate is decreased and postprandial sensations of satiation are increased in AN patients compared to HC and OB patients. In principle, these findings support the hypothesis that the physiological response to feeding is heightened in lower body weight. The improvement in gastric emptying and postprandial sensations of satiation in AN after weight rehabilitation suggest that the differences in GI motor and sensory function are unlikely to be a primary cause of abnormal body weight. Secondary causes, such as dietary habits and psychiatric comorbidities, are more likely to determine GI motor and sensory function in the investigated groups.

Abbreviations

AN: Patients with anorexia nervosa; AN2: AN at follow-up (after weight rehabilitation); BDI: Beck Depression Inventory II; BMI: Body mass index; GCSI: Gastroparesis Cardinal Symptom Index; GI: Gastrointestinal; HC: Healthy controls; LDQ: Leeds Dyspepsia Questionnaire; MRI: Magnetic resonance imaging; OB: Patients with obesity; OCTT: Oro-cecal transit time; STAI: State-Trait-Anxiety Inventory; t_{50}: Gastric content half-emptying time

Acknowledgements

The authors gratefully acknowledge Judit Valentini, Tobias Hahn and Jelena Curcic for MRI technical assistance and Simon Bütikofer for recruitment and investigation of study participants.

Funding

The study was funded by the Swiss National Science Foundation (grant 320030/125333). SB was supported by a personal grant from the Swiss National Science Foundation (P2SKP3_158649).

Authors' contributions

SB performed the recruitment of participants, data acquisition, data management and drafted the manuscript. DM performed statistical analyses and data plots. GM, MFx, OG and AS wrote the study protocol. GM, OG, MF and WS supervised the study. MFx and AS critically revised the manuscript. All authors approved the final version of the manuscript.

Competing interests

The authors declare that they have no competing interests.

Author details

[1]Division of Gastroenterology and Hepatology, University Hospital Zurich, Raemistrasse 100, CH-8091 Zurich, Switzerland. [2]Institute for Biomedical Engineering, University and ETH Zurich, Zurich, Switzerland. [3]Menne Biomed Consulting, Tuebingen, Germany. [4]Psychiatric Department, University Hospital Zurich, Zurich, Switzerland. [5]Zurich Centre for Integrative Human Physiology (ZIHP), University of Zurich, Zurich, Switzerland.

References

1. Dubois L, Ohm Kyvik K, Girard M, Tatone-Tokuda F, Perusse D, Hjelmborg J, et al. Genetic and environmental contributions to weight, height, and BMI from birth to 19 years of age: an international study of over 12,000 twin pairs. PLoS One. 2012;7(2):e30153.
2. Collins JCB, Jon E. Behavioral and psychological factors in obesity. J Lancaster General Hospital. 2009;4(4):4.
3. Schmidhauser SE, Klaus; Brügger, Urs..Environmental determinants of overweight and obesity: Extended international literature review. Final report. Study commissioned by the Federal Office of Public Health Switzerland. 2009:170.
4. Fairburn CG, Cooper Z, Doll HA, Welch SL. Risk factors for anorexia nervosa: three integrated case-control comparisons. Arch Gen Psychiatry. 1999;56(5):468–76.
5. Janssen P, Vanden Berghe P, Verschueren S, Lehmann A, Depoortere I, Tack J. Review article: the role of gastric motility in the control of food intake. Aliment Pharmacol Ther. 2011;33(8):880–94.
6. Woods SC. The control of food intake: behavioral versus molecular perspectives. Cell Metab. 2009;9(6):489–98.
7. Cummings DE, Overduin J. Gastrointestinal regulation of food intake. J Clin Invest. 2007;117(1):13–23.
8. Rui L. Brain regulation of energy balance and body weight. Rev Endocr Metab Disord. 2013;14(4):387–407.
9. Camilleri M. Integrated upper gastrointestinal response to food intake. Gastroenterology. 2006;131(2):640–58.
10. Delgado-Aros S, Cremonini F, Castillo JE, Chial HJ, Burton DD, Ferber I, et al. Independent influences of body mass and gastric volumes on satiation in humans. Gastroenterology. 2004;126(2):432–40.
11. Delgado-Aros S, Camilleri M, Castillo EJ, Cremonini F, Stephens D, Ferber I, et al. Effect of gastric volume or emptying on meal-related symptoms after liquid nutrients in obesity: a pharmacologic study. Clin Gastroenterol Hepatol. 2005;3(10):997–1006.
12. Cardoso-Junior A, Coelho LG, Savassi-Rocha PR, Vignolo MC, Abrantes MM, de Almeida AM, et al. Gastric emptying of solids and semi-solids in morbidly obese and non-obese subjects: an assessment using the 13C-octanoic acid and 13C-acetic acid breath tests. Obes Surg. 2007;17(2):236–41.
13. Wright RA, Krinsky S, Fleeman C, Trujillo J, Teague E. Gastric emptying and obesity. Gastroenterology. 1983;84(4):747–51.
14. Tosetti C, Corinaldesi R, Stanghellini V, Pasquali R, Corbelli C, Zoccoli G, et al. Gastric emptying of solids in morbid obesity. Int J Obes Relat Metab Disord. 1996;20(3):200–5.
15. Gryback P, Naslund E, Hellstrom PM, Jacobsson H, Backman L. Gastric emptying of solids in humans: improved evaluation by Kaplan-Meier plots, with special reference to obesity and gender. Eur J Nucl Med. 1996;23(12):1562–7.
16. Seimon RV, Brennan IM, Russo A, Little TJ, Jones KL, Standfield S, et al. Gastric emptying, mouth-to-cecum transit, and glycemic, insulin, incretin, and energy intake responses to a mixed-nutrient liquid in lean, overweight, and obese males. Am J Physiol Endocrinol Metab. 2013;304(3):E294–300.
17. Buchholz V, Berkenstadt H, Goitein D, Dickman R, Bernstine H, Rubin M. Gastric emptying is not prolonged in obese patients. Surg Obes Relat Dis. 2013;9(5):714–7.
18. Chiloiro M, Caroli M, Guerra V, Lodadea Piepoli A, Riezzo G. Gastric emptying in normal weight and obese children–an ultrasound study. Int J Obes Relat Metab Disord. 1999;23(12):1303–6.
19. Verdich C, Madsen JL, Toubro S, Buemann B, Holst JJ, Astrup A. Effect of obesity and major weight reduction on gastric emptying. Int J Obes Relat Metab Disord. 2000;24(7):899–905.
20. Jackson SJ, Leahy FE, McGowan AA, Bluck LJ, Coward WA, Jebb SA. Delayed gastric emptying in the obese: an assessment using the non-invasive (13)C-octanoic acid breath test. Diabetes Obes Metab. 2004;6(4):264–70.
21. Vazquez Roque MI, Camilleri M, Stephens DA, Jensen MD, Burton DD, Baxter KL, et al. Gastric sensorimotor functions and hormone profile in normal weight, overweight, and obese people. Gastroenterology. 2006;131(6):1717–24.
22. Santonicola A, Siniscalchi M, Capone P, Gallotta S, Ciacci C, Iovino P. Prevalence of functional dyspepsia and its subgroups in patients with eating disorders. World J Gastroenterol. 2012;18(32):4379–85.
23. Robinson PH. Gastric function in eating disorders. Ann N Y Acad Sci. 1989; 575:456–64. discussion 64-5.
24. Robinson PH. Perceptivity and paraceptivity during measurement of gastric emptying in anorexia and bulimia nervosa. Br J Psychiatry. 1989;154:400–5.
25. Rigaud D, Bedig G, Merrouche M, Vulpillat M, Bonfils S, Apfelbaum M. Delayed gastric emptying in anorexia nervosa is improved by completion of a renutrition program. Dig Dis Sci. 1988;33(8):919–25.
26. Waldholtz BD, Andersen AE. Gastrointestinal symptoms in anorexia nervosa. A prospective study. Gastroenterology. 1990;98(6):1415–9.
27. Benini L, Todesco T, Dalle Grave R, Deiorio F, Salandini L, Vantini I. Gastric emptying in patients with restricting and binge/purging subtypes of anorexia nervosa. Am J Gastroenterol. 2004;99(8):1448–54.
28. Hutson WR, Wald A. Gastric emptying in patients with bulimia nervosa and anorexia nervosa. Am J Gastroenterol. 1990;85(1):41–6.
29. Abell TL, Malagelada JR, Lucas AR, Brown ML, Camilleri M, Go VL, et al. Gastric electromechanical and neurohormonal function in anorexia nervosa. Gastroenterology. 1987;93(5):958–65.
30. McCallum RW, Grill BB, Lange R, Planky M, Glass EE, Greenfeld DG. Definition of a gastric emptying abnormality in patients with anorexia nervosa. Dig Dis Sci. 1985;30(8):713–22.
31. Holt S, Ford MJ, Grant S, Heading RC. Abnormal gastric emptying in primary anorexia nervosa. Br J Psychiatry. 1981;139:550–2.
32. Buchman AL, Ament ME, Weiner M, Kodner A, Mayer EA. Reversal of megaduodenum and duodenal dysmotility associated with improvement in nutritional status in primary anorexia nervosa. Dig Dis Sci. 1994;39(2):433–40.
33. Pasricha PJ, Colvin R, Yates K, Hasler WL, Abell TL, Unalp-Arida A, et al. Characteristics of patients with chronic unexplained nausea and vomiting and normal gastric emptying. Clin Gastroenterol Hepatol. 2011;9(7):567–76. e1-4.
34. Norris ML, Harrison ME, Isserlin L, Robinson A, Feder S, Sampson M.

Gastrointestinal complications associated with anorexia nervosa: A systematic review. Int J Eat Disord. 2016;49(3):216–37.

35. Eating Disorders. Core Interventions in the Treatment and Management of Anorexia Nervosa. Leicester (UK): Bulimia Nervosa and Related Eating Disorders; 2004.
36. Roy S, Fox MR, Curcic J, Schwizer W, Pal A. The gastro-esophageal reflux barrier: biophysical analysis on 3D models of anatomy from magnetic resonance imaging. Neurogastroenterol Motil. 2012;24(7):616–25. e269.
37. Kwiatek MA, Fox MR, Steingoetter A, Menne D, Pal A, Fruehauf H, et al. Effects of clonidine and sumatriptan on postprandial gastric volume response, antral contraction waves and emptying: an MRI study. Neurogastroenterol Motil. 2009;21(9):928–e71.
38. Priebe MG, Wachters-Hagedoorn RE, Landman K, Heimweg J, Elzinga H, Vonk RJ. Influence of a subsequent meal on the oro-cecal transit time of a solid test meal. Eur J Clin Investig. 2006;36(2):123–6.
39. Marciani L, Cox EF, Hoad CL, Pritchard S, Totman JJ, Foley S, et al. Postprandial changes in small bowel water content in healthy subjects and patients with irritable bowel syndrome. Gastroenterology. 2010;138(2):469–77. 77 e1.
40. Marciani L, Hall N, Pritchard SE, Cox EF, Totman JJ, Lad M, et al. Preventing gastric sieving by blending a solid/water meal enhances satiation in healthy humans. J Nutr. 2012;142(7):1253–8.
41. Kunz P, Feinle C, Schwizer W, Fried M, Boesiger P. Assessment of gastric motor function during the emptying of solid and liquid meals in humans by MRI. J Magn Reson Imaging. 1999;9(1):75–80.
42. Elashoff JD, Reedy TJ, Meyer JH. Analysis of gastric emptying data. Gastroenterology. 1982;83(6):1306–12.
43. Fraser A, Delaney BC, Ford AC, Qume M, Moayyedi P. The Short-Form Leeds Dyspepsia Questionnaire validation study. Aliment Pharmacol Ther. 2007;25(4):477–86.
44. Revicki DA, Rentz AM, Dubois D, Kahrilas P, Stanghellini V, Talley NJ, et al. Development and validation of a patient-assessed gastroparesis symptom severity measure: the Gastroparesis Cardinal Symptom Index. Aliment Pharmacol Ther. 2003;18(1):141–50.
45. Parkman HP, Yates K, Hasler WL, Nguyen L, Pasricha PJ, Snape WJ, et al. Clinical features of idiopathic gastroparesis vary with sex, body mass, symptom onset, delay in gastric emptying, and gastroparesis severity. Gastroenterology. 2011;140(1):101–15.
46. Hautzinger M, Bailer M, Worall H, Keller F. BDI Beck-Depressions-Inventar Testhandbuch. 2nd ed. Bern: Verlag Hans Huber; 1995.
47. Laux L, Glanzmann P, Schaffner P, Spielberger CD. Das State-Trait-Angstinventar. Theoretische Grundlagen und Handanweisung. Weinheim: Beltz Test GmbH; 1981.
48. Follmann DA, Proschan MA, Geller NL. Monitoring pairwise comparisons in multi-armed clinical trials. Biometrics. 1994;50(2):325–36.
49. Christensen RBP. Analysis of sensory ratings data with cumulative link models. Journal de la Société Française de Statistique. 2013;154(3):22.
50. Perez ME, Coley B, Crandall W, Di Lorenzo C, Bravender T. Effect of nutritional rehabilitation on gastric motility and somatization in adolescents with anorexia. J Pediatr. 2013;163(3):867–72. e1.
51. Glasbrenner B, Pieramico O, Brecht-Krauss D, Baur M, Malfertheiner P. Gastric emptying of solids and liquids in obesity. Clin Investig. 1993;71(7):542–6.
52. Domstad PA, Shih WJ, Humphries L, DeLand FH, Digenis GA. Radionuclide gastric emptying studies in patients with anorexia nervosa. J Nucl Med. 1987;28(5):816–9.
53. Kamal N, Chami T, Andersen A, Rosell FA, Schuster MM, Whitehead WE. Delayed gastrointestinal transit times in anorexia nervosa and bulimia nervosa. Gastroenterology. 1991;101(5):1320–4.
54. Hirakawa M, Okada T, Iida M, Tamai H, Kobayashi N, Nakagawa T, et al. Small bowel transit time measured by hydrogen breath test in patients with anorexia nervosa. Dig Dis Sci. 1990;35(6):733–6.
55. Rerksuppaphol S, Rerksuppaphol L. Rapid orocecal transit time in obese children measured by hydrogen breath test. J Med Assoc Thail. 2012;95 Suppl 12:S26–31.
56. Basilisco G, Camboni G, Bozzani A, Vita P, Doldi S, Bianchi PA. Orocecal transit delay in obese patients. Dig Dis Sci. 1989;34(4):509–12.
57. Shin HS, Ingram JR, McGill AT, Poppitt SD. Lipids, CHOs, proteins: can all macronutrients put a 'brake' on eating? Physiol Behav. 2013;120:114–23.
58. Van Citters GW, Lin HC. Ileal brake: neuropeptidergic control of intestinal transit. Curr Gastroenterol Rep. 2006;8(5):367–73.
59. Spiller RC, Trotman IF, Higgins BE, Ghatei MA, Grimble GK, Lee YC, et al. The ileal brake–inhibition of jejunal motility after ileal fat perfusion in man. Gut. 1984;25(4):365–74.
60. Fernstrom MH, Weltzin TE, Neuberger S, Srinivasagam N, Kaye WH. Twenty-four-hour food intake in patients with anorexia nervosa and in healthy control subjects. Biol Psychiatry. 1994;36(10):696–702.
61. Jauregui Lobera I, Bolanos RP. Choice of diet in patients with anorexia nervosa. Nutr Hosp. 2009;24(6):682–7.
62. Cecil JE, Francis J, Read NW. Comparison of the effects of a high-fat and high-carbohydrate soup delivered orally and intragastrically on gastric emptying, appetite, and eating behaviour. Physiol Behav. 1999;67(2):299–306.
63. Boyd KA, O'Donovan DG, Doran S, Wishart J, Chapman IM, Horowitz M, et al. High-fat diet effects on gut motility, hormone, and appetite responses to duodenal lipid in healthy men. Am J Physiol Gastrointest Liver Physiol. 2003;284(2):G188–96.
64. Seimon RV, Taylor P, Little TJ, Noakes M, Standfield S, Clifton PM, et al. Effects of acute and longer-term dietary restriction on upper gut motility, hormone, appetite, and energy-intake responses to duodenal lipid in lean and obese men. Am J Clin Nutr. 2014;99(1):24–34.
65. Cunningham KM, Daly J, Horowitz M, Read NW. Gastrointestinal adaptation to diets of differing fat composition in human volunteers. Gut. 1991;32(5):483–6.
66. Castiglione KE, Read NW, French SJ. Adaptation to high-fat diet accelerates emptying of fat but not carbohydrate test meals in humans. Am J Physiol Regul Integr Comp Physiol. 2002;282(2):R366–71.
67. Little TJ, Horowitz M, Feinle-Bisset C. Modulation by high-fat diets of gastrointestinal function and hormones associated with the regulation of energy intake: implications for the pathophysiology of obesity. Am J Clin Nutr. 2007;86(3):531–41.
68. Meyer-Gerspach AC, Wolnerhanssen B, Beglinger B, Nessenius F, Napitupulu M, Schulte FH, et al. Gastric and intestinal satiation in obese and normal weight healthy people. Physiol Behav. 2014;129:265–71.
69. Mones J, Carrio I, Calabuig R, Estorch M, Sainz S, Berna L, et al. Influence of the menstrual cycle and of menopause on the gastric emptying rate of solids in female volunteers. Eur J Nucl Med. 1993;20(7):600–2.
70. Hutson WR, Roehrkasse RL, Wald A. Influence of gender and menopause on gastric emptying and motility. Gastroenterology. 1989;96(1):11–7.
71. Knight LC, Parkman HP, Brown KL, Miller MA, Trate DM, Maurer AH, et al. Delayed gastric emptying and decreased antral contractility in normal premenopausal women compared with men. Am J Gastroenterol. 1997; 92(6):968–75.
72. Szmukler GI, Young GP, Lichtenstein M, Andrews JT. A serial study of gastric emptying in anorexia nervosa and bulimia. Aust NZ J Med. 1990;20(3):220–5.
73. Bennett EJ, Evans P, Scott AM, Badcock CA, Shuter B, Hoschl R, et al. Psychological and sex features of delayed gut transit in functional gastrointestinal disorders. Gut. 2000;46(1):83–7.
74. Germain N, Galusca B, Le Roux CW, Bossu C, Ghatei MA, Lang F, et al. Constitutional thinness and lean anorexia nervosa display opposite concentrations of peptide YY, glucagon-like peptide 1, ghrelin, and leptin. Am J Clin Nutr. 2007;85(4):967–71.
75. Atiye M, Miettunen J, Raevuori-Helkamaa A. A meta-analysis of temperament in eating disorders. Eur Eat Disord Rev. 2015;23(2):89–99.
76. Sarisoy G, Atmaca A, Ecemis G, Gumus K, Pazvantoglu O. Personality characteristics and body image in obese individuals. Asia-Pacific Psychiatry. 2014;6(2):191–9.
77. Schiesser M. Adipositaschirurgie im Wandel: Aktuelle Indikationen, Operationstechniken und Resultate. Swiss Med Forum. 2015;15(10):5.
78. Fruehauf H, Steingoetter A, Fox MR, Kwiatek MA, Boesiger P, Schwizer W, et al. Characterization of gastric volume responses and liquid emptying in functional dyspepsia and health by MRI or barostat and simultaneous C-acetate breath test. Neurogastroenterol Motil. 2009;21(7):697–e37.
79. Marciani L, Cox EF, Pritchard SE, Major G, Hoad CL, Mellows M, et al. Additive effects of gastric volumes and macronutrient composition on the sensation of postprandial fullness in humans. Eur J Clin Nutr. 2015;69(3):380–4.
80. Brennan IM, Luscombe-Marsh ND, Seimon RV, Otto B, Horowitz M, Wishart JM, et al. Effects of fat, protein, and carbohydrate and protein load on appetite, plasma cholecystokinin, peptide YY, and ghrelin, and energy intake in lean and obese men. Am J Physiol Gastrointest Liver Physiol. 2012;303(1): G129–40.
81. Kwiatek MA, Menne D, Steingoetter A, Goetze O, Forras-Kaufman Z, Kaufman E, et al. Effect of meal volume and calorie load on postprandial gastric function and emptying: studies under physiological conditions by combined fiber-optic pressure measurement and MRI. Am J Physiol Gastrointest Liver Physiol. 2009;297(5):G894–901.
82. Geeraerts B, Van Oudenhove L, Dupont P, Vanderghinste D, Bormans G, Van Laere K, et al. Different regional brain activity during physiological gastric

distension compared to balloon distension: a H2 15O-PET study. Neurogastroenterol Motil. 2011;23(6):533–e203.

83. Kanoski SE, Walls EK, Davidson TL. Interoceptive "satiety" signals produced by leptin and CCK. Peptides. 2007;28(5):988–1002.
84. Kissileff HR, Carretta JC, Geliebter A, Pi-Sunyer FX. Cholecystokinin and stomach distension combine to reduce food intake in humans. Am J Physiol Regul Integr Comp Physiol. 2003;285(5):R992–8.
85. Feinle C, D'Amato M, Read NW. Cholecystokinin-A receptors modulate gastric sensory and motor responses to gastric distension and duodenal lipid. Gastroenterology. 1996;110(5):1379–85.
86. Prince AC, Brooks SJ, Stahl D, Treasure J. Systematic review and meta-analysis of the baseline concentrations and physiologic responses of gut hormones to food in eating disorders. Am J Clin Nutr. 2009;89(3):755–65.
87. French SJ, Murray B, Rumsey RD, Fadzlin R, Read NW. Adaptation to high-fat diets: effects on eating behaviour and plasma cholecystokinin. Br J Nutr. 1995;73(2):179–89.
88. Geeraerts B, Vandenberghe J, Van Oudenhove L, Gregory LJ, Aziz Q, Dupont P, et al. Influence of experimentally induced anxiety on gastric sensorimotor function in humans. Gastroenterology. 2005;129(5):1437–44.
89. Pollatos O, Kurz AL, Albrecht J, Schreder T, Kleemann AM, Schopf V, et al. Reduced perception of bodily signals in anorexia nervosa. Eat Behav. 2008; 9(4):381–8.
90. Fassino S, Piero A, Gramaglia C, Abbate-Daga G. Clinical, psychopathological and personality correlates of interoceptive awareness in anorexia nervosa, bulimia nervosa and obesity. Psychopathology. 2004;37(4):168–74.
91. Matsumoto R, Kitabayashi Y, Narumoto J, Wada Y, Okamoto A, Ushijima Y, et al. Regional cerebral blood flow changes associated with interoceptive awareness in the recovery process of anorexia nervosa. Prog Neuro-Psychopharmacol Biol Psychiatry. 2006;30(7):1265–70.

9

Lichenoid esophagitis presenting as fatal upper gastrointestinal bleeding in a 52 year-old woman: a case diagnosed by autopsy

Andrew Mitchell* and Tony Petrella

Abstract

Background: "Lichenoid esophagitis" is a descriptive term for a lichenoid pattern of inflammation in the esophagus for which a precise histologic diagnosis cannot be established. The differential diagnosis includes lichen planus, a drug-related reaction, and viral infection. Lichenoid esophagitis causing death has not been reported previously. We describe a case, diagnosed by autopsy, of lichenoid esophagitis in which massive bleeding from generalized epithelial sloughing and a large longitudinal ulcer proved fatal.

Case presentation: A 52 year-old diabetic woman collapsed at her home in front of an acquaintance. "Bloody vomit" was noted. Despite resuscitation efforts, the patient died. A complete autopsy was performed. The middle portion of the esophagus showed a 9 cm longitudinal ulcer situated 12 cm from the esophago-gastric junction. Microscopic examination showed complete sloughing of the esophageal epithelium with a striking subepithelial lichenoid lymphocytic infiltrate extending into the muscularis mucosae. The findings were considered compatible with lichenoid esophagitis. Laboratory studies also showed the presence of diabetic ketoacidosis.

Conclusions: Lichenoid esophagitis is an appropriate diagnostic term when clinical, histologic and laboratory findings do not allow for specific categorization of lichenoid inflammation in the esophagus. As illustrated here for the first time, lichenoid esophagitis may cause ulceration and mucosal sloughing severe enough to result in massive upper gastrointestinal bleeding and death. Translating these autopsy findings to the clinical setting, it is possible that the endoscopic finding of a longitudinal mid-esophageal ulcer in the presence of proximal stricture may be indicative of underlying lichenoid esophagitis.

Keywords: Lichenoid, Esophagitis, Lichen planus, Autopsy, Case report

Background

"Lichenoid esophagitis" is a descriptive term for a lichenoid pattern of inflammation in the esophagus for which a precise histologic diagnosis cannot be established [1]. The differential diagnosis includes lichen planus (LP), a drug-related reaction, and viral infection [1]. Lichenoid esophagitis causing death has not been reported previously. We describe a case, diagnosed by autopsy, of lichenoid esophagitis in which massive bleeding from generalized epithelial sloughing and a large longitudinal ulcer proved fatal.

* Correspondence: plaines@me.com
Department of Anatomical Pathology and Cytology, Maisonneuve-Rosemont Hospital, 5415 Boulevard de L'Assomption, Montreal, Quebec H1T 2M4, Canada

Case presentation

A 52 year-old woman collapsed at her home in front of an acquaintance. "Bloody vomit" was noted. An ambulance was called and cardiopulmonary resuscitation (CPR) was begun by paramedics. The patient was transported to hospital, but she remained in cardiorespiratory arrest despite ongoing CPR. Resuscitation efforts were finally stopped.

It was later learned that several days prior to her death she had complained of unspecified upper digestive symptoms, but had steadfastly refused to seek medical advice.

The medical history included bipolar disorder for which she was apparently compliant in taking her medications. She also smoked and had type II diabetes. Her medications were the following: quetiapine, lorazepam, baclofen, glickazide, metformin, and esomeprazole.

The coroner was notified and an autopsy was requested.

Autopsy and laboratory results

A complete autopsy was performed. The pertinent anatomic findings were confined to the gastrointestinal tract. The middle portion of the esophagus showed a prominent brownish 9 cm longitudinal ulcer, with a maximal width of 0.5 cm, situated 12 cm from the esophago-gastric junction (Fig. 1). The esophago-gastric junction itself showed brownish steaks without ulceration, induration or a mass lesion. The stomach contained approximately 750 ml of dark blood; the small bowel and colon contained dark, tarry blood. There was no identifiable mucosal lesion beyond the esophagus.

Microscopic examination of numerous sections (>30) from all levels of the esophagus, including the ulcer, showed complete sloughing of the epithelium with a striking subepithelial lichenoid lymphocytic infiltrate extending into the muscularis mucosae (Fig. 2, a-e). Sections of the esophago-gastric junction showed no evidence of varices. Fungal elements and viral inclusions were absent; Periodic acid-Schiff staining for identification of fungi and immunohistochemical staining for Cytomegalovirus and Herpes simplex viruses I and II were negative.

An extensive immunohistochemical study was performed in order to characterize the immunophenotype of the lymphocytic infiltration. The following antibodies were used: CD20, CD2, CD3, CD4, CD5, CD7, CD8 and CD43. Unfortunately, marked post-mortem autolysis rendered interpretation difficult. Only CD43 staining was well preserved (Fig. 2f), showing diffuse positivity, thus demonstrating that the lymphocytic infiltrate was essentially composed of T-cells. For the other antibodies the results were less reliable, although better antigen preservation of the deeper situated lymphocytes in the muscularis mucosae was noted. Here, a high CD8/CD4 ratio was found. CD2, CD5, CD7 and CD20 were negative, but, given the absence of positive controls for these markers, interpretation was essentially impossible.

A representative formalin-fixed, paraffin-embedded tissue block was submitted for evaluation of T-cell receptor gamma chain rearrangement by polymerase chain reaction. However, amplification was not possible for technical reasons.

Laboratory results were the following: lorazepam at a therapeutic blood level; tetrahydrocannabinol metabolites were also present. Ethanol was absent. Blood acetone: 10 mmol/L (normal: 0–0.34), ocular liquid glucose: 640 mg/dL, ocular liquid lactic acid: 230 mg/dL, and ocular liquid acetone: 12 mmol/L. The results were compatible with diabetic ketoacidosis (DKA).

The final autopsy diagnoses were: 1) fatal upper gastrointestinal bleeding due to lichenoid esophagitis with diffuse mucosal sloughing and a large ulcer of the mid-esophagus, and 2) diabetic ketoacidosis.

Discussion and conclusions

To the best of our knowledge this is the first description of fatal hemorrhage due to esophagitis with a lichenoid inflammatory pattern. This is also the initial description

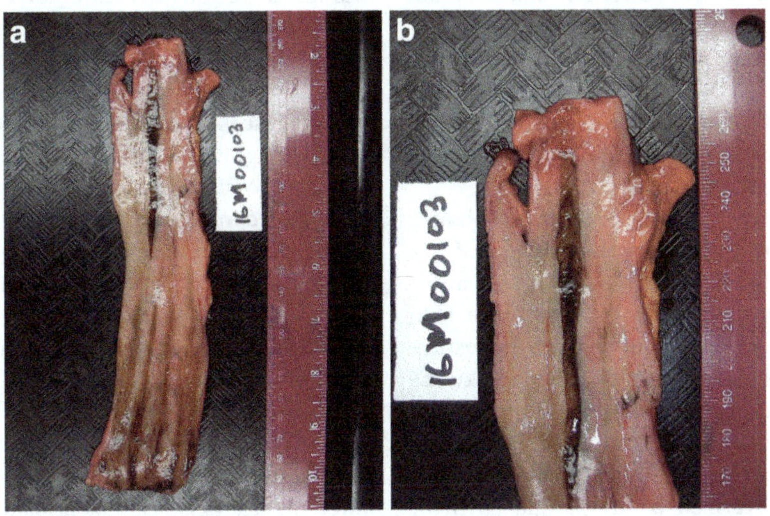

Fig. 1 Macroscopic images of the esophagus. **a** The mid-esophagus shows a 9 cm ulcer with a brown base. The esophago-gastric junction (bottom) has brownish streaks without ulceration. The rest of the esophagus is unremarkable despite the marked inflammation and complete absence of epithelium. **b** A closer view of the ulcer

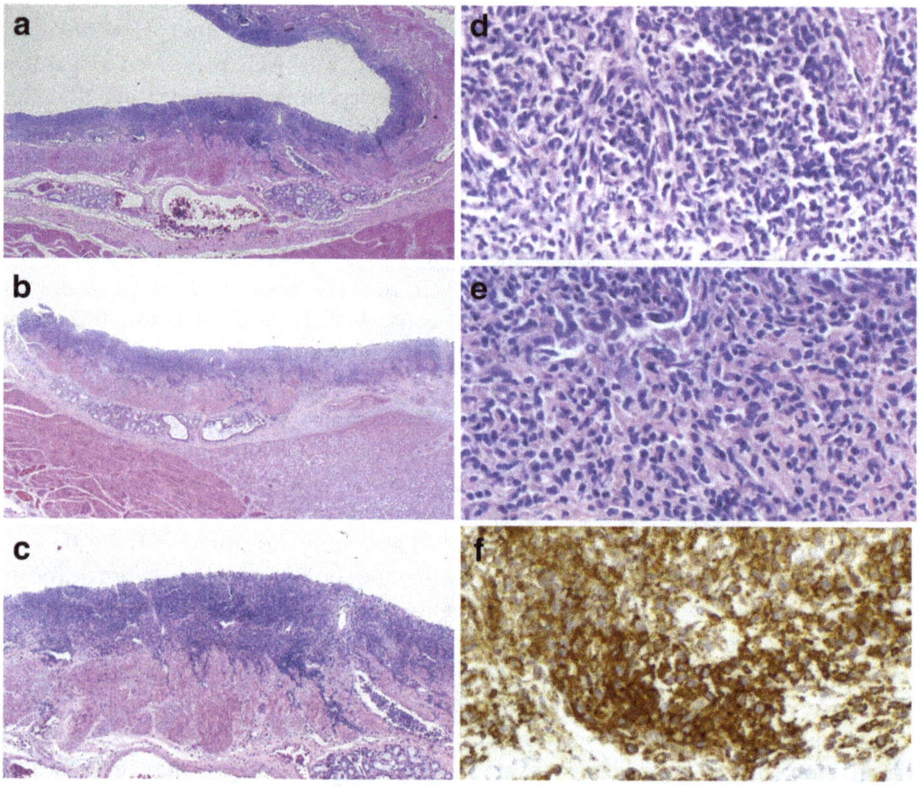

Fig. 2 Microscopic images of the esophagus. **a, b** Low power images of the esophageal wall. The epithelium has entirely sloughed off. A dense lichenoid lymphocytic infiltrate involves the lamina propria and muscularis mucosae. Esophageal glands in the submucosa are uninvolved. **c** Medium power image of the lichenoid infiltrate showing extension into the muscularis mucosae. The epithelium has entirely sloughed off. **d, e** Medium-high power images of the lymphoid infiltrate. The twisted appearance of many of the lymphocyte nuclei is typical of T-cells and does not imply atypia. **f** Medium-high power view of the lymphocytes showing uniformly strong positivity with the T-cell marker CD43

of a macroscopically distinctive mid-esophageal ulcer in this entity.

"Lichenoid esophagitis" is the descriptive term proposed by Salaria et al. [1] for a lichenoid pattern of inflammation in the esophagitis for which a precise histologic diagnosis cannot be established. This may be due to inadequate or unavailable clinical information and/or laboratory data. The differential diagnosis includes LP, a drug-related reaction, and a viral infection [1]. These entities are discussed below in regard to the present case.

LP is the prototypical lesion of the esophagus characterized by lichenoid inflammation [1–5]. LP is a mucocutaneous inflammatory disorder, likely of autoimmune cause, that most commonly affects the skin and oral mucosa [5]. Skin lesions usually resolve within a year, whereas mucosal disease tends to be chronic [5]. Although esophageal involvement is considered rare, with approximately fifty reported cases as of 2013 [3], it is likely under-recognized [1]. Clinically, esophageal LP is characterized by dysphagia (with or without odynophagia) with endoscopic findings that include mucosal sloughing and stricture, small caliber of the esophagus, and superficial ulceration [1, 4]. Chronic stricture and squamous cell carcinoma are possible complications [4, 5].

There was no known history of LP in our case. Although a perfunctory external examination of the body prior to autopsy showed no obvious skin lesions, absence of skin lesions would not rule out LP as any skin lesions may have healed [5], and esophageal LP may be the first or only disease manifestation [4]. Given the complete mucosal sloughing, histologic evaluation of the epithelium was not possible. Thus, esophageal LP could not be confirmed by clinical evaluation or histologic criteria.

The diffuse mucosal sloughing also allowed only suboptimal assessment for viral inclusions. Inclusions were not found in the viable areas of the submucosa. As noted, immunohistochemical stains for Cytomegalovirus and Herpes simplex viruses I and II were negative.

The patient took multiple (six) prescribed medications. Salaria et al. found that 62% of patients with a lichenoid pattern of esophageal inflammation were taking more than three medications [1]. 29% of patients took a proton pump inhibitor; 32% took antihypertensive medications: angiotensin converting enzyme inhibitors, beta-blockers, calcium channel blockers, hydrochlotrothiazide, or a combination.

A small number of patients in the study were receiving steroids and immune modulating medications for treatment of their esophageal disease. In the present case, as assessment of clinical and/or histologic response to withdrawal of medications was clearly not an option, it is impossible to establish if polypharmacy was responsible.

Thus, in light of the above, "lichenoid esophagitis" was considered the most appropriate term for the histologic findings.

The history of diabetes and the laboratory evidence of DKA should also be addressed, given the known association between acute esophageal necrosis (AEN), and diabetes [6–8]. AEN, also called "black esophagus" because of the endoscopic appearance of the necrotic epithelium, occurs in several critical care situations [6, 7]. Nearly 90% of patients present with upper gastrointestinal hemorrhage. There is a strong association with hyperglycemia; several cases associated with DKA have been reported. Necrotic mucosa is consistently found circumferentially at the esophago-gastric junction with varying degrees of proximal extension [6, 7]. Microscopically, there is necrosis of the mucosa and submucosa with denuded epithelium, necrotic debris and marked acute inflammation [8]. Proposed pathophysiologic mechanisms include mucosal ischemia, diminished mucosal defenses, and damage from gastric reflux [6]. Approximately 30% of patients die [6]. However, while upper gastrointestinal hemorrhage and laboratory evidence of DKA in this patient may initially suggest AEN, the pathologic findings eliminate this possibility: marked lichenoid inflammation, absence of acute inflammation, and the presence of a prominent ulcer in the mid-esophagus are not characteristic of AEN.

Finally, it is remarkable that this patient had, simultaneously, acute manifestations of two chronic conditions: severe esophageal ulceration secondary to lichenoid esophagitis and DKA complicating diabetes. Although we cannot be certain, dysphagia and bleeding from severe esophageal disease may have led to poor blood glucose control and subsequent DKA. One may also speculate as to the role of diabetes as a causative factor for lichenoid esophagitis. However, as ours is a description of a single case, further reports of this association would be needed to establish such a link.

In conclusion, lichenoid esophagitis is an appropriate diagnostic term when clinical, histologic and laboratory findings do not allow for specific categorization of lichenoid inflammation in the esophagus. This case illustrates that lichenoid esophagitis may cause ulceration and mucosal sloughing severe enough to result in massive upper gastrointestinal bleeding and death. Translating these autopsy findings to the clinical setting, it is possible that the endoscopic finding of a longitudinal mid-esophageal ulcer, especially in the presence of proximal stricture, may be indicative of underlying lichenoid esophagitis. However, further case descriptions will be necessary to provide confirmation.

Abbreviations

AEN: acute esophageal necrosis; CPR: cardiopulmonary resuscitation; DKA: diabetic ketoacidosis; LP: lichen planus

Acknowledgements

Not applicable.

Funding

No funding was provided.

Authors' contributions

AM is the main author of the manuscript, and prepared the macroscopic and microscopic images. TP provided interpretation of the histology and immunoperoxidase studies, and partially authored the pathology description. Both authors read and approved the final manuscript.

Authors' information

Not applicable.

Competing interests

The authors declare that they have no competing interests.

References

1. Salaria SN, Abu Alfa AK, Cruise MW, Wood LD, Montgomery EA. Lichenoid esophagitis-clinicopathologic overlap with established esophageal lichen planus. Am J Surg Pathol. 2013;37:1889–94.
2. Nielsen JA, Law RM, Fiman KH, Roberts CA. Esophageal lichen planus: a case report and review of the literature. World J Gastroenterol. 2013;19:2278–81.
3. Ynson ML, Forouhar F, Vaziri H. Case report and review of esophageal lichen planus treated with fluticasone. World J Gastroenterol. 2013;19:1652–16562.
4. Katzka DA, Smyrk TC, Bruce AJ, Romero Y, Alexander JA, Murray JA. Variations in presentations of esophageal involvement in lichen planus. Clin Gastroenterol Hepatol. 2010;8:777–82.
5. Le Cleach L, Chosidow O. Lichen planus. N Engl J Med. 2012;366:723–32.
6. Gurvits GE, Cherian K, Shami MN, Korabathina R, El-Nader EM, Rayapudi K, Gandolfo FJ, Alshumrany M, Patel H, Chowdhury DN, Tsiakos A. Black esophagus: new insights and multicenter international experience in 2014. Dig Dis Sci. 2015;60:444–53.
7. Galtés I, Gallego MA, Esgueva R, Martin-Fumadó C. Acute oesophageal necrosis (black oesophagus). Rev Esp Enferm Dig. 2016;108:154–5.
8. Rigolon R, Fossa I, Rodella L, Targher G. Black esophagus syndrome associated with diabetic ketoacidosis. World J Clin Cases. 2016;4:56–9.

10

'Pre-endoscopy point of care test (Simtomax- IgA/IgG-Deamidated Gliadin Peptide) for coeliac disease in iron deficiency anaemia: diagnostic accuracy and a cost saving economic model'

Michelle Shui Yee Lau[1*], Peter D. Mooney[1], William L. White[1], Victoria Appleby[2], Sulleman Moreea[2], Ismail Haythem[3], Joshua E. Elias[4], Kiran Bundhoo[4], Gareth D. Corbett[4], Liam Wong[5], Her Hsin Tsai[5], Simon S. Cross[6], John M. Hebden[7], Sami Hoque[3] and David S. Sanders[1]

Abstract

Background: International guidelines recommend coeliac serology in iron deficiency anaemia, and duodenal biopsy for those tested positive to detect coeliac disease. However, pre-endoscopy serology is often unavailable, thus committing endoscopists to take routine duodenal biopsies. Some endoscopists consider duodenal biopsy mandatory in anaemia to exclude other pathologies. We hypothesise that using a point of care test at endoscopy could fill this gap, by providing rapid results to target anaemic patients who require biopsies, and save costs by biopsy avoidance. We therefore assessed three key aspects to this hypothesis: 1) the availability of pre-endoscopy serology in anaemia; 2) the sensitivities and cost effectiveness of pre-endoscopy coeliac screening with Simtomax in anaemia; 3) whether other anaemia-related pathologies could be missed by this targeted-biopsy approach.

Methods: Group 1: pre-endoscopy serology availability was retrospectively analysed in a multicentre cohort of 934 anaemic patients at 4 UK hospitals. Group 2: the sensitivities of Simtomax, endomysial and tissue-transglutaminase antibodies were compared in 133 prospectively recruited patients with iron deficiency anaemia attending for a gastroscopy. The sensitivities were measured against duodenal histology as the reference standard in all patients. The cost effectiveness of Simtomax was calculated based on the number of biopsies that could have been avoided compared to an all-biopsy approach. Group 3: the duodenal histology of 153 patients presenting to a separate iron deficiency anaemia clinic were retrospectively reviewed.

Results: In group 1, serology was available in 361 (33.8 %) patients. In group 2, the sensitivity and negative predictive value (NPV) were 100 % and 100 % for Simtomax, 96.2 % and 98.9 % for IgA-TTG, and 84.6 % and 96.4 % for EMA respectively. In group 3, the duodenal histology found no causes for anaemia other than coeliac disease.
(Continued on next page)

* Correspondence: michellelau@doctors.org.uk
[1]Academic Department of Gastroenterology, Royal Hallamshire Hospital, Sheffield Teaching Hospitals, Sheffield, UK
Full list of author information is available at the end of the article

(Continued from previous page)

Conclusion: Simtomax had excellent diagnostic accuracy in iron deficiency anaemia and was comparable to conventional serology. Duodenal biopsy did not identify any causes other than coeliac disease for iron deficiency anaemia, suggesting that biopsy avoidance in Simtomax negative anaemic patients is unlikely to miss other anaemia-related pathologies. Due to its 100 % NPV, Simtomax could reduce unnecessary biopsies by 66 % if only those with a positive Simtomax were biopsied, potentially saving £3690/100 gastroscopies.

Keywords: Coeliac disease, Small intestine, Endoscopy, Histopathology, Iron deficiency anaemia, Diagnostic tests, Health economics, Screening

Background

The prevalence of coeliac disease is approximately 1 % [1–5]. However, 75 % of cases remain undiagnosed [6], possibly due to its insidious onset, and patients do not always have symptoms. Moreover, the sensitivities of the endoscopic features of coeliac disease are limited as they may not always be present or easily recognised [7, 8]. One of the common presenting symptoms is anaemia, affecting 15–26.8 % of untreated patients [9, 10]. It usually results from malabsorption, leading to iron, folate, and B12 deficiency [11]. One way to increase the detection of coeliac disease is by screening individuals with iron deficiency anaemia, which affects 2–5 % of the general population in the developed world [12, 13]. At the endoscopy setting, 2.6–8.7 % of patients presenting with anaemia are diagnosed with coeliac disease, although the data is sparse and mainly from small cohorts [10, 14–18]. The current British Society of Gastroenterology (BSG) iron deficiency anaemia guidelines recommend routine screening for coeliac disease with tissue transglutaminase (TTG) and/or endomysial antibodies (EMA). This is based on the excellent negative predictive value of modern serological tests for coeliac disease. Individuals who are tested positive should then undergo a gastroscopy for duodenal biopsy to confirm the presence of coeliac disease [19]. Anecdotally, the availability and utilisation of coeliac serology prior to endoscopy appears to be highly variable, thus committing clinicians to take duodenal biopsies if serology results are unavailable. However, this is an expensive way of case detection. A recent Swedish study [10] showed that a routine duodenal biopsy strategy was ineffective, with a number needed to biopsy of 577 to detect one case of coeliac disease, spending more than €30,000 per case. In an attempt to target patients who require a duodenal biopsy, Hopper et al. [20] devised a clinical decision tool using a combination of pre-endoscopy serological testing and symptom assessment. This algorithm had a 100 % sensitivity and negative predictive value in detecting coeliac disease when applied to 2000 prospectively recruited patients. Yet, the lack of serology availability prior to endoscopy in real clinical practice seemed to have precluded the widespread utilisation of this effective and cost saving clinical decision tool.

One method of filling the gap of unavailable serology is by using a point of care test at the point of endoscopy. Several point of care tests are now commercially available for clinicians and patients to purchase, mostly detecting TTG antibodies. Simtomax, a new point of care test for coeliac disease, is a finger prick test that provides rapid results within ten minutes. Simtomax detects coeliac disease with a unique combination of immunoglobulin A (IgA) and immunoglobulin G (IgG) antibodies against deamidated gliadin peptides (DGP) as well as the total level of IgA [21]. This ensures that results are not affected by patients with IgA deficiency, which is more common in people with coeliac disease than the general population (2.6 % versus 0.14–0.2 %) [22].

In this study, our aim was to evaluate the role of utilising a pre-endoscopy point of care test for coeliac disease, Simtomax, in iron deficiency anaemia in a cost saving model. Firstly, we reviewed the rates of adherence to the BSG guidelines on coeliac serological screening in iron deficiency anaemia in real clinical practice, to demonstrate the pre-endoscopy availability of serology. We then ascertained the sensitivities of Simtomax in detecting coeliac disease in iron deficiency, and established the economic impact of using Simtomax as a screening tool to target biopsy taking only in those tested positive for Simtomax. Finally, we explored whether routine duodenal biopsy would yield any alternative causes for iron deficiency anaemia other than coeliac disease, in order to evaluate whether using Simtomax to target biopsies only in Simtomax positive anaemic patients would miss other duodenal pathologies causing anaemia. We chose to review the duodenal histology of patients from the general population attending a non-coeliac specialised iron deficiency anaemia clinic at the Northern General Hospital, because the results would represent real world data without tertiary referral bias.

Methods

Study design and participants

Group 1 was a multicentre retrospective analysis of all patients with anaemia attending a gastroscopy with duodenal biopsy at four UK hospitals (Addenbrooke's, Bradford, Hull and Whipps Cross) over a 12 month period ranging from 2012 to 2014. The availability of coeliac serology prior to gastroscopy was reviewed.

Group 2 was a prospective study comparing the sensitivities of Simtomax to conventional serology in an iron deficient cohort. We prospectively recruited 133 consecutive patients (age range: 18–89 years, median 53) with iron deficiency with or without anaemia attending a single coeliac disease research endoscopy list at the tertiary referral centre Royal Hallamshire Hospital between 2013 and 2015. All recruited patients were consented for the study prior to the gastroscopy. The patients concurrently undertook the point of care test, Simtomax, conventional coeliac serology (IgA-TTG, IgA-EMA) and total IgA levels at the endoscopy unit. All patients then had a gastroscopy with quadrantic duodenal biopsy from the second part of the duodenum and at least one duodenal bulb biopsy. Patients were excluded from the study if they were known to have coeliac disease or were on a gluten free diet. Patients with coagulopathy, active gastrointestinal bleeding or a suspected carcinoma observed during the examination were also excluded. Clinical information of the patients was available to the endoscopist, however the endoscopist was blinded to the results of the Simtomax test.

Group 3 was a retrospective histological analysis of patients attending a separate non-coeliac specific iron deficiency anaemia clinic at the Northern General Hospital in 2013–2014. We reviewed their duodenal histology and hospital case notes to determine the yield of alternative causes other than coeliac disease in the context of iron deficiency anaemia.

Point of care test, Simtomax

Simtomax is a point of care test for coeliac disease manufactured by Augurix Diagnostics, Switzerland. It detects both IgA and IgG antibodies to DGP, as well as the total IgA level. The assay is based on lateral flow immunochromatography using colloidal gold antihuman antibodies as a signal detector. A sample of 25 μl of capillary venous blood is required which can be obtained through a simple finger prick technique. The assay can also be performed using a plasma sample either in ethylenediaminetetraacetic acid (EDTA) or heparin as well as a separated serum sample, although a smaller sample volume of 20 μl is required. The blood sample is then applied to the test device, followed by the application of 5 drops of the provided buffer solution. The result can be read after 10 min. Positive results are indicated by the presence of a solid red test line for IgA and/or IgG-DGP positivity. A second single red line indicates the presence of IgA. An in-built red control line ensures a correctly functioning test.

Serology

Total IgA was measured on a Behring BN2 nephelometer. IgA-TTG antibodies were evaluated using enzyme-linked immunosorbent assay kits (Aesku Diagnostics, Wendelsheim, Germany). An IgA-TTG titre of > 15 U/ml before 20/5/2014, a new cut off level of >9 U/ml from 20/5-11/12/2014, and then >7 U/ml from 12/12/2014 onwards, were regarded as positive as per the manufacturer's guidance. IgA-EMA was detected by immunofluorescence on primate oesophagus sections (Binding Site, Birmingham, UK).

Biopsies and histology

In total, at least five biopsies were taken from the duodenum, including at least one from the duodenal bulb, with each biopsy fixed in formalin at the time of the gastroscopy. Specimens were then processed, orientated and embedded in paraffin wax by the pathology department. Standard 3 μm thick sections at three levels were stained with haematoxylin and eosin, and reported by gastrointestinal histopathologists without knowledge of the Simtomax results. Villous atrophy was graded according to the modified Marsh criteria.

Diagnosis of coeliac disease

The presence of villous atrophy (Marsh 3a-3c) on histology with a positive IgA-EMA or IgA-TTG were required for the diagnosis of coeliac disease. In cases of seronegative villous atrophy, human leucocyte antigen (HLA) genotyping was performed, with a negative HLA DQ2 or DQ8 phenotype used to rule out coeliac disease. Supporting information such as family history and response to a gluten free diet were also taken into account.

Ethics

The study protocol was approved by the Yorkshire and the Humber Research Ethics committee and registered with the local research and development department of Sheffield Teaching Hospital NHS Foundation Trust under the registration number STH15416. Written consent was obtained from all participants.

Statistical analysis

The sensitivity, specificity, positive (PPV) and negative predictive values (NPV) of Simtomax, IgA-EMA and IgA-TTG were measured against duodenal histology as the reference standard. As the PPV and NPV of a test are influenced by the pre-test probability, positive (PLR) and negative likelihood ratios (NLR) were also calculated as these are less prone to influence by disease prevalence.

Exact Clopper-Pearson method was used to calculate the confidence intervals for the diagnostic test sensitivities.

Cost analysis

In the UK, the Health Resource Group tariff (payment from the National Health Service [NHS] commissioners to hospitals for providing a service) for a gastroscopy with duodenal biopsy and a gastroscopy alone are £382 and £344 respectively. This means that £38 would be saved for the NHS budget if a duodenal biopsy was avoided for each gastroscopy performed. On the other hand, there is cross charging between departments for each service provided. At the Royal Hallamshire Hospital, the histopathology department charges the gastroenterology department £86 for the service of analysing four D2 biopsies and one D1 biopsy (local tariff may vary among different trusts). We will demonstrate the financial impact at a local and national level if Simtomax were to be used to target biopsies in iron deficient patients with a positive Simtomax test, as opposed to a routine biopsy strategy.

Results

In group 1, a total of 934 patients with anaemia underwent a gastroscopy with duodenal biopsy at four UK hospitals. Coeliac serology was only available in 315 patients (33.8 %) prior to endoscopy. Forty-four (14 %) serology samples were performed in primary care.

In group 2, 133 patients (88 females) with iron deficiency attending for a gastroscopy at the tertiary referral centre Royal Hallamshire Hospital were prospectively recruited. Twenty-six patients (19.5 %) were diagnosed with coeliac disease. Simtomax correctly identified all cases of coeliac disease, defined by a combination of a positive serology (IgA-EMA/IgA-TTG) and Marsh grade 3a-c villous atrophy. The results are shown in Tables 1 and 2. There was one case of a 38 year old Zambian lady with seronegative villous atrophy secondary to tuberculosis. The sensitivity, specificity, PPV and NPV of Simtomax were 100 %, 82.2 %, 57.8 % and 100 % respectively. A comparison of the sensitivities of Simtomax, IgA-TTG and IgA-EMA are shown in Table 3. Please refer to Fig. 1 for the flow diagram of group 2. There were no invalid Simtomax results. No adverse events occurred with the Simtomax tests or gastroscopies.

In group 3, 215 patients with iron deficiency anaemia attended a separate non-coeliac specialised anaemia clinic at the Northern General Hospital for investigation from 2013–2014. A total of 175 patients underwent a gastroscopy, and 153 of those had a duodenal biopsy. The duodenal histology samples of these 153 patients were analysed. Two patients had Marsh grade 3 villous atrophy on histology- one had a positive coeliac serology and hence was diagnosed with coeliac disease; the other patient was found to have a colonic tumour during the course of the IDA investigation and subsequently died. He never had coeliac serology or HLA genotyping to confirm the diagnosis. Assuming the latter case to be coeliac disease, the prevalence of coeliac disease in group 3 would be 1.3 %. One hundred and forty-one patients (92.2 %) had normal duodenal histology. Seven patients (4.6 %) had lymphocytic duodenosis (Marsh grade 1) on their histology, all of whom had negative coeliac serology. We reviewed their hospital case notes and screened for drug causes for lymphocytic duodenosis such as aspirin, proton pump inhibitors, olmesartan, non steroidal anti-inflammatories and chemotherapy; autoimmune associations such as type 1 diabetes, thyroid disorders etc; and infections such as Helicobacter pylori, Whipple's, Giardia etc. Six of these patients had a cause for or association with lymphocytic duodenosis: vitiligo, autoimmune hypothyroidism, multiple sclerosis, aspirin use, proton pump inhibitor use and Helicobacter pylori infection respectively. We could not find a cause attributable to the lymphocytic duodenosis in the remaining one patient, whose helicobacter status was unknown. Three patients had reactive changes, chronic duodenitis and submucosal haemangioma respectively on their duodenal histology which were not the cause for their iron deficiency anaemia. Please refer to Fig. 2 for the flow chart of group 3 patients.

Cost saving economic model

In our group 2 cohort, 88 out of 133 patients had a negative Simtomax test. Based on the 100 % sensitivity and NPV of Simtomax, a duodenal biopsy could have been avoided in these 88 patients (66.2 %). At the Royal Hallamshire Hospital, the cost of having duodenal biopsies reported (four D2 and one D1 biopsy) is £86, and the price of each Simtomax test kit is £20. The cost saving from avoided biopsies in this cohort would be £7568 (£86x88). After taking into account the cost of using Simtomax on all patients (£20x133 = £2660), the overall cost saving in this cohort would be £4908

Table 1 Group 2 patient characteristics and corresponding results

	Simtomax positive	EMA positive	TTG positive	M[a]0	M1	M2	M3a	M3b	M3c	Coeliac disease
Iron deficiency anaemia ($n = 81$)	30	13	19	55	7	1	2[b]	5	10	16 (19.8 %)
Iron deficiency without anaemia ($n = 52$)	15	10	15	33	8	1	2	2	6	10 (19.2 %)

[a]Marsh grade
[b]One patient had seronegative Marsh grade 3a villous atrophy which was secondary to tuberculosis instead of coeliac disease

Table 2 Cross tabulation of Simtomax results by serology and duodenal histology results

	Simtomax positive	Simtomax negative
Coeliac disease (positive serology and Marsh 3 histology)	26	0
No coeliac disease (negative serology and/or Marsh 0-2 histology)	19	88

(£7568–£2660) for the gastroenterology department. This equates to a potential cost saving of £3690 per 100 gastroscopies. At a national level, the difference in the HRG tariff between a gastroscopy alone and a gastroscopy with duodenal biopsy paid by the clinical commissioners to the trust is £38. This equates to a cost saving of £2514/100 gastroscopies for the NHS budget (£38x88/133x100).

Discussion

Principal findings

We demonstrated with real life data that the availability of coeliac serology in anaemia prior to gastroscopy was low (33.8 %). This result is consistent with a study conducted by Wiland et al. in 2013 demonstrating that only one third of patients suspected to have coeliac disease had serology available prior to endoscopy [23].

To our knowledge, this is the first study showing that a combined IgA/IgG-DGP based point of care test, Simtomax, had 100 % sensitivity and negative predictive value in detecting coeliac disease in iron deficient patients. The positive and negative likelihood ratios were 5.63 and 0 respectively, indicating a negative Simtomax test effectively rules out coeliac disease in iron deficient patients. This compares to the results from the study by Mooney et al. which demonstrated a slightly lower but still excellent sensitivity of Simtomax at 92.7 % in an unselected cohort of 508 patients attending for a gastroscopy [24]. The higher sensitivity of Simtomax in this study could be due to the specific target population with iron deficiency anaemia causing a positive ascertainment bias. Although the pre-test probability in group 2 was relatively high, it is similar to that of Mooney et al.'s study at 13.4 %.

Our group 3 duodenal histology review revealed no alternative causes for iron deficiency anaemia other than villous atrophy secondary to coeliac disease. With a 100 % NPV, taking a duodenal biopsy in patients with a negative Simtomax test would be highly unlikely to yield any diagnosis for iron deficiency in routine clinical practice, and hence could be avoided in patients presenting with iron deficiency with or without anaemia.

The local cost saving of £3690/100 gastroscopies was based on the coeliac disease prevalence of 19.5 % in our coeliac enriched group 2 cohort. In a lower prevalence population, the potential cost saving would be greater. If we base our calculations on the average coeliac disease prevalence of 5 % in iron deficient cohorts, [14–18] the potential cost saving for the gastroenterology department would be £5826/100 gastroscopies, assuming the same tariff was applied; and £3456/100 gastroscopies would be saved at a national level for the NHS budget. This is excluding a wide range of intangible savings from the positive knock on effects, such as cost savings from not using biopsy pots and forceps, staff time and workload for both the endoscopy and histopathology departments.

Strengths and weaknesses

The strength of our prospective study (group 2) is that the sensitivities of Simtomax were measured against duodenal histology rather than serology as the reference standard. Furthermore, in order to reduce selection bias, all patients underwent duodenal biopsies irrespective of their serology or Simtomax results. This sets our study apart from the three out of four published Simtomax studies, [25–27] where only patients with a positive serology or Simtomax test went on to have duodenal biopsies, which could potentially lead to a positive ascertainment bias and falsely elevated sensitivities. This limitation is also common in previous studies on the sensitivities of coeliac serology. A meta-analysis [28] published in 2010 on studies comparing IgA-DGP serology to IgA-TTG serology showed that only two [29, 30] out of eleven studies were unlikely to have ascertainment bias, where both of these studies also biopsied controls.

One of the limitations of our study is the relatively high pre-test probability in group 2 being investigated at our tertiary referral centre for coeliac disease, giving a coeliac disease prevalence of 19.5 %. This referral bias may falsely increase the positive predictive value of Simtomax, although the weight of its negative predictive value may be strengthened.

Another limitation is that even though the non-specialist group 3 cohort represented real life data from

Table 3 A comparison of the sensitivities of Simtomax, IgA-TTG and IgA-EMA in group 2

	Sensitivity, % (95 % CI)	Specificity, % (95 % CI)	PPV, % (95 % CI)	NPV, % (95 % CI)
Simtomax	100 (86.8–100.0)	82.2 (73.7–89.0)	57.8 (42.2–72.3)	100 (95.9–100.0)
IgA-TTG	96.2 (80.4–99.9)	91.5 (84.5–96.4)	73.5 (55.6–87.1)	99.0 (94.5–100.0)
IgA-EMA	84.6 (65.1–95.6)	99.1 (94.9–100.0)	95.7 (78.1–99.9)	96.4 (91.0–99.0)

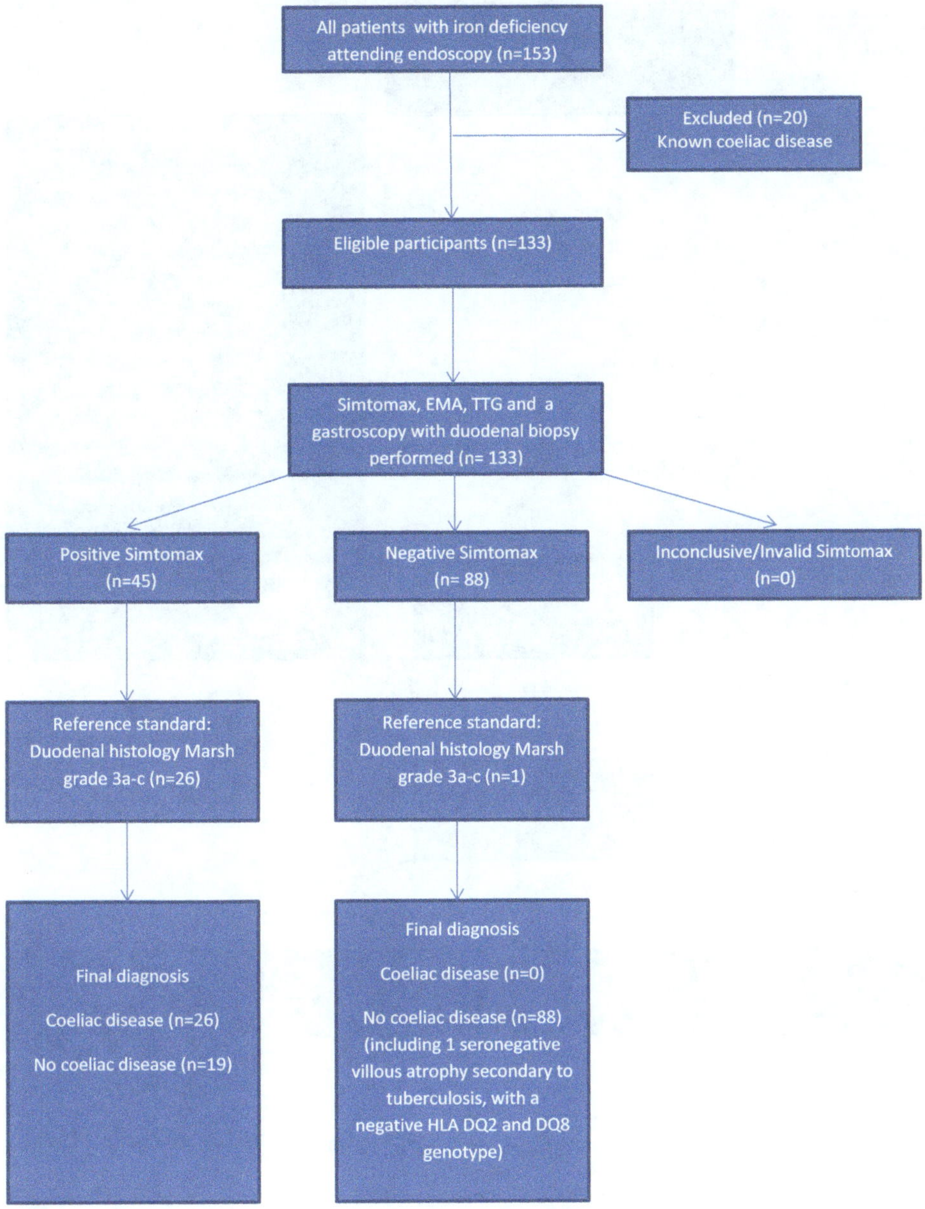

Fig. 1 Flow of participants in group 2 study

the general population where no other causes for anaemia apart from coeliac disease were found on duodenal histology, it is a relatively small cohort and may not be representative of other populations. For instance, infective causes may be seen in other cohorts, and their prevalence varies from different populations and geographical regions. Two Turkish studies reported a 2 % prevalence of Giardia found on duodenal biopsies in their cohorts with iron deficiency anaemia [31, 32]. On the other hand, a German study found a 0.2 % prevalence of Giardiasis on routine duodenal biopsy in 1000 unselected patients attending for a gastroscopy, [33] and a study from the U.S. had a 0.3 % yield of Giardiasis on routine duodenal biopsy in 300 patients presenting with abdominal pain [34]. Therefore, the cost saving economic model through biopsy avoidance in iron deficient patients with a negative Simtomax test may not be applicable to populations where parasitic infections are common, as infective diagnoses may be missed.

In our group 2 tertiary centre iron deficient cohort, there was one case of seronegative villous atrophy secondary to tuberculosis. This is a rare cause of seronegative villous atrophy. It must be emphasised that the group 2 cohort does not reflect what is normally seen in routine clinical practice, as the Royal Hallamshire Hospital is a tertiary referral centre. Apart from coeliac disease and

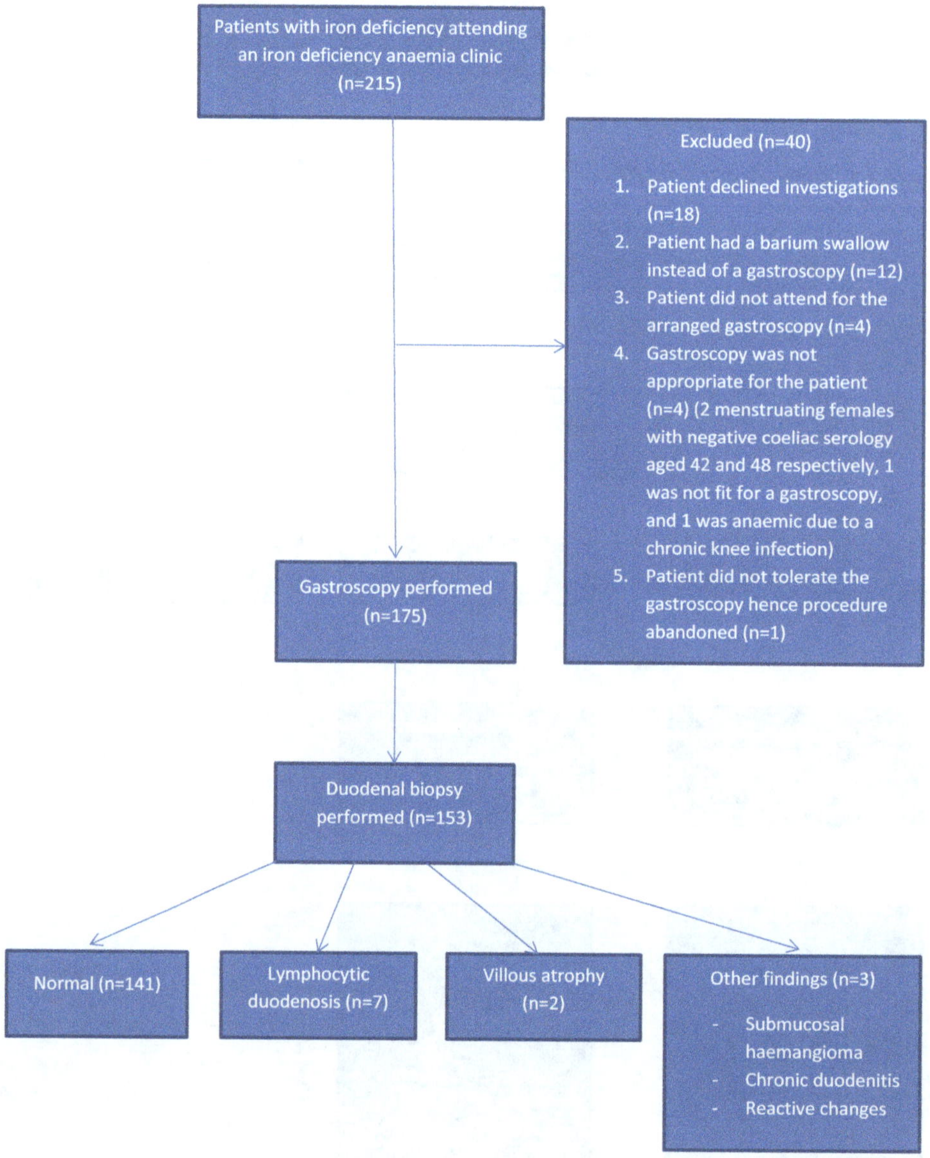

Fig. 2 Flow chart for group 3 cohort analysis

parasitic infections, rarer malabsorptive enteropathies with villous atrophy have been reported in other studies, such as in patients with Whipple's disease, [35] graft versus host disease, [36] common variable immunodeficiency, [37, 38] autoimmune enteropathy, [39], and olmesartan associated enteropathy [40]. The literature has shown that patients with gastrointestinal parasitic infections and other rare enteropathies described above typically present with significant symptoms such as diarrhoea, abdominal pain and malnutrition, rather than solely with iron deficency anaemia [34, 37–39]. Therefore, in iron deficient patients where there is a high index of suspicion for other enteropathies, such as malasborptive symptoms or high risk ethnicities, the threshold for taking duodenal biopsies should be lowered.

Our study demonstrated excellent sensitivity and negative predictive value of Simtomax in iron deficiency, and its performance was comparable to both IgA-EMA and IgA-TTG. This is consistent with two other studies testing Simtomax in high risk groups performed by Benkebil et al. in 2013 [26] (100 % sensitivity for coeliac disease in a high risk population) and Bienvenu et al. in 2014 [27] (100 % sensitivity and NPV for coeliac disease in IgA deficient children, median age 8.4). However, Bienvenu et al. 2012 [25] showed that the sensitivity of Simtomax to be slightly lower at 93.1 % when tested on a paediatric population with clinical suspicion of coeliac disease, although it should be noted that this sensitivity was measured against TTG as the reference standard rather than duodenal histology.

Conclusion

This is the first study that demonstrated the excellent diagnostic accuracy of Simtomax in iron deficiency, which was comparable to conventional serological testing. With a 100 % sensitivity and negative predictive value, Simtomax could be used judiciously by clinicians as an effective and cost saving screening test for coeliac disease in the endoscopic setting, by avoiding duodenal biopsies in patients presenting with iron deficiency with a negative Simtomax test.

Abbreviations

BSG: British society of gastroenterology; DGP: Deamidated gliadin peptide antibodies; EDTA: Ethylenediaminetetraacetic acid; EMA: Endomysial antibodies; HLA: Human leucocyte antigen; IgA: Immunoglobulin A; IgG: Immunoglobulin G; NHS: National Health Service; NLR: Negative likelihood ratio; NPV: Negative predictive value; PLR: Positive likelihood ratio; PPV: Positive predictive value; TTG: Tissue transglutaminase antibodies

Acknowledgement

Not applicable.

Funding

Not applicable.

Authors' contribution

Specific author contributions: MSL recruited patients, collected, analysed and interpreted data, drafted and reviewed the final version of the manuscript. PDM helped design the study, recruited patients, collected, analysed data and helped draft the manuscript; DSS designed the study, recruited, analysed data and reviewed the final version of the manuscript; WLW, VA, SM, IH, SH, JE, KB, GC, LW, HHT, JMH helped recruit patients and collect data; WLW helped recruit patients and analysed data; SSC reviewed histopathology specimens and helped analyse data; All authors have read and approved of the final manuscript.

Competing interests

Professor David Sanders has received funding from Tillotts Pharma for investigator-led studies into point of care testing for coeliac disease. Tillott's Pharma did not have any input in the study design, access to study data, interpretation of the findings or drafting of the manuscript. The remaining authors disclosed no conflicts of interests.

Author details

[1]Academic Department of Gastroenterology, Royal Hallamshire Hospital, Sheffield Teaching Hospitals, Sheffield, UK. [2]Department of Gastroenterology, Bradford Royal Infirmary, Bradford, UK. [3]Department of Gastroenterology, Whipps Cross University Hospital, London, UK. [4]Department of Gastroenterology, Addenbrooke's Hospital, Cambridge, UK. [5]Department of Gastroenterology, Hull Royal Infirmary, Hull, UK. [6]Academic Unit of Pathology, Department of Neuroscience, Faculty of Medicine, Dentistry & Health, The University of Sheffield, Sheffield, UK. [7]Department of Gastroenterology, Northern General Hospital, Sheffield Teaching Hospitals, Sheffield, UK.

References

1. Fasano A, Berti I, Gerarduzzi T, Not T, Colletti RB, Drago S, et al. Prevalence of celiac disease in at-risk and not-at-risk groups in the United States: a large multicenter study. Arch Intern Med. 2003;163(3):286–92.
2. Mustalahti K, Catassi C, Reunanen A, Fabiani E, Heier M, McMillan S, et al. The prevalence of celiac disease in Europe: results of a centralized, international mass screening project. Ann Med. 2010;42(8):587–95.
3. West J, Logan RF, Hill PG, Lloyd A, Lewis S, Hubbard R, et al. Seroprevalence, correlates, and characteristics of undetected coeliac disease in England. Gut. 2003;52(7):960–5.
4. Cook HB, Burt MJ, Collett JA, Whitehead MR, Frampton CM, Chapman BA. Adult coeliac disease: prevalence and clinical significance. J Gastroenterol Hepatol. 2000;15(9):1032–6.
5. Bingley PJ, Williams AJ, Norcross AJ, Unsworth DJ, Lock RJ, Ness AR, et al. Undiagnosed coeliac disease at age seven: population based prospective birth cohort study. BMJ. 2004;328(7435):322–3.
6. West J, Fleming KM, Tata LJ, Card TR, Crooks CJ. Incidence and prevalence of celiac disease and dermatitis herpetiformis in the UK over two decades: population-based study. Am J Gastroenterol. 2014;109(5):757–68.
7. William D. Endoscopic markers for celiac disease. Nat Clin Pract Gastroenterol Hepatol. 2006;3(10):546.
8. Olds G, McLoughlin R, Morian C, Sivak MV. Celiac disease for the endoscopist. Gastrointest Endosc. 2002;56(3):407–15.
9. Leffler DA, Green PH, Fasano A. Extraintestinal manifestations of coeliac disease. Nat Rev Gastroenterol Hepatol. 2015;12(10):561–71.
10. Burger JP, Meijer JW, Wahab PJ. Routine duodenal biopsy to screen for coeliac disease is not effective. Neth J Med. 2013;71(6):308–12.
11. Halfdanarson TR, Litzow MR, Murray JA. Hematologic manifestations of celiac disease. Blood. 2007;109(2):412–21.
12. McLean E, Cogswell M, Egli I, Wojdyla D, de Benoist B. Worldwide prevalence of anaemia, WHO Vitamin and Mineral Nutrition Information System, 1993-2005. Public Health Nutr. 2009;12(4):444–54.
13. Guralnik JM, Eisenstaedt RS, Ferrucci L, Klein HG, Woodman RC. Prevalence of anemia in persons 65 years and older in the United States: evidence for a high rate of unexplained anemia. Blood. 2004;104(8):2263–8.
14. McIntyre AS, Long RG. Prospective survey of investigations in outpatients referred with iron deficiency anaemia. Gut. 1993;34(8):1102–7.
15. Corazza GR, Valentini RA, Andreani ML, D'Anchino M, Leva MT, Ginaldi L, et al. Subclinical coeliac disease is a frequent cause of iron-deficiency anaemia. Scand J Gastroenterol. 1995;30(2):153–6.
16. Unsworth DJ, Lock RJ, Harvey RF. Improving the diagnosis of coeliac disease in anaemic women. Br J Haematol. 2000;111(3):898–901.
17. Howard MR, Turnbull AJ, Morley P, Hollier P, Webb R, Clarke A. A prospective study of the prevalence of undiagnosed coeliac disease in laboratory defined iron and folate deficiency. J Clin Pathol. 2002;55(10):754–7.
18. Grisolano SW, Oxentenko AS, Murray JA, Burgart LJ, Dierkhising RA, Alexander JA. The usefulness of routine small bowel biopsies in evaluation of iron deficiency anemia. J Clin Gastroenterol. 2004;38(9):756–60.
19. Goddard AF, James MW, McIntyre AS, Scott BB, Gastroenterology BSo. Guidelines for the management of iron deficiency anaemia. Gut. 2011;60(10):1309–16.
20. Hopper AD, Cross SS, Hurlstone DP, McAlindon ME, Lobo AJ, Hadjivassiliou M, et al. Pre-endoscopy serological testing for coeliac disease: evaluation of a clinical decision tool. BMJ. 2007;334(7596):729.
21. Mooney PD, Kurien M, Sanders DS. Simtomax, a novel point of care test for coeliac disease. Expert Opin Med Diagn. 2013;7(6):645–51.
22. Cataldo F, Marino V, Ventura A, Bottaro G, Corazza GR. Prevalence and clinical features of selective immunoglobulin A deficiency in coeliac disease: an Italian multicentre study. Italian Society of Paediatric Gastroenterology and Hepatology (SIGEP) and "Club del Tenue" Working Groups on Coeliac Disease. Gut. 1998;42(3):362–5.
23. Wiland HO, Henricks WH, Daly TM. Limited utilization of serologic testing in patients undergoing duodenal biopsy for celiac disease. BMC Gastroenterol. 2013;13:156.
24. Mooney PD, Wong SH, Johnston AJ, Kurien M, Avgerinos A, Sanders DS. Increased Detection of Celiac Disease With Measurement of Deamidated Gliadin Peptide Antibody Before Endoscopy. Clin Gastroenterol Hepatol. 2015;13(7):1278–84. e1.
25. Bienvenu F, Besson Duvanel C, Seignovert C, Rouzaire P, Lachaux A, Bienvenu J. Evaluation of a point-of-care test based on deamidated gliadin peptides for celiac disease screening in a large pediatric population. Eur J Gastroenterol Hepatol. 2012;24(12):1418–23.
26. Benkebil F, Combescure C, Anghel SI, Besson Duvanel C, Schäppi MG. Diagnostic accuracy of a new point-of-care screening assay for celiac disease. World J Gastroenterol. 2013;19(31):5111–7.
27. Bienvenu F, Anghel SI, Besson Duvanel C, Guillemaud J, Garnier L, Renosi F, et al. Early diagnosis of celiac disease in IgA deficient children: contribution of a point-of-care test. BMC Gastroenterol. 2014;14:186.
28. Lewis NR, Scott BB. Meta-analysis: deamidated gliadin peptide antibody and tissue transglutaminase antibody compared as screening tests for coeliac disease. Aliment Pharmacol Ther. 2010;31(1):73–81.

29. Niveloni S, Sugai E, Cabanne A, Vazquez H, Argonz J, Smecuol E, et al. Antibodies against synthetic deamidated gliadin peptides as predictors of celiac disease: prospective assessment in an adult population with a high pretest probability of disease. Clin Chem. 2007;53(12):2186–92.
30. Rashtak S, Ettore MW, Homburger HA, Murray JA. Comparative usefulness of deamidated gliadin antibodies in the diagnosis of celiac disease. Clin Gastroenterol Hepatol. 2008;6(4):426–32. quiz 370.
31. Gonen. Diagnostic yield of routine duodenal biopsies in iron deficiency anaemia: a study from Western Anatolia. Eur J Gastroenterol Hepatol. 2007;19(1):37–41.
32. Gulen H, Kasirga E, Yildirim SA, Kader S, Sahin G, Ayhan S. Diagnostic yield of upper gastrointestinal endoscopy in the evaluation of iron deficiency anemia in older children and adolescents. Pediatr Hematol Oncol. 2011;28(8):694–701.
33. Tischendorf JJ, Wopp K, Streetz KL, Bach J, Meyer M, Tischendorf S, et al. The value of duodenal biopsy within routine upper endoscopy: a prospective study in 1000 patients. Z Gastroenterol. 2008;46(8):771–5.
34. Dubin SM, Kwong W, Kalmaz D, Savides T. Low yield of routine duodenal biopsies for evaluation of abdominal pain. World J Gastroenterol. 2015;21(24):7495–9.
35. Bai JC, Mazure RM, Vazquez H, Niveloni SI, Smecuol E, Pedreira S, et al. Whipple's disease. Clin Gastroenterol Hepatol. 2004;2(10):849–60.
36. Patey-Mariaud de Serre N, Reijasse D, Verkarre V, Canioni D, Colomb V, Haddad E, et al. Chronic intestinal graft-versus-host disease: clinical, histological and immunohistochemical analysis of 17 children. Bone Marrow Transplant. 2002;29(3):223–30.
37. Luzi G, Zullo A, Iebba F, Rinaldi V, Sanchez Mete L, Muscaritoli M, et al. Duodenal pathology and clinical-immunological implications in common variable immunodeficiency patients. Am J Gastroenterol. 2003;98(1):118–21.
38. Khodadad A, Aghamohammadi A, Parvaneh N, Rezaei N, Mahjoob F, Bashashati M, et al. Gastrointestinal manifestations in patients with common variable immunodeficiency. Dig Dis Sci. 2007;52(11):2977–83.
39. Masia R, Peyton S, Lauwers GY, Brown I. Gastrointestinal biopsy findings of autoimmune enteropathy: a review of 25 cases. Am J Surg Pathol. 2014;38(10):1319–29.
40. Marthey L, Cadiot G, Seksik P, Pouderoux P, Lacroute J, Skinazi F, et al. Olmesartan-associated enteropathy: results of a national survey. Aliment Pharmacol Ther. 2014;40(9):1103–9.

11

Determination of the appropriate propofol infusion rate for outpatient upper gastrointestinal endoscopy

Qiongzhen Li[1†], Qinghe Zhou[2†], Wangpin Xiao[2] and Hongmei Zhou[2*]

Abstract

Background: Pain and discomfort related to endoscopy sessions can be alleviated by sedation, which minimizes anxiety and allows safe examination. For outpatient endoscopy, reliable short-term sedation without secondary effects is required. This study aimed to assess the effects of intravenous propofol rates on sedation in outpatients undergoing upper gastrointestinal endoscopy.

Methods: This randomized prospective study evaluated 300 outpatients submitted to upper gastrointestinal endoscopy. Patients received propofol at 500, 1000 or 2000 ml/h. The primary outcome assessed was hypoxemia incidence. In addition, time to sedation and incidence of hypotension, deep sedation, extremity motor activity, cough, nausea, hiccough, and awareness were evaluated.

Results: Recovery time and incidence of hypoxemia, hypotension, and deep sedation were significantly increased in individuals treated at 2000 ml/h in comparison with values obtained for 500 and 1000 ml/h groups ($P < 0.01$). Compared with the 500 ml/h group, motor activity of the extremities, cough, nausea, hiccough, and awareness were significantly decreased and the mean scores for endoscopist's and patients' satisfaction were significantly increased in the 1000 and 2000 ml/h groups ($P < 0.01$).

Conclusion: Propofol infused at 1000 ml/h appeared to be the most suitable infusion rate for outpatient upper gastrointestinal endoscopy.

Keywords: Propofol, Outpatient, Upper gastrointestinal endoscopy, Sedation, Complications

Background

Pain and discomfort related to endoscopy sessions can be alleviated by sedation, which minimizes anxiety and allows safe examination [1]. Over 98 % of endoscopies are performed under sedation [2, 3]. For outpatient endoscopic procedures, reliable short term sedation without secondary effects is required. Intravenous (IV) propofol is frequently used [4, 5].

* Correspondence: zhouhongmei120@sina.com
†Equal contributors
[2]Department of Anesthesia, Second Hospital, Jiaxing Medical College, No. 1518, North Huancheng Road, Jianshe Street, Nanhu District, Jiaxing 314000, Zhejiang, China
Full list of author information is available at the end of the article

Propofol (2, 6-diisopropylphenol) is a hypnotic agent that induces anesthesia in about 50 s at standard doses [6]. Propofol is characterized by short half-life, rapid onset, important volume of distribution, and absence of active metabolites, leading to rapid recovery and discharge. These properties make propofol suitable for outpatient gastrointestinal endoscopy.

Using the same dose, the final blood concentrations of propofol depend on patient sex, age and weight, and drug dose, administration rate, and cardiac output [7–10]. Previous studies have shown that the required doses for anesthesia onset are affected by changes in the rate of injection [7, 10, 11]. A previous study has shown that the hypnotic peak effect of propofol is lower using a very slow injection rate (240 s), but there was no difference when using clinically-used injection rates (5–120 s) [12]. Another study showed that the sleep dose of propofol is reduced using slower infusion rates, while fast infusion rates resulted in greater decreases in heart rate and higher incidence of apnea [13]. The use of a slow infusion rate results in longer induction duration, but requires a lower total dose, and results in a lower incidence of apnea and a lesser decrease in blood pressure [14]. However, the appropriate injection rate in an outpatient setting is still controversial.

This study aimed to identify the most suitable propofol infusion rate for outpatients submitted to upper gastrointestinal endoscopy that resulted in the lowest adverse effect incidence and was associated with the highest patient satisfaction.

Methods

Study design

This randomized, parallel, controlled study was performed at the Department of Anesthesia, Second Hospital, Jiaxing Medical College (Jiaxing, Zhejiang, China) between June 2014 and August 2014 (registration number ChiCTR-TRC-14004786). The procedures were approved by the ethics review board of the Second Affiliated Hospital of Jiaxing College, chaired by Professor Liqin Jiang (number CZJ 65). Written informed consent was obtained from each patient prior to participation.

Patients

For patient inclusion, the following criteria were set: 1) American Society of Anesthesiologists (ASA) class I-III; 2) upper gastrointestinal endoscopy; and 3) age 18–65 years. Exclusion criteria were: 1) pregnancy; 2) allergies to eggs, beans, or latex; 3) history of alcohol or sedative overdose [15]; 4) history of adverse events associated with propofol; 5) sleep apnea or acute gastrointestinal hemorrhage; or 6) recent abnormalities of the central nervous system such as stroke.

Intervention

The patients were randomized to one of three groups using a random number table. Patients were administered oxygen at a rate of 2–3 L/min using a nasal catheter before induction. Propofol (Xi'an Libang Shaanxi, China; batch number: 1405282) was administered as an IV bolus by a sub-senior anesthesiologist (13 years of experience) at 500 (500 ml/h group), 1000 (1000 ml/h group) or 2000 ml/h (2000 ml/h group) to unconsciousness. Upon loss of consciousness, rapid infusion was stopped. If the patient still had body movements after infusion, an additional 20–30 mg of propofol was administered to avoid body movements during the procedure. The same senior endoscopist (18 years of experience) performed all procedures with the help of the same supervisor nurse (15 years of experience). The endoscopist had no access to grouping information. The anesthesiologist that administered the additional propofol was blinded to patient's history and initial induction infusion rate.

The target depth of sedation was loss of consciousness, no response to call, and eyelashes reflection. At this moment, propofol was stopped and the endoscope was inserted. If the patients had a body response upon endoscope insertion, propofol was added. The depth of sedation was evaluated according to body response and bispectral index (BIS) values.

Monitoring

An arm vein of the patient was intubated with a 22G infusion catheter, and non-invasive monitoring of the arterial pressure was performed with the contralateral arm. Heart, respiratory, and oxygen saturation (SpO_2) rates were continuously monitored. Induction dose corresponded to the drug amount delivered, and the rate was recorded (Smiths WZ-50F6 two-way injection pump; Zhejiang Smith Medical Instruments Co., Ltd., Ningxia, China). Any excitatory effects or periods of apnea (>30 s) after induction were recorded. Recovery time reflected the period from endoscopy end to full orientation (the patient was able to provide his/her correct date of birth).

The level of sedation was evaluated using BIS monitoring [16–18]. After skin disinfection, disposable electrodes were placed on the forehead, with the leads connected to a BIS Aspect monitor (Medical System, USA), whose output was assessed throughout the operation and recovery. BIS ≤65, 66–85, and >85 indicated deep, conscious, and mild sedation states, respectively. BIS levels were recorded at the following times: baseline, loss of consciousness, endoscope reaching the glottis, endoscope reaching the duodenum, end of endoscopy, and recovery. An independent observer (resident doctor, 3 years of experience, blind to grouping) was responsible for monitoring the patients including level of consciousness and adverse reactions (hypoxemia, bradycardia, hypotension, body movements, cough, nausea, hiccough, awareness) and for data collection (drugs, doses, and onset of cardiorespiratory events).

Adverse events were: hypoxemia (hypoxemia was defined SpO2 falling below 90 %), hypotension (systolic or diastolic blood pressure values decreasing by 20 % or more) and bradycardia (heart rate less than 50 bpm). Severe hypoxemia was defined as SpO2 declining below 90 %, while mild hypoxemia was defined as SpO2 declining below 90 % but rising to above 90 % after more than 30 s of jaw thrust maneuver.

As described by Cohen [19], we compared the three groups with respect to the time to induction (time period from first drug bolus dose to procedure initiation) and the time to recovery (time elapsed from endoscope removal to final evaluation). A patient was discharged only when BIS levels exceeded 90 and when there was no complaint of pain or discomfort.

At hospital discharge, a 10-point visual analogue scale (VAS) was used to evaluate patient satisfaction, from 1 to 10, representing least and most satisfied, respectively. Additionally, a VAS was used by the endoscopist to record his level of satisfaction with the sedation regimen. Respondents had to circle the number that corresponded the best to their experience. The endoscopist's VAS was scored as 1–3, 4–7, and 8–10 for considerable, minor, and no difficulty in performing the procedure; respectively.

Data collection

Age, sex, weight, height, ASA physical status, complications and adverse reactions during endoscopy, patient VAS score, and endoscopist VAS score were recorded. The following parameters were recorded during endoscopy: time to unconsciousness, total propofol dose, propofol dose (mg.kg^{-1}), duration of endoscopy, recovery time, and BIS value at baseline, loss of consciousness, endoscope reaching the glottis, endoscope reaching the duodenum, end of endoscopy and recovery.

Endpoints

The primary endpoint was the incidence of hypoxemia. The secondary endpoints were: incidence of adverse events other than hypoxemia (bradycardia, hypotension, body movement, cough, nausea, hiccough and, awareness); satisfaction of the endoscopist with sedation; BIS values; time to loss of consciousness; total propofol dose; pain during injection; endoscopy duration; and recovery time.

Statistical analysis

Based on our preliminary experiments, the mean frequency of hypoxemia (primary outcome) was approximately 12 % during gastrointestinal endoscopy, and the sample size was calculated based on reducing this frequency by 50 %. To achieve 90 % power at an α level of 0.05 to detect a two-tailed difference, at least 88 patients were required in each group.

Data were analyzed using SPSS 19.0 (IBM, Armonk, NY, USA). Continuous data are mean ± standard deviation (SD). Categorical data were reported as frequencies. One-way analysis of variance (ANOVA) was employed for group comparisons, with the post hoc Bonferroni multiple comparison test. Categorical variables were assessed by the Pearson's chi-square test. Two-tailed P-value ≤0.05 was considered statistically significant. Statistical review of this study was performed by a biomedical statistician (Tao Zhu).

Results

Characteristics of the patients

A total of 368 individuals were enrolled, with 41 not meeting the inclusion criteria; 18 withdrew from the study and 9 were excluded for unknown reasons. All patients underwent endoscopy for diagnostic procedures. The remaining 300 patients were randomized into one of the three groups (Fig. 1). Table 1 presents the characteristics of the patients. Patients were aged 50.1 ± 13.1, 52.0 ± 11.3 and 51.0 ± 11.3 years in the 500, 1000 and 2000 ml/h groups, respectively, and the proportion of females was 68.4, 72.2 and 64.3 %, respectively (all $P > 0.05$). There was no difference in weight, height, ASA class, body mass index (BMI), and endoscopy history (all $P > 0.05$).

Time to loss of conscious, dose, duration of endoscopy, and recovery time

Time to loss of consciousness was significantly longer with the slower infusion rates (86.4 ± 6.0 vs. 54.1 ± 4.8 vs. 32.4 ± 5.2 s at 500, 1000 and 2000 ml/h, respectively; all $P < 0.01$). Total (induction dose + eventual additional doses) and weight-related induction doses were significantly less with 500 and 1000 ml/h compared with 2000 ml/h (2.4 ± 0.4 and 2.4 ± 0.3 vs. 2.9 ± 0.5 mg/kg, $P < 0.01$). In comparison with patients treated at 500 ml/h, the duration of endoscopy was decreased in the 1000 and 2000 ml/h groups ($P < 0.05$). However, in comparison with individuals treated with propofol at 2000 ml/h, recovery times were shorter in the 500 and 1000 ml/h groups (18.1 ± 2.0 vs. 13.2 ± 1.6 and 13.1 ± 1.6 min, $P < 0.05$) (Table 2).

Bispectral index values

Compared with the 500 and 1000 ml/h groups, BIS values were significantly decreased in patients receiving propofol at 2000 ml/h at loss of consciousness, endoscope reaching the glottis, endoscope reaching the duodenum and end of endoscopy ($P < 0.01$) (Table 3).

Complications and adverse reactions

In comparison with the 2000 ml/h group, the frequencies of hypotension and hypoxemia were significantly decreased in patients administered propofol at 500 and 1000 ml/h ($P < 0.01$). However, no statistically significant differences were obtained between groups regarding arrhythmia and pain during injection (Tables 4 and 5). Compared with the 1000 and 2000 ml/h groups, the frequencies of extremity motor activity, cough, nausea, hiccough and awareness were significantly increased in patients treated at 500 ml/h ($P < 0.01$) (Table 4). Deep sedation rate was significantly increased after propofol administration at 2000 ml/h

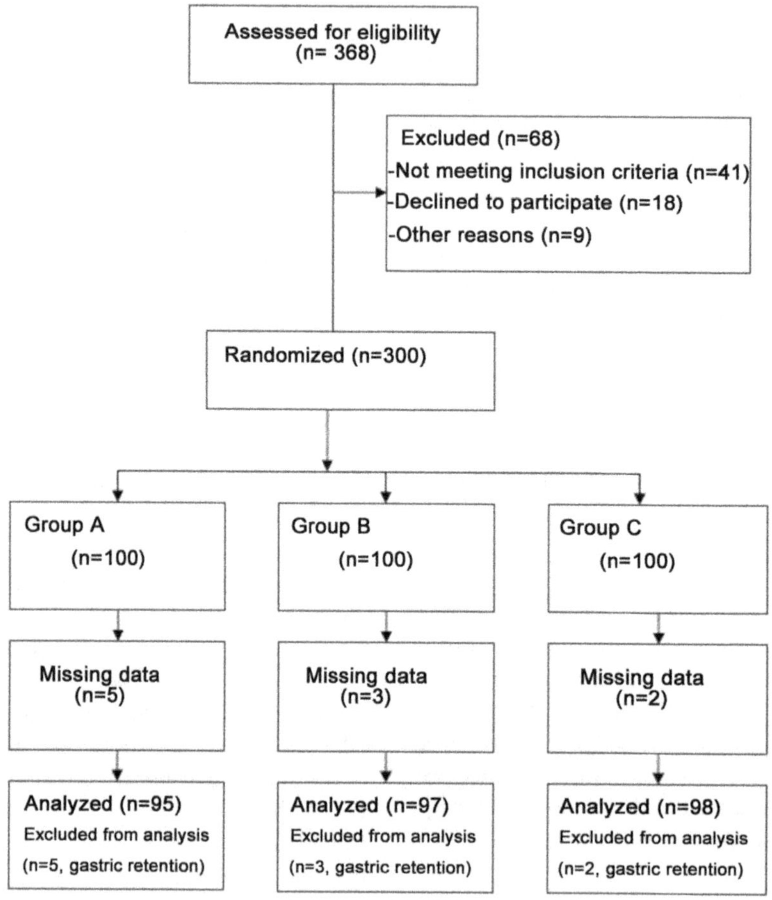

Fig. 1 Patient flowchart

compared with the 500 and 1000 ml/h groups ($P < 0.01$) (Table 4).

Satisfaction

Mean VAS scores were significantly decreased in patients treated with propofol at 500 ml/h in comparison with those receiving the drug at 1000 ml/h ($P < 0.01$) and 2000 ml/h ($P < 0.05$). Average VAS scores for endoscopist's satisfaction were significantly increased in the 1000 and 2000 ml/h groups compared with the 500 ml/h group ($P < 0.01$) (Table 5).

Discussion

This study aimed to assess three infusion rates of propofol for their impact on sedation and adverse effects for outpatient upper gastrointestinal endoscopy. Results showed that the incidences of hypoxemia, hypotension, and deep sedation and the recovery times were significantly increased in patients treated at 2000 ml/h in comparison with the 500 and 1000 ml/h groups. Compared with the 500 ml/h group, motor activity of the extremities, cough, nausea, hiccough, and awareness were significantly decreased and the mean scores on the visual analogue scale for endoscopist's and

Table 1 Characteristics of the patients

Variables	500 ml/h (*n* = 95)	1000 ml/h (*n* = 97)	2000 ml/h (*n* = 98)	*P*-value
Age (years)	50.1 ± 13.1	52 ± 11.3	51 ± 11.3	>0.05
Sex (M/F)	65/30	70/27	63/35	>0.05
Weight (kg)	63.6 ± 11.7	62.5 ± 8.1	61.9 ± 8.8	>0.05
Height (cm)	162.7 ± 7.1	161.9 ± 6.6	161.6 ± 6.7	>0.05
ASA class I/II/III	60/30/5	63/26/8	58/34/6	>0.05
BMI <16 or BMI >30 (kg m^{-2})	2/5	1/2	3/3	>0.05
Endoscopy history	65	72	70	>0.05

Data are expressed as means ± SD or number of patients. *ASA* American Society of Anesthesiologists

Table 2 Time to loss of consciousness, dosage, duration of endoscopy, and recovery time

Variables	500 ml/h	1000 ml/h	2000 ml/h
Time to loss of consciousness	86.4 ± 6.0	54.1 ± 4.8*	32.4 ± 5.2*, **
Total propofol dose (induction dose + additional doses) (mg)	155.1 ± 15.4	150.8 ± 12.1	180.1 ± 19.5*, **
Propofol dose (mg.kg^{-1})	2.4 ± 0.4	2.4 ± 0.3	2.9 ± 0.5*, **
Duration of endoscopy (min)	4.0 ± 0.6	3.4 ± 0.6*	3.5 ± 0.6*
Recovery times (min)	13.2 ± 1.6	13.1 ± 1.6	18.1 ± 2.0*, **

Data are expressed as means ± SD
*$P < 0.01$ vs. 500 ml/h
**$P < 0.01$ vs. 1000 ml/h

patients' satisfaction were significantly increased in the 1000 and 2000 ml/h groups.

Here, BIS was used as a new way to assess deep sedation frequency. To improve the sensitivity and specificity, deep sedation was defined as BIS ≤65 [16–18, 20]. Based on this definition, deep sedation occurred in 18, 16 and 51 % of the patients in the 500, 1000 and 2000 ml/h groups, respectively. Although propofol was administered at rates targeting conscious sedation, deep sedation was often obtained at 2000 ml/h. However, it should be noted that BIS monitoring accuracy for detecting deep sedation is still controversial [17]. Differences in BIS values were observed between the groups at loss of consciousness, endoscope reaching the glottis, endoscope reaching the duodenum and the end of endoscopy. In addition, a greater decrease in BIS was observed after treatment at 2000 ml/h in comparison with the 500 and 1000 ml/h groups. Prior to these time points, BIS values were similar between the three groups. Therefore, it may be assumed that these differences might result from the propofol dose used for induction (2.9 mg kg^{-1}) during procedure initiation. The BIS recordings are reflective of the previous 15 s of brain activity [18], and BIS values exhibit good correlation with consciousness [9]. Deep sedation associated adverse effects were readily alleviated with common clinical procedures. Although brain propofol amounts were not measured here, the delay from infusion completion and complete response suppression in the 2000 ml/h group might corroborate findings in sheep by Ludbrook et al. [21]. Our method eliminated spuriously high BIS scores that arise from patient stimulation during modified observer's assessment of alertness/sedation (MOAA/S) scale evaluation. By frequently stimulating the patient for MOAA/S, the sedation target might require more medication and a higher MOAA/S score than if the MOAA/S score were assessed less frequently. The drug dose and sedation depth were similar when the two methods were used [22]. In the present study, the patients were evaluated, and the drugs were adjusted according to BIS rather than MOAA/S score. BIS is superior to MOAA/S in simplicity, offering more continuous measurements. It therefore objectively evaluate sedation in individuals submitted to endoscopy [16].

Low infusion rates in the 500 ml/h group did not abolish patient reflexes although eyelids remained closed, which probably led to the difference in endoscopy duration since less movements results in an easier procedure. Our findings indicate that increased propofol infusion rate is associated with decreased BIS values, in agreement with previous studies [20, 23]. Insufficient propofol administration results in patient excitement, and additional propofol must be given for endotracheal intubation. Therefore, there is a need for proper anesthetic amounts during endoscopy, prior to the procedure. Slow induction is more likely to cause excitatory side effects. In the present study,

Table 3 Bispectral index value at different time points

Time points	500 ml/h	1000 ml/h	2000 ml/h
Baseline	96.0 ± 1.7	96.5 ± 1.5	96.1 ± 1.8
Loss of consciousness	80.0 ± 3.8	79.1 ± 3.7	75.9 ± 4.0*, **
Endoscope reaching the glottis	75.8 ± 3.9	74.9 ± 3.5	69.0 ± 2.7*, **
Endoscope reaching the duodenum	67.0 ± 2.9	68.0 ± 3.0	62.9 ± 4.5*, **
End of endoscopy	71.2 ± 5.6	72.0 ± 5.4	67.8 ± 3.1*, **
Recovery	87.6 ± 1.5	87.8 ± 1.5	87.5 ± 1.5

Data are expressed as means ± SD
*$P < 0.01$ vs. 500 ml/h
**$P < 0.01$ vs. 1000 ml/h

Table 4 Complications and adverse reactions during endoscopy

Complications and adverse reactions	500 ml/h	1000 ml/h	2000 ml/h
Hypoxemia	10 (10.5)	15 (15.4)	40 (40.8)*, **
Arrhythmia	0 (0.0)	1 (1.0)	3 (3.1)
Systolic hypotension	10 (10.5)	14 (14.4)	30 (30.6)*, **
Diastolic hypotension	16 (16.8)	19 (19.6)	45 (45.9)*, **
Extremity motor activity	33 (34.7)	9 (9.3)*	7 (7.1)*
Cough	16 (16.8)	5 (5.2)*	2 (2.0)*
Nausea	19 (20.0)	7 (7.2)*	4 (4.1)*
Hiccough	15 (15.8)	4 (4.1)*	3 (3.1)*
Awareness	17 (17.9)	2 (2.1)*	1 (1.0)*
Deep sedation	18 (18.9)	16 (16.5)	51 (52.0)*, **

Data are expressed as number (%)
*$P < 0.01$ vs. 500 ml/h
**$P < 0.01$ vs. 1000 ml/h

Table 5 Pain during injection and satisfaction

Variable	500 ml/h	1000 ml/h	2000 ml/h
Pain during injection	7 (7.4)	10 (10.3)	9 (9.2)
Patients' VAS	9.5 ± 0.6	9.8 ± 0.4*	9.7 ± 0.5**
Endoscopist's VAS	8.0 ± 0.8	9.3 ± 0.9*	9.4 ± 0.8*

Data are expressed as means ± SD or number (%)
*$P < 0.01$ vs. 500 ml/h
**$P < 0.05$ vs. 1000 ml/h

deeper anesthesia was achieved with faster injection, as indicated by the loss of the eyelash reflex.

Fanti et al. [24] have reported that the most common complications in gastrointestinal endoscopy were related to the sedation and not to the procedure itself. These complications include cardio-respiratory adverse events such as hypoxemia, hypoventilation, apnea, dysrhythmias, hypotension and vasovagal episodes [24]. As shown above, no differences in heart rates among the three groups were observed.

Hypoxemia incidence rates were 10, 15 and 40 % in the 500 ml/h, 1000 ml/h and 2000 ml/h groups, respectively, making it the most common complication. However, hypoxemia responded to oxygen supplementation. Relatively high transient mild hypoxemia rates in all groups might result from the close patient monitoring during sedation. Such data contribute to fueling the debate on the routine administration of supplemental oxygen during upper gastrointestinal endoscopy. The overall incidence of apnea was 22.4 % as shown above, in agreement with previous studies (20–30 %) [25, 26] assessing younger subjects with apnea defined as a ventilatory pause >40 s.

Mild hypotension is a frequent complication of propofol sedation. The reduction in hypotension frequency in the 500 and 1000 ml/h groups compared with the 2000 ml/h group is consistent with the results of previous studies [7–10, 12–14, 27]. This mild hypotension rarely has adverse clinical consequences and usually requires no intervention. The hypotensive episodes in the present study were transient and did not require pharmacological treatment.

Studies have demonstrated that a slower propofol injection rate decreases cardiovascular effects ([12–14, 28, 29]. However, slow injection rates might result in longer induction times [12–14, 30]. As shown above, increased induction times were observed with lower injection speeds, corroborating previous studies [12–14, 30, 31]. Here, lower infusion rates caused increased induction times, resulting in reduced induction doses of propofol, without differences in the total propofol dose at induction end. Propofol was administered at 2.4 mg/kg in average at 500 and 1000 ml/h, which is in the standard range of 2–2.5 mg/kg [32].

This study has some potential limitations. First, the patients were exclusively Chinese individuals, and some conclusions might not be globally generalized. Second, we did not evaluate the economics or the side effects of the regimens after the patients were discharged. Third, all patients received oxygen before induction, and the controversy about routine oxygen administration [33, 34] could not be addressed by the present study. Fourth, men and women were included, and it is well known that there are gender differences in anesthesia [35]. Fifth, different levels of sedation depth could be associated different rates of adverse effects, which could confound the results. Sixth, only mild/moderate sedation was studied, and the results may not apply to deep sedation. Seventh, no cost-effectiveness analysis was performed, but it may be assumes that optimizing the sedation process should lead to decrease costs. Eighth, some patients had a history of endoscopy, which could influence their experience of subsequent procedures. Finally, we did not follow-up the patients after discharge to monitor eventual longer-term adverse effects.

The present study suggests that a propofol infusion rate of 1000 ml/h appears to be the most appropriate rate for upper gastrointestinal endoscopy anesthesia, resulting in fewer adverse effects and improved satisfaction. Therefore, this rate should be used for upper gastrointestinal endoscopy anesthesia in selected patients corresponding to the inclusion criteria of this study. These results suggests that it is possible to optimize propofol administration in these patients. Nevertheless, further studies are necessary to broaden the generalisability of these results.

Conclusion

In conclusion, a propofol infusion rate of 1000 ml/h appears to be the most appropriate rate for upper gastrointestinal endoscopy anesthesia. This rate resulted in fewer complications and adverse reactions during endoscopy, as well as in improved endoscopist satisfaction.

Abbreviations

IV: intravenous; VAS: visual analogue scale.

Competing interests

The authors declare that they have no competing interests.

Authors' contributions

QZL, QHZ and HMZ contributed to conception and design; QZL, QHZ, WPX and HMZ contributed to acquisition of data, or analysis and interpretation of data; QZL, QHZ and HMZ have been involved in drafting the manuscript or revising it critically for important intellectual content; all authors have given final approval of the version to be published.

Acknowledgements
This work was supported by the Second Affiliated Hospital of Jiaxing College, Jiaxing, China. The authors thank the nurses in the recovery room and the gastroscopy department for their help in observing the study subjects and collecting the data.

Author details
[1]Department of Anesthesia, Shanghai Chest Hospital, Shanghai Jiao Tong University, Shanghai, China. [2]Department of Anesthesia, Second Hospital, Jiaxing Medical College, No. 1518, North Huancheng Road, Jianshe Street, Nanhu District, Jiaxing 314000, Zhejiang, China.

References

1. Lichtenstein DR, Jagannath S, Baron TH, Anderson MA, Banerjee S, Dominitz JA, et al. Standards of Practice Committee of the American Society for Gastrointestinal, Endoscopy. Sedation and anesthesia in GI endoscopy. Gastrointest Endosc. 2008;68:815–26.
2. McQuaid KR, Laine L. A systematic review and meta-analysis of randomized, controlled trials of moderate sedation for routine endoscopic procedures. Gastrointest Endosc. 2008;67:910–23.
3. Cohen LB, Wecsler JS, Gaetano JN, Benson AA, Miller KM, Durkalski V, et al. Endoscopic sedation in the United States: results from a nationwide survey. Am J Gastroenterol. 2006;101:967–74.
4. Dumonceau JM, Riphaus A, Aparicio JR, Beilenhoff U, Knape JT, Ortmann M, et al. European Society of Gastrointestinal Endoscopy, European Society of Gastroenterology and Endoscopy Nurses and Associates, and the European Society of Anaesthesiology Guideline: Non-anaesthesiologist administration of propofol for GI endoscopy. Eur J Anaesthesiol. 2010;27:1016–30.
5. Liu SY, Poon CM, Leung TL, Wong CW, Chan YL, Leung TC, et al. Nurse-administered propofol-alfentanil sedation using a patient-controlled analgesia pump compared with opioid-benzodiazepine sedation for outpatient colonoscopy. Endoscopy. 2009;41:522–8.
6. Coll-Vinent B, Sala X, Fernandez C, Bragulat E, Espinosa G, Miro O, et al. Sedation for cardioversion in the emergency department: analysis of effectiveness in four protocols. Ann Emerg Med. 2003;42:767–72.
7. Kazama T, Ikeda K, Morita K, Ikeda T, Kikura M, Sato S. Relation between initial blood distribution volume and propofol induction dose requirement. Anesthesiology. 2001;94:205–10.
8. Kazama T, Ikeda K, Morita K, Kikura M, Ikeda T, Kurita T, et al. Investigation of effective anesthesia induction doses using a wide range of infusion rates with undiluted and diluted propofol. Anesthesiology. 2000;92:1017–28.
9. Adachi YU, Higuchi H. Prediction of propofol induction dose using multiple regression analysis. Anesthesiology. 2002;96:518–9.
10. Adachi YU, Watanabe K, Higuchi H, Satoh T. The determinants of propofol induction of anesthesia dose. Anesth Analg. 2001;92:656–61.
11. Rolly G, Versichelen L, Zubair NA. Use of ICI 35868 as an anesthetic induction agent. Acta Anaesthesiol Belg. 1980;31:241–7.
12. Blum J, Kochs E, Forster N, Schneider G. The influence of injection rate on the hypnotic effect of propofol during anesthesia: a randomized trial. PLoS Clin Trials. 2006;1:e17.
13. Stokes DN, Hutton P. Rate-dependent induction phenomena with propofol: implications for the relative potency of intravenous anesthetics. Anesth Analg. 1991;72:578–83.
14. Peacock JE, Lewis RP, Reilly CS, Nimmo WS. Effect of different rates of infusion of propofol for induction of anaesthesia in elderly patients. Br J Anaesth. 1990;65:346–52.
15. Santos ME L d, Maluf-Filho F, Chaves DM, Matuguma SE, Ide E, Luz Gde O, et al. Deep sedation during gastrointestinal endoscopy: propofol-fentanyl and midazolam-fentanyl regimens. World J Gastroenterol. 2013;19:3439–46.
16. Moses PL, Vargo JJ, Mitty RD, Pleskow DK, Walker JA, Rex DK. BIS values correlate with clinical sedation scores during midazolam/narcotic or propofol sedation for endoscopy. Gastrointest Endosc. 2004;59:P130.
17. Qadeer MA, Vargo JJ, Patel S, Dumot JA, Lopez AR, Trolli PA, et al. Bispectral index monitoring of conscious sedation with the combination of meperidine and midazolam during endoscopy. Clin Gastroenterol Hepatol. 2008;6:102–8.
18. Johansen JW. Update on bispectral index monitoring. Best Pract Res Clin Anaesthesiol. 2006;20:81–99.
19. Cohen LB, Hightower CD, Wood DA, Miller KM, Aisenberg J. Moderate level sedation during endoscopy: a prospective study using low-dose propofol, meperidine/fentanyl, and midazolam. Gastrointest Endosc. 2004;59:795–803.
20. Gale T, Leslie K, Kluger M. Propofol anaesthesia via target controlled infusion or manually controlled infusion: effects on the bispectral index as a measure of anaesthetic depth. Anaesth Intensive Care. 2001;29:579–84.
21. Ludbrook GL, Upton RN, Grant C, Martinez A. The effect of rate of administration on brain concentrations of propofol in sheep. Anesth Analg. 1998;86:1301–6.
22. Miner JR, Danahy M, Moch A, Biros M. Randomized clinical trial of etomidate versus propofol for procedural sedation in the emergency department. Ann Emerg Med. 2007;49:15–22.
23. Rudner R, Jalowiecki P, Kawecki P, Gonciarz M, Mularczyk A, Petelenz M. Conscious analgesia/sedation with remifentanil and propofol versus total intravenous anesthesia with fentanyl, midazolam, and propofol for outpatient colonoscopy. Gastrointest Endosc. 2003;57:657–63.
24. Fanti L, Testoni PA. Sedation and analgesia in gastrointestinal endoscopy: what's new? World J Gastroenterol. 2010;16:2451–7.
25. Sanderson JH, Blades JF. Multicentre study of propofol in day case surgery. Anaesthesia. 1988;43(Suppl):70–3.
26. Redfem N, Srafford MA, Brooker J, Hull CJ. Incremental propofol for minor gynaecological procedures. Postgrad Med J. 1985;61:127–8.
27. Claeys MA, Gepts E, Camu F. Haemodynamic changes during anaesthesia induced and maintained with propofol. Br J Anaesth. 1988;60:3–9.
28. Kanto J, Gepts E. Pharmacokinetic implications for the clinical use of propofol. Clin Pharmacokinet. 1989;17:308–26.
29. Wagner BK, Berman SL, Devitt PA, O'Hara DA. Retrospective analysis of postoperative nausea and vomiting to determine antiemetic activity of droperidol added to propofol: a possible drug interaction. Pharmacotherapy. 1994;14:586–91.
30. Rolly G, Versichelen L, Huyghe L, Mungroop H. Effect of speed of injection on induction of anaesthesia using propofol. Br J Anaesth. 1985;57:743–6.
31. Gillies GW, Lees NW. The effects of speed of injection on induction with propofol. A comparison with etomidate. Anaesthesia. 1989;44:386–8.
32. Cummings GC, Dixon J, Kay NH, Windsor JP, Major E, Morgan M, et al. Dose requirements of ICI 35,868 (propofol, 'Diprivan') in a new formulation for induction of anaesthesia. Anaesthesia. 1984;39:1168–71.
33. Zed PJ, Abu-Laban RB, Chan WW, Harrison DW. Efficacy, safety and patient satisfaction of propofol for procedural sedation and analgesia in the emergency department: a prospective study. CJEM. 2007;9:421–7.
34. Tohda G, Higashi S, Wakahara S, Morikawa M, Sakumoto H, Kane T. Propofol sedation during endoscopic procedures: safe and effective administration by registered nurses supervised by endoscopists. Endoscopy. 2006;38:360–7.
35. Pleym H, Spigset O, Kharasch ED, Dale O. Gender differences in drug effects: implications for anesthesiologists. Acta Anaesthesiol Scand. 2003;47:241–59.

12

Association between polymorphisms of *TAS2R16* and susceptibility to colorectal cancer

Jonathan Barontini[1], Marco Antinucci[1], Sergio Tofanelli[1], Maurizio Cammalleri[1], Massimo Dal Monte[1], Federica Gemignani[1], Pavel Vodicka[2,3,4], Roberto Marangoni[1], Ludmila Vodickova[2,3,4], Juozas Kupcinskas[5], Veronika Vymetalkova[2,3], Asta Forsti[6], Federico Canzian[7], Angelika Stein[7], Victor Moreno[8], Nicola Mastrodonato[9], Francesca Tavano[9], Anna Panza[9], Roberto Barale[1], Stefano Landi[1*] and Daniele Campa[1]

Abstract

Background: Genetics plays an important role in the susceptibility to sporadic colorectal cancer (CRC). In the last 10 years genome-wide association studies (GWAS) have identified over 40 independent low penetrance polymorphic variants. However, these loci only explain around 1-4% of CRC heritability, highlighting the dire need of identifying novel risk loci. In this study, we focused our attention on the genetic variability of the *TAS2R16* gene, encoding for one of the bitter taste receptors that selectively binds to salicin, a natural antipyretic that resembles aspirin. Given the importance of inflammation in CRC, we tested whether polymorphic variants in this gene could affect the risk of developing this neoplasia hypothesizing a role of *TAS2R16* in modulating chronic inflammation within the gut.

Methods: We performed an association study using 6 tagging SNPs, (rs860170, rs978739, rs1357949, rs1525489, rs6466849, rs10268496) that cover all *TAS2R16* genetic variability. The study was carried out on 1902 CRC cases and 1532 control individuals from four European countries.

Results: We did not find any statistically significant association between risk of developing CRC and selected SNPs. However, after stratification by histology (colon vs. rectum) we found that rs1525489 was associated with increased risk of rectal cancer with a (P_{trend} of = 0.0071).

Conclusions: Our data suggest that polymorphisms within *TAS2R16* gene do not have a strong influence on colon cancer susceptibility, but a possible role in rectal cancer should be further evaluated in larger cohorts.

Keywords: Taste receptors, *TAS2R16*, Polymorphisms, Colon cancer, Rectal cancer, Colorectal cancer, Cancer risk, Genetic association study

Background

Colorectal cancer (CRC) is the third most commonly diagnosed cancer worldwide [1]. Several environmental/life style risk factors have been identified for CRC, such as obesity, sedentary behavior, high red meat consumption, high intake of hyper caloric foods, diets rich in fat and poor in fiber, tobacco smoking, alcohol consumption and diabetes [2]. In addition gut inflammation, due to chronic conditions such as ulcerative colitis and Crohn's disease, is an established risk factor [2]. Also genetics is hypothesized to play an important role for the sporadic form. In the last 10 years genome-wide association studies (GWAS) have identified over 40 independent low penetrance polymorphic variants [3]. Besides GWAS, an overwhelming number of hypothesis-driven studies carried out on specific candidate genes highlighted variants belonging to multiple pathways to be connected to CRC risk. The majority of the studies focused on SNPs within DNA repair genes [4], xenobiotic metabolism and transport genes [5–14], inflammatory response genes [15–17], hormone metabolisms [18, 19] and more recently miRNAs [20, 21]. Our group and others have also analyzed the possible involvement of taste receptor genes in CRC risk [22–24]. In the human genome, there

* Correspondence: stefano.landi@unipi.it
[1]Department of Biology, University of Pisa, Via Derna 1, 56100 Pisa, Italy
Full list of author information is available at the end of the article

are 25 functional genes and 11 pseudogenes belonging to the *TAS2Rs* gene family. It has already been ascertained that polymorphic variants in these genes are responsible for the variability observed in several human phenotypes and life habits such as alcohol consumption [25, 26], and nicotine dependence [27]. However, taste receptors seem to have also less obvious functions. In fact taste receptors certainly do not only have a role in taste perception, as documented by their ectopic expression in a variety of extra-oral tissues including gut [28–31]. In this study we focused our attention on the genetic variability of the *TAS2R16* gene whose encoded receptor selectively binds to salicin [32], a natural anti-inflammatory and analgesic agent extracted from willow bark and resembling aspirin [33]. Given the similarities between salicin and aspirin it is reasonable to postulate that variants within the *TAS2R16* gene could affect the receptor activity following its binding with ligands such as salicin or aspirin. In particular, aspirin intake is an established factor reducing the risk to develop CRC. In fact, there are evidences from case-control and cohort studies indicating benefit from long term use of aspirin at low dose in colorectal cancer chemoprevention [34]. This effect could be elicited through an anti-inflammatory activity or to the binding to specific receptors in the gut. Furthermore, there are indications that regular use of aspirin is associated with improved survival for patients with colorectal cancer [35]. The hypothesis is corroborated by a previous study (Campbell and colleagues) conducted on two different African populations, describing that the polymorphic variant rs846664 within TAS2R16 confers different sensitivities to salicin [36]. Unfortunately, this finding could not be replicated among Caucasians since this SNP is monomorphic in this population. However, according to this base of knowledge, it could be hypothesized that *TAS2R16* could modulate chronic inflammation in the gut. Alternatively, the receptor, upon binding with its natural ligands, could affect the individual risk of cancer with mechanisms similar to those observed following a long term aspirin intake. Thus, in the present work we tested whether polymorphic variants within *TAS2R16* could affect the risk of developing CRC. The study was carried out in a large cohort of European individuals.

Methods

Study population

A total of 2252 CRC case subjects and 1630 controls were collected in four European countries (Czech Republic, Italy, Lithuania and Spain). CRC patients had histological verification of colorectal adenocarcinoma. Controls were collected in the same hospitals and in the same time frame as the cases among hospitalized individuals without neoplastic diseases. A more detailed description of the sampling and collection methods has been provided elsewhere [9, 37–39]. For the cases we collected information about gender, age at diagnosis, tumor localization (colon or rectum), while for the controls we have information on gender and age at sampling.

SNPs selection

We used tagging SNPs to cover all the common genetic variability of *TAS2R16*. We selected the gene region and added 4 k base pairs on the 5 prime and 3 prime directions. According to HapMap 3 database, within the selected region there are 24 known common SNPs with a MAF > 0.05 among Caucasians. Using the software Haploview [40] we selected six tagging SNPs by setting the LD threshold at $r^2 \geq 0.8$. The final selection of the SNPs resulted in rs860170, rs978739, rs1357949, rs1525489, rs6466849, and rs10268496 covering 87% of the common genetic variability.

Sample preparation and genotyping

DNA was extracted from whole blood. Samples were kept frozen until used. Genotyping was performed on 384 well plates using the KASP (LGC, Teddington, UK) and TaqMan (Thermo Fisher, Waltham, MA USA) genotyping chemistry. In each plate there was DNA from cases and controls in order to avoid bias due to genotyping. We included a mean of 15 duplicated samples for plate to be used as quality controls. After the PCR the plates were "read" via the spectrophotometer Fluostar Omega (Ω) (BMG.LABTECH®) and genotyping calls were done using the KlusterCaller software (LGC Group Teddington, UK).

Statistical analysis

The observed genotype frequencies of all SNPs were tested for deviation from Hardy–Weinberg equilibrium (HWE) in controls. The association between the genotypes of all polymorphisms and CRC risk was estimated using an unconditional logistic regression computing odds ratios (OR), 95% confidence intervals (95% CIs) and *P*-values. The common allele among the controls was assigned as the reference category and the co-dominant inheritance model was assessed. All analyses were adjusted for age (at diagnosis for cases and at sampling for controls), gender and country origin. We also performed stratified analyses for country of origin and tumor site. The significance level in each test was adjusted according to the Bonferroni's correction, namely adjusted $P = \alpha/$ number of individual tests ($0.05/6 = 0.008$).

Bioinformatic tools

We carried out bioinformatic analyses to assess the possible functional effect of the studied polymorphisms, for example to detect if the nucleotide sequences of the polymorphisms are targets of transcription factors or if they are situated in DNase sensitivity region. Specifically we have used RegulomeDB V1.1 [41] and Haploreg V4.1 [42]; to test whether the polymorphisms could have a known regulatory impact. Additionally, we used the data available in the GTEx project V6 to identify expression of quantitative trait loci (eQTLs) [43].

Results

Data filtering and quality control

We examined 6 SNPs belonging to the *TAS2R16* gene to assess their possible role in the risk of developing CRC. We have genotyped up to 3882 individuals (2252 CRC cases and 1630 controls) enrolled in the Czech Republic, Lithuania, Italy and Spain. The distributions of the genotype frequencies for all the variants included in the study were in accordance with HWE. Four hundred forty-eight (448) subjects (346 CRC cases 102 controls) for which we did not have covariates data or that did not pass quality control (call rate < 75%) were removed from subsequent analyses, leaving a total of 3434 subjects (1902 CRC cases and 1532 controls) for statistical analysis. All the relevant characteristics of the population used in the analyses are shown in Table 1. The average SNP call rate was 96.24% with a minimum of 98.16% (rs1525489) and a maximum of 99.66% (rs10268496). The analysis of the samples duplicated for quality control showed a concordance greater than 99%. All the frequencies, call rate and HWE values of each polymorphism are reported in Additional file 1: Table S1.

Effect of SNPs on colorectal cancer risk

Overall, we did not observe any statistically significant association between selected SNPs and risk of CRC. The polymorphism with the lowest *p*-value was rs1525489 showing a p-trend of $P = 0.084$. Following the stratification by tumor site (colon / rectum) we found that rs1525489 showed a marginal/borderline significance with increased risk of rectal cancer at nominal level of ($P_{trend} = 0.0071$), while the associations between the SNPs and colon cancer were similar to those considering the two strata together (Table 2). However, performing a case-case analysis (colon vs. rectum) we did not observe any heterogeneity. When stratifying for country of origin we obtained one marginally significant value. In the Lithuanian case control study subjects the minor (C) allele of rs1525489 was associated with an increased risk of developing CRC with a nominal $P_{trend} = 0.047$. We observed the same trend also in the Spanish sub-population ($P = 0.051$). The stratified analyses are reported in Additional file 2: Table S2, Additional file 3: Table S3, Additional file 4: Table S4, and Additional file 5: Table S5.

Bioinformatic analysis

We used three bioinformatic tools to identify possible functional properties of rs1525489, the SNP showing the best results from a statistical point of view. RegulomeDB showed a score of six (which means minimal binding evidence). Using HaploReg we did not observe any potentially relevant data. GTEx database did not show any statistically significant eQTLs between the SNP and nearby genes in any of the tissues present in the database.

Discussion

To further expand our knowledge on CRC genetic susceptibility we investigated whether polymorphic variants within *TAS2R16* could have a role in the etiology of the disease. Our hypothesis finds its rationale on several epidemiologic evidences that polymorphic variants within taste receptor genes could be associated with risk of cancer development. For instance *TAS2R38* SNPs were found to be associated with risk of developing CRC in two different populations of Caucasian origin [23], while SNPs within *TAS2R38* and *TAS1Rs* were associated with increased risk of gastric cancer [44, 45]. In this study we examined the genetic variability of *TAS2R16* gene because the receptor binds different compounds including salicin, a natural anti-inflammatory substance which is very similar to aspirin [32, 33]. One of the strongest risk factors for CRC is represented by chronic inflammation especially arisen from diseases that trigger a continuous inflammatory responses such as ulcerative colitis and Crohn's disease [2]. Aspirin treatment reduces the risk of CRC [2] and therefore genetic variants that modulate the efficiency or the expression of the receptor may play a role in CRC development. Since polymorphisms in taste genes are generally functional as reflected in their effect in a multitude of phenotypes, it is reasonable to hypothesize a possible link between *TAS2R16* allelic

Table 1 Population in study

Country of origin	Colorectal Cancer Cases				Controls			
	Males	Females	Total	Mean Age	Males	Females	Total	Mean Age
Czech Republic	588	400	988	61.92	393	296	689	54.87
Lithuania	102	76	178	67.04	91	92	183	57.29
Italy	179	142	321	65.97	252	94	346	51.94
Spain	248	167	415	66.35	166	148	314	65.34
Total	**1117**	**785**	**1902**	**64.09**	**902**	**630**	**1532**	**56.69**

Table 2 Association between colorectal cancer risk and SNPs in the *TAS2R16* region stratified by histology

SNP	Alleles (Major/ minor)	Site	Case/Control[a]			MM vs Mm[b]	*P value*	MM vs mm[b]	*P value*	MM vs Mm +mm[b]	*P value*	MM + Mm vs mm[b]	P value	P trend
			MM	Mm	mm									
rs860170	A/G	All	785/653	846/ 681	245/ 184	1.04(0.9–1.22)	0.57	1.05(0.83–1.32)	0.69	1.05(0.9–1.21)	0.55	1.03(0.83–1.27)	0.82	0.37
		Colon	447/653	487/ 681	141/ 184	1.03(0.87–1.23)	0.73	1.07(0.82–1.4)	0.52	1.04(0.88–1.23)	0.64	1.06(0.82–1.35)	0.67	0.37
		Rectum	231/653	256/ 681	68/ 184	1.06(0.85–1.32)	0.61	1.02(0.74–1.43)	0.89	1.05(0.85–1.29)	0.64	0.99(0.73–1.36)	0.97	0.65
rs978739	A/G	All	830/693	777/ 678	182/ 156	0.97(0.83–1.13)	0.67	0.98(0.77–1.26)	0.89	0.97(0.84–1.12)	0.68	1(0.79–1.27)	0.99	0.65
		Colon	487/693	422/ 678	97/ 156	0.9(0.75–1.07)	0.22	0.88(0.65–1.17)	0.37	0.89(0.75–1.05)	0.18	0.92(0.7–1.22)	0.58	0.18
		Rectum	240/693	222/ 678	71/ 156	0.97(0.78–1.22)	0.82	1.36(0.97–1.9)	0.08	1.04(0.85–1.29)	0.68	1.37(1–1.89)	0.05	0.30
rs1357949	T/C	All	927/719	761/ 659	180/ 145	0.91(0.78–1.05)	0.20	0.95(0.74–1.23)	0.71	0.91(0.79–1.06)	0.22	1(0.78–1.27)	0.99	0.31
		Colon	512/719	443/ 659	110/ 145	0.97(0.81–1.15)	0.72	1.09(0.82–1.46)	0.54	0.99(0.84–1.17)	0.92	1.11(0.84–1.46)	0.46	0.98
		Rectum	292/719	211/ 659	50/ 145	0.78(0.63–0.97)	0.03	0.82(0.57–1.19)	0.30	0.79(0.64–0.97)	0.02	0.92(0.65–1.32)	0.66	0.06
rs1525489	T/C	All	1728/ 956	145/ 62	1/0	1.24(0.88–1.73)	0.22	-	-	1.22(0.88–1.70)	0.23	-	-	0.08
		Colon	992/956	77/62	0/0	1.22(0.83–1.8)	0.30	-	-	1.22(0.83–1.8)	0.30	-	-	0.31
		Rectum	505/956	53/62	1/0	1.59(1.03–2.43)	0.03	-	-	1.62(1.06–2.47)	0.03	-	-	**0.007**
rs6466849	G/A	All	1276/ 1024	524/ 452	62/52	0.97(0.83–1.14)	0.75	1.01(0.68–1.51)	0.95	0.98(0.84–1.14)	0.78	1.02(0.69–1.51)	0.92	0.40
		Colon	748/ 1024	284/ 452	36/52	0.88(0.73–1.05)	0.16	0.97(0.61–1.53)	0.88	0.88(0.74–1.06)	0.18	1(0.64–1.58)	0.99	0.16
		Rectum	376/ 1024	156/ 452	22/52	1(0.8–1.26)	0.97	1.25(0.73–2.15)	0.42	1.03(0.83–1.28)	0.79	1.25(0.73–2.13)	0.42	0.92
rs10268496	T/G	All	1200/ 951	596/ 510	100/ 70	0.92(0.79–1.07)	0.28	1.07(0.77–1.49)	0.70	0.94(0.81–1.08)	0.38	1.1(0.79–1.53)	0.57	0.81
		Colon	678/951	342/ 510	62/70	0.94(0.79–1.12)	0.49	1.18(0.81–1.71)	0.39	0.97(0.82–1.15)	0.72	1.2(0.83–1.74)	0.33	0.79
		Rectum	364/951	175/ 510	25/70	0.88(0.7–1.09)	0.24	0.86(0.53–1.41)	0.55	0.87(0.71–1.08)	0.21	0.9(0.55–1.46)	0.67	0.37

[a]Numbers may not add up 100% to genotyping failure, covariate missing values or DNA depletion

[b]MM vs Mm = Common homozygous carriers vs heterozygous; MM vs mm = Common homozygous vs rare homozygous; MM vs Mm + mm = Common homozygous vs heterozygous + rare homozygous (Dominant Model); MM + Mm vs mm = Common homozygous + heterozygous vs rare homozygous. Odds Ratio (95% confidence interval).All analysis are adjusted for age, gender and country of origin

variants and CRC risk. To perform our analysis 6 SNPs tagging the common variants present in the region of the gene under examination were chosen. The selection was mainly based on linkage disequilibrium scores between all the variants of the region. Our results seem to suggest no association between the selected polymorphism and risk of developing CRC. The signal closest to the significance threshold of $P < 0.05$ was observed for rs1525489. For this SNP stratifying the analysis for country of origin we found in the Lithuanian and in the Spanish sub-populations a tendency for individuals with at least 1 C allele of the rs1525489 polymorphism to have and increased risk of developing CRC (P 0.047 and $P = 0.051$, respectively). However, these associations were not statistically significant following Bonferroni's correction. A possible explanation for this association is that this SNP interact with a lifestyle factor or a dietary habit a factor that we do not account for in the analysis. However, this difference maybe just due to statistical fluctuations. Schembre and colleagues have performed a study investigating two *TAS2R16* polymorphic variants (rs846672 and rs846664) in relation to the risk of developing colorectal adenoma [24]. Even though the study is rather small (914 cases of three different ethnic groups) their results are concordant with ours, suggesting an overall no effect of the two variants in the disease. The rs846664 SNP is monomorphic in Caucasian and therefore was not typed in our study while rs846672 is in complete LD with rs860170 that was used in the present study (r^2 = 1 in European Hapmap Ceu). When analyzing separately colon and rectum, we observed an association between the minor allele of the rs1525489 and an increased risk of developing specifically rectal cancer. This association was showed to have a marginal/borderline statistically significance also after Bonferroni's correction (P = 0.0071). However, this finding must be taken with caution since it is the result of a stratified analysis, on a limited sample size, and it is also difficult to explain from a biological point of view. In fact, the bioinformatics tools did not reveal any possible functional effect for this SNP nor for the variants in LD with it. We acknowledge that the present study has several limitations. We could not collect information on aspirin use and therefore we could not analyze any possible interaction with the SNP analyzed. Moreover, cases and controls are not individually matched for age and gender, however we have adjusted all the analyses for these two variables to minimize their possible effect. We had a power greater than 80% (considering an alpha of 0.05/6 = 0.008) to find an association with an OR of 1.25 or higher for all the SNPs in analysis with the exception of rs1525489 that had a low MAF and for which we had the power to find OR greater than 1.53. An OR of 1.25 is compatible with the ORs found by GWAS in CRC [3]. Using a tagging approach, we have covered most of the common variability of the gene region excluding the possibility of having missed an association with a common but un-typed variant.

Conclusions

Thus, although we have to be very cautious with the results, our data suggest that polymorphisms of the *TAS2R16* gene do not have a strong influence on colon cancer susceptibility, but that the study should be replicated in large cohorts to better evaluate the effect of rs1525489 on the risk of rectal cancer.

Additional files

Additional file 1: Table S1. Description of data stratified analysis frequencies, call rate and Hardy-Weinberg equilibrium values of each polymorphism.

Additional file 2: Table S2. Description of data Association between colon/rectal cancer risk and SNPs in the *TAS2R16* region considering only the Czech Republic.

Additional file 3: Table S3. Description of data Association between colon/rectalcancer risk and SNPs in the *TAS2R16* region considering only Lithuania.

Additional file 4: Table S4. Description of data Association between colon/rectalcancer risk and SNPs in the *TAS2R16* region considering only Italy.

Additional file 5: Table S5. Description of data Association between colon/rectal cancer risk and SNPs in the *TAS2R16* region considering only Spain.

Abbreviations

CI: Confidence interval; CRC: Colorectal cancer; eQTL: Expression quantitative trait loci; GWAS: Genome-wide association studies; HWE: Hardy-Weinberg equilibrium; LD: Linkage disequilibrium; MAF: Minor allele frequency; OR: Odds ratio; SNP: Single nucleotide polymorphism

Acknowledgements

Not applicable.

Funding

This work was supported by the University of Pisa PRA 2016 Grant. VM was supported by Instituto de Salud Carlos III, co-funded by FEDER funds –a way to build Europe– PI1400616 and Catalan Government DURSI grant 2014SGR647. PV was supported by Grant AZV MZCR: 15–27,580 by the Czech Ministry of Health.

Authors' contributions

JB performed the genotyping the statistical analyses and drafted the manuscript; MA performed in silico analyses; ST, MC, MDM, FG, RM, RB, SL, DC planned the study; PV, LV, JK, VV, AF, FC, AS, VM, NM, FT, AP, collected the samples and worked in the collection of the clinical and epidemiologic data. All authors read and approved the final manuscript.

Competing interests

The authors declare that they have no competing interests.

Author details

[1]Department of Biology, University of Pisa, Via Derna 1, 56100 Pisa, Italy. [2]Department of Molecular Biology of Cancer, Institute of Experimental Medicine, Academy of Science of Czech Republic, Prague, Czech Republic. [3]Institute of Biology and Medical Genetics, 1st Medical Faculty, Charles University, Prague, Czech Republic. [4]Biomedical Centre, Medical School Pilsen, Charles University in Prague, Pilsen, Czech Republic. [5]Department of Gastroenterology, Lithuanian University of Health Sciences, Kaunas, Lithuania. [6]Genomic Epidemiology Group, German Cancer Research Center (DKFZ), Heidelberg, Germany. [7]Division of Molecular Genetic Epidemiology, German Cancer Research Center (DKFZ), Heidelberg, Germany. [8]Cancer Prevention and Control Program, Catalan Institute of Oncology (ICO), IDIBELL, CIBERESP and Department of Clinical Sciences, Faculty of Medicine, University of Barcelona, Barcelona, Spain. [9]Division of Gastroenterology and Research Laboratory, IRCCS Scientific Institute and Regional General Hospital "Casa Sollievo della Sofferenza", San Giovanni Rotondo, Italy.

References

1. Ervik FLM, Ferlay J, Mery L, Soerjomataram I, Bray F. Cancer Today. Lyon: International Agency for Research on Cancer; 2016. Available from: http://gco.iarc.fr/today. Accessed 20 Mar 2017.
2. Marley AR, Nan H. Epidemiology of colorectal cancer. Int J Mol Epidemiol Genet. 2016;7(3):105–14.
3. Peters U, Bien S, Zubair N. Genetic architecture of colorectal cancer. Gut. 2015;64(10):1623–36.
4. Vymetalkova V, Pardini B, Rosa F, Di Gaetano C, Novotny J, Levy M, Buchler T, Slyskova J, Vodickova L, Naccarati A, et al. Variations in mismatch repair genes and colorectal cancer risk and clinical outcome. Mutagenesis. 2014;29(4):259–65.

5. Andersen V, Egeberg R, Tjonneland A, Vogel U. ABCC2 transporter gene polymorphisms, diet and risk of colorectal cancer: a Danish prospective cohort study. Scand J Gastroenterol. 2012;47(5):572–4.
6. Andersen V, Vogel U. Interactions between meat intake and genetic variation in relation to colorectal cancer. Genes Nutr. 2015;10(1):448.
7. Campa D, Pardini B, Naccarati A, Vodickova L, Novotny J, Forsti A, Hemminki K, Barale R, Vodicka P, Canzian F. A gene-wide investigation on polymorphisms in the ABCG2/BRCP transporter and susceptibility to colorectal cancer. Mutat Res. 2008;645(1–2):56–60.
8. Campa D, Pardini B, Naccarati A, Vodickova L, Novotny J, Steinke V, Rahner N, Holinski-Feder E, Morak M, Schackert HK, et al. Polymorphisms of genes coding for ghrelin and its receptor in relation to colorectal cancer risk: a two-step gene-wide case-control study. BMC Gastroenterol. 2010;10:112.
9. Campa D, Sainz J, Pardini B, Vodickova L, Naccarati A, Rudolph A, Novotny J, Forsti A, Buch S, von Schonfels W, et al. A comprehensive investigation on common polymorphisms in the MDR1/ABCB1 transporter gene and susceptibility to colorectal cancer. PLoS One. 2012;7(3):e32784.
10. Campa D, Vodicka P, Pardini B, Novotny J, Forsti A, Hemminki K, Barale R, Canzian F. Could polymorphisms in ATP-binding cassette C3/multidrug resistance associated protein 3 (ABCC3/MRP3) modify colorectal cancer risk? Eur J Cancer. 2008;44(6):854–7.
11. Dik VK, Bueno-de-Mesquita HB, Van Oijen MG, Siersema PD, Uiterwaal CS, Van Gils CH, Van Duijnhoven FJ, Cauchi S, Yengo L, Froguel P, et al. Coffee and tea consumption, genotype-based CYP1A2 and NAT2 activity and colorectal cancer risk-results from the EPIC cohort study. Int J Cancer. 2014; 135(2):401–12.
12. Ferrari P, McKay JD, Jenab M, Brennan P, Canzian F, Vogel U, Tjonneland A, Overvad K, Tolstrup JS, Boutron-Ruault MC, et al. Alcohol dehydrogenase and aldehyde dehydrogenase gene polymorphisms, alcohol intake and the risk of colorectal cancer in the European prospective investigation into cancer and nutrition study. Eur J Clin Nutr. 2012;66(12):1303–8.
13. Kopp TI, Andersen V, Tjonneland A, Vogel U. Polymorphisms in ATP-binding cassette transporter genes and interaction with diet and life style factors in relation to colorectal cancer in a Danish prospective case-cohort study. Scand J Gastroenterol. 2015;50(12):1469–81.
14. Liao LH, Zhang H, Lai MP, Lau KW, Lai AK, Zhang JH, Wang Q, Wei W, Chai JH, Lung ML, et al. The association of CYP2C9 gene polymorphisms with colorectal carcinoma in Han Chinese. Clin Chim Acta. 2007;380(1–2):191–6.
15. Landi S, Bottari F, Gemignani F, Gioia-Patricola L, Guino E, Osorio A, de Oca J, Capella G, Canzian F, Moreno V. Interleukin-4 and interleukin-4 receptor polymorphisms and colorectal cancer risk. Eur J Cancer. 2007;43(4):762–8.
16. Landi S, Gemignani F, Bottari F, Gioia-Patricola L, Guino E, Cambray M, Biondo S, Capella G, Boldrini L, Canzian F, et al. Polymorphisms within inflammatory genes and colorectal cancer. J Nega Results Biomed. 2006;5:15.
17. Vogel LK, Saebo M, Hoyer H, Kopp TI, Vogel U, Godiksen S, Frenzel FB, Hamfjord J, Bowitz-Lothe IM, Johnson E, et al. Intestinal PTGS2 mRNA levels, PTGS2 gene polymorphisms, and colorectal carcinogenesis. PLoS One. 2014; 9(8):e105254.
18. Rudolph A, Sainz J, Hein R, Hoffmeister M, Frank B, Forsti A, Brenner H, Hemminki K, Chang-Claude J. Modification of menopausal hormone therapy-associated colorectal cancer risk by polymorphisms in sex steroid signaling, metabolism and transport related genes. Endocr Relat Cancer. 2011;18(3):371–84.
19. Sainz J, Rudolph A, Hoffmeister M, Frank B, Brenner H, Chang-Claude J, Hemminki K, Forsti A. Effect of type 2 diabetes predisposing genetic variants on colorectal cancer risk. J Clin Endocrinol Metab. 2012;97(5):E845–51.
20. Landi D, Gemignani F, Landi S. Role of variations within microRNA-binding sites in cancer. Mutagenesis. 2012;27(2):205–10.
21. Landi D, Gemignani F, Pardini B, Naccarati A, Garritano S, Vodicka P, Vodickova L, Canzian F, Novotny J, Barale R, et al. Identification of candidate genes carrying polymorphisms associated with the risk of colorectal cancer by analyzing the colorectal mutome and microRNAome. Cancer. 2012; 118(19):4670–80.
22. Campa D, Vodicka P, Pardini B, Naccarati A, Carrai M, Vodickova L, Novotny J, Hemminki K, Forsti A, Barale R, et al. A gene-wide investigation on polymorphisms in the taste receptor 2R14 (TAS2R14) and susceptibility to colorectal cancer. BMC Med Genet. 2010;11:88.
23. Carrai M, Steinke V, Vodicka P, Pardini B, Rahner N, Holinski-Feder E, Morak M, Schackert HK, Gorgens H, Stemmler S, et al. Association between TAS2R38 gene polymorphisms and colorectal cancer risk: a case-control study in two independent populations of Caucasian origin. PLoS One. 2011;6(6):e20464.
24. Schembre SM, Cheng I, Wilkens LR, Albright CL, Marchand le L. Variations in bitter-taste receptor genes, dietary intake, and colorectal adenoma risk. Nutr Cancer. 2013;65(7):982–90.
25. Hinrichs AL, Wang JC, Bufe B, Kwon JM, Budde J, Allen R, Bertelsen S, Evans W, Dick D, Rice J, et al. Functional variant in a bitter-taste receptor (hTAS2R16) influences risk of alcohol dependence. Am J Hum Genet. 2006; 78(1):103–11.
26. Wang JC, Hinrichs AL, Bertelsen S, Stock H, Budde JP, Dick DM, Bucholz KK, Rice J, Saccone N, Edenberg HJ, et al. Functional variants in TAS2R38 and TAS2R16 influence alcohol consumption in high-risk families of African-American origin. Alcohol Clin Exp Res. 2007;31(2):209–15.
27. Mangold JE, Payne TJ, Ma JZ, Chen G, Li MD. Bitter taste receptor gene polymorphisms are an important factor in the development of nicotine dependence in African Americans. J Med Genet. 2008;45(9):578–82.
28. Behrens M, Meyerhof W. Oral and extraoral bitter taste receptors. Results Probl Cell Differ. 2010;52:87–99.
29. Clark AA, Liggett SB, Munger SD. Extraoral bitter taste receptors as mediators of off-target drug effects. FASEB J. 2012;26(12):4827–31.
30. Rozengurt E, Sternini C. Taste receptor signaling in the mammalian gut. Curr Opin Pharmacol. 2007;7(6):557–62.
31. Sternini C. Taste receptors in the gastrointestinal tract. IV. Functional implications of bitter taste receptors in gastrointestinal chemosensing. Am J Physiol Gastrointest Liver Physiol. 2007;292(2):G457–61.
32. Bufe B, Hofmann T, Krautwurst D, Raguse JD, Meyerhof W. The human TAS2R16 receptor mediates bitter taste in response to beta-glucopyranosides. Nat Genet. 2002;32(3):397–401.
33. Vane JR. The fight against rheumatism: from willow bark to COX-1 sparing drugs. J Physiol Pharmacol. 2000;51(4 Pt 1):573–86.
34. Singh Ranger G. The role of aspirin in colorectal cancer chemoprevention. Crit Rev Oncol Hematol. 2016;104:87–90.
35. Hua X, Phipps AI, Burnett-Hartman AN, Adams SV, Hardikar S, Cohen SA, Kocarnik JM, Ahnen DJ, Lindor NM, Baron JA, et al. Timing of aspirin and other nonsteroidal anti-inflammatory drug use among patients with colorectal cancer in relation to tumor markers and survival. J Clin Oncol. 2017. JCO.2017.2072.3569.
36. Campbell MC, Ranciaro A, Zinshteyn D, Rawlings-Goss R, Hirbo J, Thompson S, Woldemeskel D, Froment A, Rucker JB, Omar SA, et al. Origin and differential selection of allelic variation at TAS2R16 associated with salicin bitter taste sensitivity in Africa. Mol Biol Evol. 2014;31(2):288–302.
37. Kupcinskas J, Bruzaite I, Juzenas S, Gyvyte U, Jonaitis L, Kiudelis G, Skieceviciene J, Leja M, Pauzas H, Tamelis A, et al. Lack of association between miR-27a, miR-146a, miR-196a-2, miR-492 and miR-608 gene polymorphisms and colorectal cancer. Sci Rep. 2014;4:5993.
38. Kupcinskas J, Gyvyte U, Bruzaite I, Leja M, Kupcinskaite-Noreikiene R, Pauzas H, Tamelis A, Jonaitis L, Skieceviciene J, Kiudelis G. Common genetic variants of PSCA, MUC1 and PLCE1 genes are not associated with colorectal cancer. Asian Pac J Cancer Prev. 2015;16(14):6027–32.
39. Moreno V, Gemignani F, Landi S, Gioia-Patricola L, Chabrier A, Blanco I, Gonzalez S, Guino E, Capella G, Canzian F. Polymorphisms in genes of nucleotide and base excision repair: risk and prognosis of colorectal cancer. Clin Cancer Res. 2006;12(7 Pt 1):2101–8.
40. Barrett JC, Fry B, Maller J, Daly MJ. Haploview: analysis and visualization of LD and haplotype maps. Bioinformatics. 2005;21(2):263–5.

13

Quality of life of early stage colorectal cancer patients in Morocco

Hind Mrabti[1*], Mounia Amziren[1], Ibrahim ElGhissassi[1], Youssef Bensouda[1], Narjiss Berrada[1], Halima Abahssain[1], Saber Boutayeb[1], Samira El Fakir[2], Chakib Nejjari[2], Abdellatif Benider[3], Nawfel Mellas[4], Omar El Mesbahi[4], Maria Bennani[5], Rachid Bekkali[5], Ahmed Zidouh[5] and Hassan Errihani[1]

Abstract

Background: A multicentre cohort study was held in Morocco, designed to evaluate the quality of life of cancer patients. The aim of this paper is to report the assessment of the quality of life of early colorectal cancer patients, before and after cancer treatment, to identify other factors which are related to this quality of life.

Methods: We used the third version of the QLQ-C30 questionnaire of the European organization for Research and treatment of Cancer (EORTC) after a transcultural validation. The Data collection was done at inclusion and then every twelve weeks to achieve one year of follow up.

Results: Overall 294 patients presented with early colorectal cancer, the median age was 56 years (range: 21–88). The male–female sex ratio was 1.17. At inclusion, the global health status was the most affected functional dimension. For symptoms: financial difficulties and fatigue scores were the highest ones. Emotional and social functions were significantly worse in rectal cancer. Most symptoms were more present in rectal cancer. At inclusion, global health status score was significantly worse in stage III. Anorexia was significantly more important among colorectal female patients. For Patients over 70 years-old, the difference was statistically significant for the physical function item which was lower. Overall, Functional dimensions scores were improved after chemotherapy. The symptoms scores did not differ significantly for patients treated by radiotherapy, between inclusion and at one year.

Conclusion: Our EORTC QLQ C30 scores are overall comparable to the reference values. Neither chemotherapy, nor radiotherapy worsened the quality of life at one year.

Keywords: Quality of life, EORTC QLQ C30, Early, Colorectal cancer

Background

Colorectal cancer is frequent in western countries, it represents the third most common cancer in France, with approximately 40 000 new cases per year [1]. According to Moroccan registries, it represents the first gastro-intestinal cancer before gastric cancer, and the fourth most common cancer, with an incidence of 8,4/100 000 habitants in 2007 [2]. This incidence have increased these last years (it was 6.9/100 000 habitants in 2005) [2]. This could be explained by the fact that Morocco has experienced, over the past 5 years, considerable progress in the detection, diagnosis and treatment of cancer. Many anticancer centers, equipped with the latest technologies have been constructed, most of anti-cancer drugs are available, and a national cancer plan (2010–2019) has been established.

When improving treatment of cancer, quality of life (QOL) becomes an important parameter to assess. It permits the evaluation of the impact of cancer and its treatment on the overall life of patients.

A multicentre cohort study was held in Morocco, designed to evaluate the quality of life of Moroccan cancer patients, including colorectal, cervical, breast and lung cancer [3, 4]. It is a prospective multicentre cohort study, performed in the ten existing oncological centers in Morocco.

* Correspondence: mrabti_h@yahoo.fr
[1]Department of Medical Oncology, National Institute of Oncology, University Hospital, Rabat, Morocco
Full list of author information is available at the end of the article

The aim of this paper is to report the assessment of the quality of life of early colorectal cancer patients, before and after specific cancer treatment (chemotherapy and/or radiotherapy), to identify other factors which are related to this quality of life (age, sex, localization: colon or rectum, performance status, disease stage), to describe Moroccan cancer patients characteristics.

Methods

Study design and study population

This is a Moroccan multicentre prospective cohort study. Patients were included, between December 2009 and December 2011, in the ten existing cancer centers in Morocco: seven public institutions (National Institute of oncology and Mohammed V military hospital in Rabat, Ibn rochd University hospital in Casablanca, Oujda, Agadir, Marrakech, Fez) and 3 private cancer clinics (Al Kindy and le Littoral in Casablanca, Nakhil in Rabat).

All patients were adults of 18 years or older, newly diagnosed with a histologically proven colorectal cancer. The diagnosis had to be made in less than three months before inclusion. Patients operated for their cancers within 3 months before inclusion were eligible to enter the study. A written informed consent was required for enrolment in the study, after the patient has received all the informations regarding the conditions of the study. Ethical approval was obtained from the ethics committees of the University Hospital Center Hassan II in Fez. Patients who received a specific treatment, chemotherapy or radiotherapy, and those with major neuropsychological defect were excluded.

In this paper we report quality of life assessment of early stage colorectal cancer patients which was defined by localized, stage I-II and III, colorectal cancer. Metastatic colorectal cancer (stage IV) was excluded, and will be separately analyzed, because patients are treated in a palliative setting, with systemic therapy and all patients remain under treatment at one year.

Collection data procedure

Questionnaires and data collection

We used the third version of the QLQ-C30 questionnaire of the European organization for Research and treatment of Cancer (EORTC). It is a validated tool for the assessment of QoL in cancer patients. It contains 14 items: 5 of them are related to activity (Physical, professional and leisure, cognitive, emotional and social functioning), 3 of them to symptoms (Asthenia, pain, nauseas and vomiting) and the remaining six are independent items evaluating other symptoms (dyspnea, insomnia, appetite loss, constipation, diarrhea, and financial difficulties). The QLQ-C30 was used after a transcultural validation [3]. It was developed according to Beaton and al recommendations [5].

The QLQ-C30 is a self-reporting questionnaire; however it was administered to illiterate patients by trained interviewers. The Data collection was done at inclusion and then every three months to each patient, until one year of follow-up.

All socio-demographic, economic and therapeutic data were extracted for colorectal cancer : age, gender, geographic origin, marital status, profession, income, level of education, medical insurance, localization, histological subtype, Tumor-Node-Metastasis (TNM) staging, evaluation of performance status according to Eastern Cooperative Oncology Group (ECOG) criteria, treatment (surgery, pre-operative radiotherapy or concurrent chemo-radiation for rectal cancer, adjuvant chemotherapy).

Statistical methods

- Calculation of EORTC QLQ-C30 scores [6]:

Scores of the items were linearly transformed to a scale from 0 to 100. A high score for a functional scale represents a healthy level of functioning, a high score for the global health status represents a high quality of life, but a high score for a symptom item represents a high level of symptomatology.

- Descriptive analysis

Descriptive analysis was performed for sociodemographic and clinical features, with a confidence interval defined at 95 %. To describe the quality of life scores, we calculated the means and standard deviations, minimum and maximum.

- Univariate analysis:

At inclusion, a global analysis was conducted in the whole population of early colorectal patients. Subgroup analyses were performed according to some variables: age, gender, tumor location (colon versus rectum), performance status (PS ≤ 1 versus >1) and stage. The comparison between subgroups was performed by t-tests and one-way ANOVA. A p-value of less than 0.05 was considered as statistically significant. To assess the scores variability of quality of life between inclusion (before treatment: chemotherapy or radiotherapy) and at 1 year (after treatment), we used the paired Student's t-test. The statistical analysis was performed by SPSS, version 17.0, software.

Results

Overall 2903 cancer patients were recruited, among whom 461 patients presented with colorectal cancer, 294 (63.7 %) were diagnosed at an early stage (I, II or III).

Socio-demographic and clinical characteristics of early colorectal cancer patients

Two hundred ninety-four patients with an early stage colorectal cancer were included in the study, of which there were 161 colon cancers (54.7 %) and 133 rectal cancers (45.3 %). The median age at diagnosis was 56 years (range: 21–88). The male–female sex ratio was 1.17. Majority of patients came from urban areas (78.2 %), a significant number were illiterate (49 %), and only 7.5 % had a high level of education. 32.7 % of patients were professionally active, but the majority of them had a low-intermediate socio-economic status. About 60 % of patients had no medical insurance. Eighty percent were married (see Table 1).

Tumor-node-metastasis staging system was as follows: Stage I = 19 (6.5 %), stage II = 80 (27.2 %), stage III = 195 (66.3 %). One hundred and ninety eight patients (67.3 %) patients received adjuvant chemotherapy based on the combination of capecitabin and Oxaliplatin every three weeks, during 6 months (eight cycles). Among rectal cancer patients (133), 50 (37.5 %) received pre-operative radiotherapy, which was concomitant to chemotherapy in 40 patients. (See Table 2).

This study have some limitations: mainly data concerning surgery are missed. The surgery have been performed, in majority of patients (223) (except those treated by pre-operative radiotherapy) before inclusion in the study. At inclusion, 50 patients presenting with rectal cancer have not been operated because they were candidate for pre-operative radiotherapy. The surgical procedure was unknown in 37 % of patients (Table 2). Therefore, the QOL have not been assessed before surgical treatment.

QOL assessment

At inclusion, all patients were assessed before receiving any specific treatment: radiotherapy or chemotherapy.

At inclusion, the global health status was the most affected functional dimension (score 62.84). For symptoms: financial difficulties and fatigue scores were the highest ones (61.72 and 38.21 respectively). The scores at inclusion are summarized in Tables 3 and 4.

Localization specific scores

The global health status had the lowest score at inclusion for both colon and rectal cancer patients. The less affected dimension was the cognitive function (scores 86 and 85 for colon and rectal cancers respectively). Differences were statistically significant between the two localizations for emotional and social functions. They were worse in rectal cancer (61 vs 68 and 76 vs 85 respectively) (see Table 3).

Most symptoms were more present in rectal cancer. The difference was statistically significant for Nauseas, pain, insomnia, anorexia, constipation and diarrhea (See Table 4).

Table 1 Sociodemographic characteristics of colorectal cancer patients at inclusion, Morocco, 2009–2011

	No (total 294)	%
Age (median)	56 years (range : 21–88)	
Sex		
• Male	159	54.1
• Female	135	45.9
Living environment		
• Urban	204	78.2
• Rural	57	21.8
Residency		
• Casablanca	29	10.2
• Rabat	33	11.6
• Agadir	9	3.2
• Meknes	9	3.2
• Kenitra	9	3.2
• Marrakech	35	12.3
• Others	170	57.9
Education		
• Illiterate	144	49.0
• Primary school	55	18.7
• College	73	24.8
• High school	22	7.5
Marital status		
• Single	32	10.9
• Married	235	80
• Divorced	10	3.4
• Widower	17	5.8
Professional Status		
• Working	96	32.7
• Retired	41	13.9
• Without profession	49	16.7
• Housewife	106	36.1
• Student	2	0.7
Socioeconomic Status		
• Low	142	48.3
• Intermediate	141	48.0
• High	11	3.7
Medical insurance		
• Public health-insurance	108	36.7
• Private insurance	10	3.4
• No medical insurance	176	59.9

Stage specific scores

At inclusion, global health status score was significantly worse in stage III ($p = 0.003$). Moreover, Role, emotional and cognitive functions were more altered in stage III

Table 2 Clinical features of early colorectal cancer patients, Morocco, 2009–2011

	No (total 294)	%
Localization		
• Colon	161	54.7
• Rectum	133	45.3
TNM Staging		
• Stage I	19	6.5
• Stage II	80	27.2
• Stage III	195	66.3
Surgery		
• Radical surgery	113	38.4
• Conservative surgery	67	22.8
• Palliative surgery	5	1.7
• Unknown	109	37.1
Radiotherapy (rectal cancer)	133	
• Performed	50	37.5
• Not performed	83	62.5
Adjuvant chemotherapy		
• Performed	198	67.3
• Not performed	77	26.2
• Unknown	19	6.5

colorectal cancer but the difference was not statistically significant (see Table 3). In addition to financial difficulties, the prominent symptom in all stages was the fatigue. The scores were 37, 39 and 36 for stages I, II and III respectively. Curiously, nausea was significantly higher in stage I (See Table 4).

Sex specific scores

Overall, women had more altered functional functions and more permanent symptoms (see stables 3 and 4). Anorexia was significantly more prevalent among colorectal female patients (28 versus 37) (see Table 4).

Age specific scores

Patients over 70 years-old had lower scores, for global health status, physical role and cognitive functions. The difference was statistically significant for the physical function item (see Table 3). Major symptoms in all age subgroups were financial difficulties (scores ranges between 57 and 65) and fatigue (scores 36 to 44). There was no significant difference between symptoms according to the age range. Nevertheless, descriptive data suggested that patients of more than 70 years-old had higher scores of pain, dyspnea and constipation. Patients between 60 and 69 years-old had more diarrheas while patients less than 50 years-old had higher scores of nauseas and insomnia (see Table 4).

Performance status (PS) specific scores

Majority of patients had PS >1 (67.9 %) at inclusion (see Table 2). Except for the emotional function, all of the functional dimensions were significantly more altered in patients with PS > 1 (see Table 3). In the same way, most symptoms scores were higher in "PS > 1" patients. The difference was statistically significant apart from dyspnea, diarrhea and financial difficulties (see Table 4).

Evolution according to treatment

Overall, Functional dimensions scores were improved after the end of chemotherapy. However, this improvement was significant only for global health status and role functioning (66.93 vs 73.4 and 70 vs 79.8 respectively) (Fig. 1). A trend to an improvement was also seen for symptoms. The scores of fatigue, pain, appetite loss, constipation and diarrhea significantly decreased after completion of chemotherapy (Fig. 2).

Curiously, the cognitive function was the only dimension which had a statistically significant variation. The cognitive capacities were altered after treatment by radiotherapy (91 vs 80 $p = 0.04$) (Fig. 3). Likewise, except for constipation, the symptoms scores did not differ significantly for patients treated by radiotherapy, between inclusion and at one year (Fig. 4). The constipation score fell from 38 to 13.33 ($p = 0.005$). Moreover, there was a borderline trend to an improvement in pain scores (40 vs 24.16 $p = 0.054$) (Fig. 4).

When we look to the evolution of QOL scores every three months: overall, functional dimensions were stable at 12 weeks and have started to improve thereafter. The global health status began to improve after inclusion, whereas social function has slightly worsened at 12 weeks and increased thereafter (Fig. 5). Majority of symptoms were also stable at 12 weeks and decreased with time. Some symptoms have started to improve at 12 weeks like pain and constipation. Nausea was the only symptom that worsened at 12 weeks and improved thereafter (Fig. 6).

Discussion

This is the first large prospective study assessing the quality of life of early colorectal cancer patients, in Morocco, and also in North Africa. The objective of this study was also to compare quality of life, before and after specific cancer treatment (chemotherapy and/or radiotherapy), at one year, when acute treatment effects are expected to have declined, to identify other factors which are related to this quality of life (age, sex, localization: colon or rectum, performance status, disease stage), to describe Moroccan cancer patients characteristics. In our study, the global health status was the most affected functional dimension at inclusion. For symptoms: financial difficulties and fatigue scores were

Table 3 Inclusion mean scores of functional dimensions according to sex, age, localization, stage and Performance status, among colorectal cancer patients, Morocco, 2009–2011

Subgroup	Global health status	Physical function	Role function	Emotional function	Cognitive function	Social function
All	62.8499	71.6667	67.5641	65.6595	86.0051	81.9338
Localization						
Colon	63.4199	70.6494	67.9825	68.7049*	86.5801	85.6061*
Rectum	62.0370	73.1308	66.9753	61.3169	85.1852	76.6975
				$p = 0.022$		$p = 0.005$
Stage						
I	66.6667	69.8148	74.0741	68.5185	91.6667	88.8889
II	68.3824	72.9657	67.1642	69.2402	89.9510	81.3725
III	60.3220*	71.3524	67.0476	63.9836	83.9015	81.4394
	$p = 0.003$					
Sex						
Male	64,0443	71,4085	69,4836	67.4825	85.5478	83.3333
Female	61,4146	71,9748	65,2542	63.4687	86.5546	80.2521
Age						
< 50	63.5294	74.5490*	71.7647	65.3595	85.2941	83.9216
50–60	63.5294	72.2603	65.9722	65.0304	89.2694	84.2466
60–69	62.9944	73.6782	70.3390	67.0904	85.3107	77.1186
≥ 70	58.8889	62.6667	58.3333	65.3704	82.9630	80.7407
		$p = 0.033$				
PS						
< 1	70.2236*	80.8333*	79.2683*	69.9864	90.8537*	92.6829*
≥ 1	59.4907	67.4674	62.1723	63.6883	83.7963	77.0370
	$p < 0.001$	$p < 0.001$	$p < 0.001$		$p < 0.001$	$p < 0.001$

*: statistically significant

the main factors affecting colorectal cancer patient's Qol. The most important factors affecting Qol were: rectal location, advanced disease (stage III). The impact of age and gender on Qol was less important, mainly the impact of advanced age was equivocal.

The data on socio-demographic characteristics of the Moroccan population are important to describe, they may explain some Qol aspects. About one third of patients were less than 50 years old, the median age at diagnosis was comparable to the one found in a study assessing quality of life of Malaysian colorectal cancer patients [7] but it was lower than the European average [8]. There was also a slight male predominance, which is in agreement with other studies [7–9]. This study reports the socio-economic characteristics of Moroccan colorectal cancer patients; they are consistent with the results of previous studies examining psychosocial characteristics of Moroccan cancer patients [10, 11]. Most of patients are illiterate, have low income. However the rate of medical insurance is higher in this study (40 %) while it was not exceeding 15 % in previous Moroccan cohorts [10, 11], this could be explained by a new health policy of the Moroccan government. Moreover, majority of patients came from urban areas (78 %), in contradiction with previous studies where this rate was between 30 and 40 % [8, 9], and this could be explained, by the availability of new structures treating cancers in most of Moroccan regions.

It was interesting to assess the quality of life of Moroccan cancer patients in this particular context of poverty and illiteracy, while the health system, and in particular management of cancer is improving. Another proof of better fight against cancer is the diagnosis of colorectal cancer at a non-metastatic stage in more than 60 % of cases, while this percentage was previously found for metastatic disease. However most of patients had a stage III disease (66.3 %), which is comparable to the results of Malaysian and Chinese studies [7, 12]. In developed countries, earlier stages, I and II, are the most frequent [13]. This could be explained by the absence of a screening program in Morocco, in addition to the other socioeconomic characteristics of Moroccan patients. The proportion of rectal cancers (45 %) is high in this study, as it was reported in Moroccan registries, in comparison with European studies. In a French cohort, examining colorectal cancer quality of life, rectal cancer represented 36 % [1].

Table 4 Inclusion mean scores of symptoms according to sex, age, localization, stage and Performance status, among colorectal cancer patients, Morocco, 2009–2011

Subgroup	Fatigue	Nausea	Pain	Dyspnea	Insomnia	Anorexia	Constipation	Diarrhea	Financial difficulties
All	38.2103	11.3868	30.1527	15.2672	32.3116	32.3116	20.4835	18.3206	61.7188
Localization									
Colon	35.7504	8.9827*	25.3247*	13.4199	21.8615*	28.5714*	14.9351*	14.5022	62.6398
Rectum	41.7181	14.8148	37.0370	17.9012	35.1852	37.6947	28.3951	23.7654	60.4361
		p =0.028	p =0.001		p =0.001	$p = 0.024$	$p < 0.001$	$p = 0.006$	
Stage									
I	37.0370	15.7407*	23.1481	11.1111	25.9259	29.6296	18.5185	18.5185	61.1111*
II	35.8660	4.4118	26.7157	12.2549	22.5490	28.9216	13.7255	18.1373	52.0202
III	39.2361	13.6364	32.1970	16.8561	29.3561	33.9048	23.2955	18.3712	65.5039
		$p = 0.006$							$p = 0.033$
Sex									
Male	36.2082	11.6550	27.3893	14.6853	26.3403	28.4038*	18.1818	19.8135	61.2293
Female	40.6162	11.0644	33.4734	15.9664	36.9748	36.9748	23.2493	16.5266	62.3188
						$p = 0.032$			
Age									
< 50	36.4052	13.1373	30.3922	16.4706	30.5882	35.3175	23.1373	18.0392	65.4618
50–60	36.5297	8.9041	27.3973	11.8721	27.3973	27.3973	17.3516	20.5479	60.0939
60–69	38.4181	11.2994	31.6384	13.5593	23.1638	34.4633	16.3842	16.9492	57.4713
≥ 70	44.0741	12.2222	32.2222	20.7407	26.6667	31.8519	25.9259	17.0370	62.8788
PS									
< 1	26,8970*	6,5041*	20,5285*	11,3821*	17.0732	24.7967*	11.7886*	15.4472	65.0407
≥ 1	43,3642	13,6111	34,5370	17,0370	32.0370	35.7542	24.4444	19.6296	60.1533
	$p < 0.001$	$p = 0.012$	$p < 0.001$	$p < 0.001$		$p = 0.01$	$p = 0.001$		

*: statistically significant

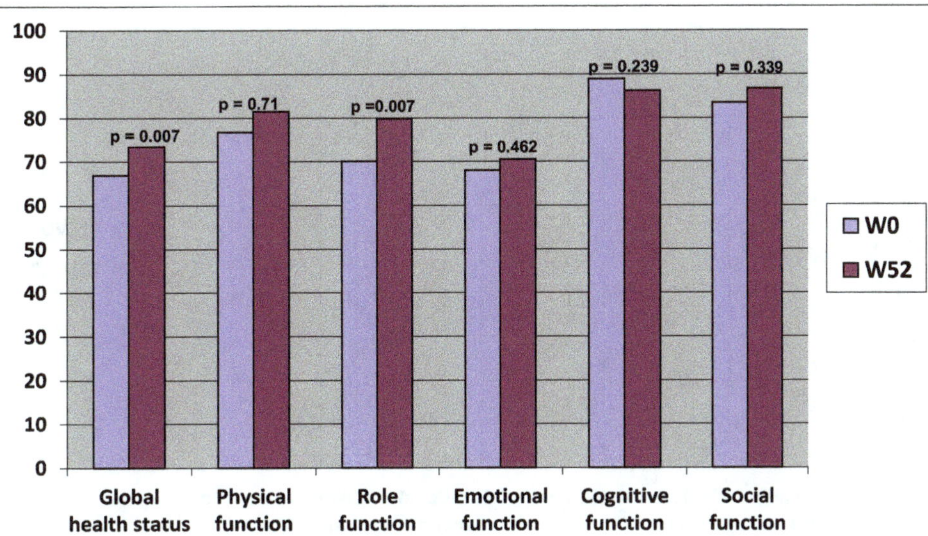

Fig. 1 QLQ C30 functional scores before and after treatment by chemotherapy, among colorectal cancer patients, Morocco, 2009–2011

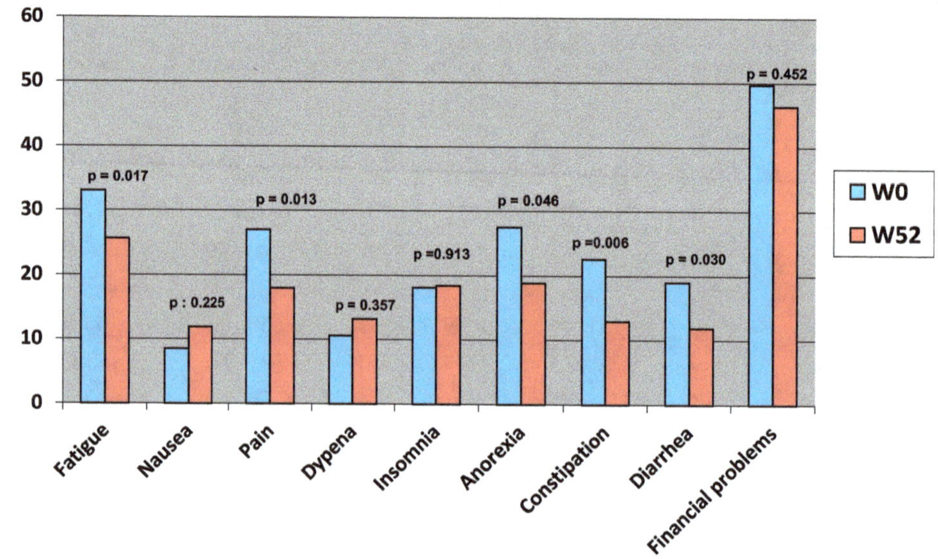

Fig. 2 QLQ C30 symptoms scores before and after treatment by chemotherapy, among colorectal cancer patients, Morocco, 2009–2011

At inclusion, the global health status was comparable to an American population [9] and the EORTC reference values [8]. However, it was lower than a Malaysian population. (See Table 5).

Physical, role and emotional functions scores are lower than those of other populations but they remain close to the EORTC reference values [8]. All these parameters may be related, to the socioeconomic status of Moroccan patients.

The social function score is well above American and European ones [1, 8, 9]. This could be due to the Moroccan culture that promotes social and family relationships [10, 11].

The financial difficulties are, by far, more present in the Moroccan population. This is because of the low socioeconomic status and the lack of medical insurance. The lowest score are found in the European's, whose health system is very well designed [1, 8].

The other symptoms scores are higher than those of the Malaysian population, in spite of the fact that the Malaysian study included stage IV colorectal cancer [7]. Moroccan scores are close to EORTC reference values except for nauseas, pain and appetite losses, suggesting a need for better supportive care for our patients.

Emotional and social functions were significantly worse in rectal cancer. Most symptoms were more present in

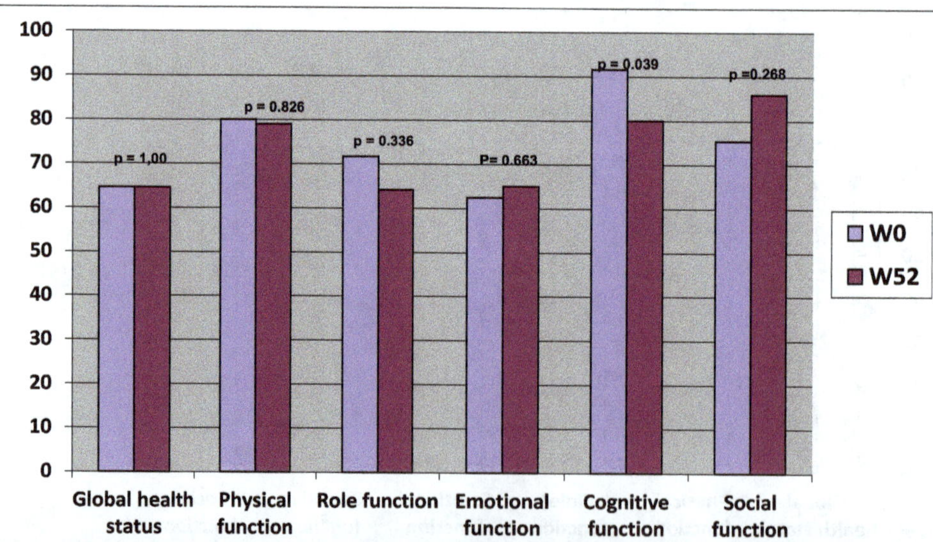

Fig. 3 QLQ C30 functional scores before and after treatment by radiotherapy, among colorectal cancer patients, Morocco, 2009–2011

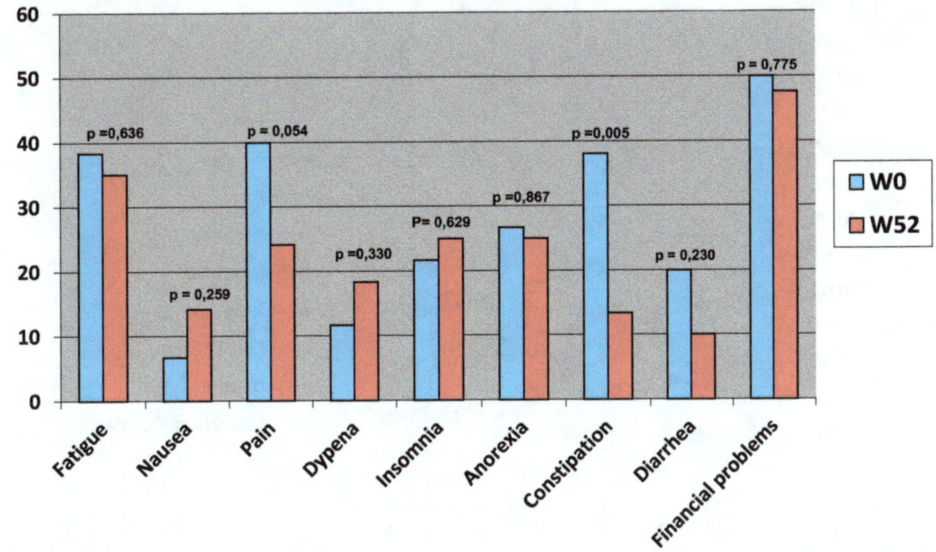

Fig. 4 QLQ C30 symptoms scores before and after treatment by radiotherapy, among colorectal cancer patients, Morocco, 2009–2011

rectal cancer. The difference was statistically significant for Nauseas, pain, insomnia, anorexia, constipation and diarrhea. At inclusion, global health status score was significantly worse in stage III. Anorexia was the only parameter which was significantly more important among colorectal female patients. A german study, didn't find significant differences, between patients with colon and rectal cancer, neither differences between male nor female [13]. An Austrian study focused on the Qol impact of gender and found no gender-specific reaction to disease [14].

For Patients over 70 years-old, the difference was statistically significant for the physical function item which was lower. The influence of age on the impact of the disease is equivocal. Older people certainly have a higher morbidity associated with the disease. However, studies have shown that they better accept the deterioration of their health. Younger patients may be more impaired quality of life especially in relation to the psychological impact of the disease and some symptoms that are seen more significantly [13]. In our study, patients less than 50 years-old had higher scores of nauseas and insomnia.

Overall, Functional dimensions scores were improved after the end of chemotherapy. The symptoms scores did not differ significantly for patients treated by radiotherapy, between inclusion and at one year. When we look to the evolution of QOL scores every three months: overall, functional dimensions and symptoms were stable at 12 weeks and have started to improve thereafter, so even during treatments, as chemotherapy or radiotherapy, the QOL was maintained. Nausea was the only symptom

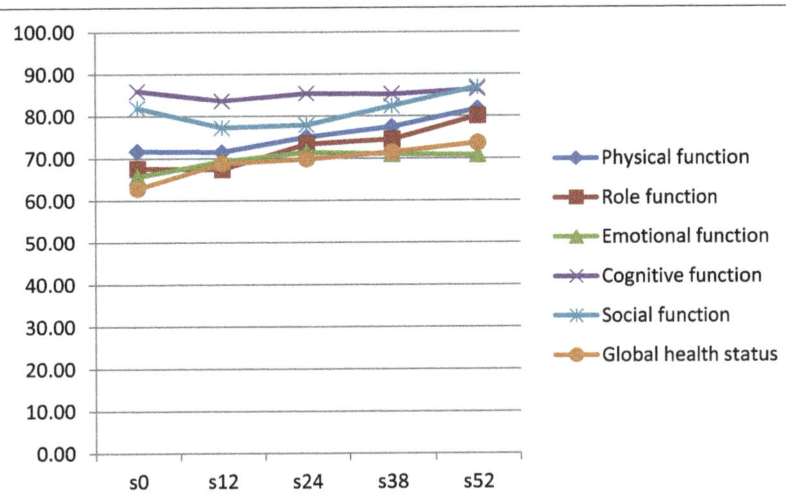

Fig. 5 Evolution of functional dimensions every three months

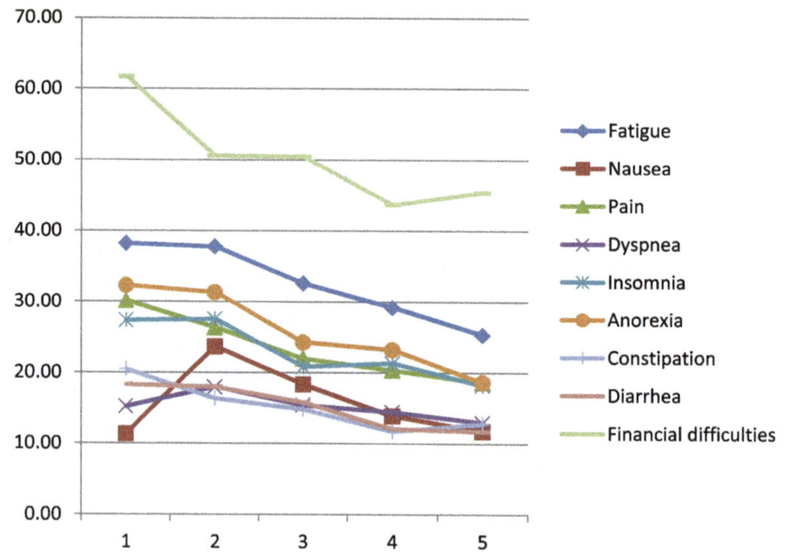

Fig. 6 Evolution of symptoms every three months

that worsened at 12 weeks and improved thereafter, since it is the main symptom of which patients undergoing chemotherapy complain. This finding is consistent with a german study, where adjuvant chemotherapy didn't alter long term's quality of life of early colorectal cancer patients, at one year [13]. In the subgroup treated by adjuvant chemotherapy, a significant improvement was seen in the global health status, role function, fatigue, pain, anorexia, constipation and diarrhea [13]. Several studies showed that with actual management of adjuvant chemotherapy, the Qol can decrease during treatement, but in a non statistically significant manner. However patients quickly recover their quality of life scores before treatment within a few months after completion of therapy [15, 16].

In the radiotherapy subgroup, the only significant change for functional dimensions was observed in the cognitive function. Unfortunately, we could not find any reasonable explanation. Moreover, constipation was significantly and largely improved, according to EORTC criteria [17–19]. Pre-operative radiotherapy or chemoradiation didn't impact quality of life of early colorectal cancer patients. The main limitation of this study is the lack of Qol assessment before surgery, mainly for colon cancer. QOL effects seen could be due to the surgery or

Table 5 Comparison of QLQ-C30 scores at inclusion between Moroccan colorectal cancer patients and patients of three others populations

Item	Moroccan population	Malaysian population	American population	EORTC reference values
Global health status	62.8	79	62.6	60.7
Physical function	71	83	78.6	79.2
Role function	67	79	70.3	70.4
Emotional function	65.65	86.4	70.6	68.9
Cognitive function	86	92.2	79.7	85.2
Social function	81	88.2	68.4	76
Fatigue	38.2	16.6	38.8	34.7
Nauseas	11.3	4	13.4	7.3
Pain	30.15	17.2	29.3	24
Dyspnea	15.26	8.7	19.5	17.4
Insomnia	32.3	20.7	33.7	30.5
Appetite loss	32.6	18	25.2	19.1
Constipation	20.4	8.67	17.5	15.8
Diarrhea	18.3	10.3	15.4	16.6
Financial difficulties	61.7	26	32.5	13.6

the subsequent treatments. The strengths of the reported study are in related with its multicentre characteristic, including all Moroccan oncology centers and using a reliable tool of quality of life assessment.

Conclusion

This study shows that Moroccan colorectal cancer patients are a young population. A screening program and more generalized medical insurance may help diagnosing colorectal cancer at an earlier stage. QLQ C30 scores are overall comparable to the EORTC QLQ C30 reference values except for some symptoms, which could be improved by more supportive care. Neither chemotherapy, nor radiotherapy worsened the long term quality of life of early colorectal cancer patients. The management of colorectal cancer, in addition to specific treatments, must take into account the patients quality of life, to overcome some insufficiencies.

Abbreviations

EORTC: European organization for Research and treatment of Cancer; PS: Performance status; QOL: Quality of life

Acknowledgments

To The Foundation Lalla Salma-Prevention and treatment of cancer and "Roche Laboratories" for their support.

Authors' contributions

HM has contributed to conception and design, acquisition of data, analysis and interpretation of data, wrote the manuscript; MA have been involved in drafting the manuscript; IE has contributed to acquisition of data; YB has contributed to acquisition of data; NB has contributed to acquisition of data; HA has contributed to acquisition of data; SB has contributed to acquisition of data; SF has contributed to conception and design, acquisition of data, analysis and interpretation of data, CN has contributed to conception and design, analysis and interpretation of data, has been involved in revising critically the manuscript for important intellectual content and has given final approval of the version to be published; AB has made substantial contributions to conception and design of data; NM has contributed to acquisition of data, OM has contributed to acquisition of data; MB has contributed to conception and design of data; RB has contributed to conception and design of data; AZ has contributed to conception and design; HE has contributed to conception and design of data, acquisition of data, has been involved in revising critically the manuscript for important intellectual content and has given final approval of the version to be published. All authors read and approved the final manuscript.

Competing interests

The authors declare that they have no competing interests.

Author details

[1]Department of Medical Oncology, National Institute of Oncology, University Hospital, Rabat, Morocco. [2]Department of Epidemiology and Public health, Faculty of Medicine, Fez, Morocco. [3]Department of Radiotherapy, Ibn Rochd University Hospital, Casablanca, Morocco. [4]Department of Medical Oncology, Hassan II University Hospital, Fez, Morocco. [5]Lalla Salma Foundation-Prevention and Treatment of Cancers, Rabat, Morocco.

References

1. Caravati-Jouvenceaux A, Launoy G, Klein D, Henry-Amar M, Abeilard E, Danzon A, Pozet A, Velten M, Mercier M. Health-related quality of life among long-term survivors of colorectal cancer: a population-based study. Oncologist. 2011;16(11):1626–36.
2. Cancer Registry of Grand Casablanca region: 2005-2006-2007. Edition 2012
3. Nejjari C, El Fakir S, Bendahhou K, El Rhazi K, Abda N, Zidouh A, Benider A, Errihani H, Bekkali R. Translation and validation of European organization for research and treatment of cancer quality of life questionnaire -C30 into Moroccan version for cancer patients in Morocco. BMC Res Notes. 2014;7:228.
4. El Fakir S, Abda N, Bendahhou K, Zidouh A, Bennani M, Errihani H, Benider A, Bekkali R, Nejjari C. The European Organization for Research and Treatment of Cancer quality of life questionnaire-BR23 Breast Cancer-Specific Quality of Life Questionnaire: psychometric properties in a Moroccan sample of breast cancer patients. BMC Res Notes. 2014;7:53.
5. Beaton D, Bombardier C, Guillemin F, Ferraz MB. Guidelines for the process of cross-cultural adaptation of self-report measures. SPINE. 2000;25(24):3186–91.
6. Fayers PM, Aaronson NK, Bjordal K, Groenvold M, Curran D, Bottomley A, et al. The EORTC QLQ-C30 Scoring Manual. 3rd ed. Brussels: European Organisation for Research and Treatment of Cancer; 2001.
7. Natrah MS, Ezat Sharifa WP, Syed MA, Rizal Mohd MA, Saperi S. Quality of life in Malaysian colorectal cancer patients: a preliminary result. Asian Pacific J Cancer Prev. 2012;13:957–62.
8. Neil W Scott, Peter M Fayers, Neil K Aaronson, Andrew Bottomley, Alexander de Graeff, Mogens Groenvold, Chad Gundy, Michael Koller, Morten A Petersen, Mirjam AG « EORTC QLQ-C30 Reference Values ».EORTC Quality of Life group July 2008.
9. Braun Braun DP, Gupta D, Grutsch JF. Can changes in health related quality of life scores predict survival in stages III and IV colorectal cancer? Health Qual Life Outcomes. 2011;9:2–8.
10. Errihani H, Mrabti H, Sbitti Y, Kaikani W, El Ghissassi I, Afqir S, Boutayeb S, Farik M, Riadi A, Hammoudi M, Chergui H. Psycho-social and religious impact of cancer diagnosis on Moroccan patients: experience from the National Oncology Center of Rabat. Bull Cancer. 2010;97(4):461–8.
11. Errihani H, Mrabti H, Boutayeb S, El Ghissassi I, El Mesbahi O, Hammoudi M, Chergui H, Riadi A. Impact of cancer on Moslem patients in Morocco. Psychooncology. 2008;17(1):98–100.
12. Peng J, Shi D, Goodman KA, Goldstein D, Xiao C, Guan Z, Cai S. Early results of quality of life for curatively treated rectal cancers in Chinese patients with EORTC QLQ-CR29. Radiat Oncol. 2011;6:93.
13. Arndt V, Merx H, Stegmaier C, Ziegler H, Brenner H. Quality of life in patients with colorectal cancer 1 year after diagnosis compared with the general population: a population-based study. J Clin Oncol. 2004;22:4829–36.
14. Giesinger J1, Kemmler G, Mueller V, Zabernigg A, Mayrbaeurl B, Thaler J, Ofner D, Pegger C, Rumpold G, Weber B, Sperner-Unterweger B, Holzner B. Are gender-associated differences in quality of life in colorectal cancer patients disease-specific? Qual Life Res. 2009 Jun;18(5):547–55. doi: 10.1007/s11136-009-9468-0. Epub 2009 Apr 1.
15. Zaniboni A, Labianca R, Marsoni S, et al.: GIVIO-SITAC 01: A randomized trial of adjuvant 5-fluorouracil and folinic acid administered to patients with colon carcinoma—long term results and evaluation of the indicators of healthrelated quality of life.
16. Gruppo Italiano Valutazione Interventi in Oncologia. Studio Italiano Terapia Adiuvante Colon. Cancer. 1998;82(34):2135–44.
17. Guren MG, Dueland S, Skovlund E, et al. Quality of life during radiotherapy for rectal cancer. Eur J Cancer. 2003;39:587–594.
18. Uwer L, Rotonda C, Guillemin F, Miny J, Kaminsky M-C, Mercier M, Tournier-Rangeard L, Leonard I, Montcuquet P, Rauch P, Conroy T. Responsiveness of EORTC QLQ-C30, QLQ-CR38 and FACT-C quality of life questionnaires in patients with colorectal cancer. Health Qual Life Outcomes. 2011;9:70.
19. Osoba D, Rodrigues G, Myles J, Zee B, Pater J. Interpreting the significance of changes in health-related quality-of-life scores. J Clin Oncol. 1998;16:139–44.

14

Successful sofosbuvir treatment with ribavirin dose reduction for chronic hepatitis C virus genotype 2 infection in a patient with ulcerative colitis

Yuki Ohta[1], Tatsuo Kanda[1*], Tatsuro Katsuno[1], Shin Yasui[1], Yuki Haga[1], Reina Sasaki[1], Masato Nakamura[1], Shuang Wu[1], Shingo Nakamoto[2], Makoto Arai[1] and Osamu Yokosuka[1]

Abstract

Background: Ulcerative colitis is a lifelong, immunologically mediated disease. Direct-acting antivirals (DAAs) are now available for the treatment of chronic hepatitis C virus (HCV) infection. An interferon-free regimen appears useful, safe and effective for many patients for whom interferon-based treatment is contraindicated.

Case presentation: We studied a 56-year-old treatment-naïve Japanese man with chronic HCV genotype 2b infection who had ulcerative colitis. This patient was treated with sofosbuvir and ribavirin for 12 weeks. During treatment, diarrhoea and bloody faeces were frequent. After ribavirin was reduced to 400 mg daily, these symptoms decreased. Finally, the patient achieved a sustained virologic response 12 weeks after the stoppage of the treatment.

Conclusion: Clinicians should pay careful attention to the ribavirin dose in the treatment of certain HCV patients with inflammatory bowel disease who are receiving sofosbuvir plus ribavirin.

Keywords: Case report, Direct-acting antiviral (DAA), Hepatitis C virus (HCV), Interferon-free, Ribavirin, Ulcerative colitis

Background

Inflammatory bowel disease (IBD), which comprises ulcerative colitis and Crohn's disease, is a chronic immunologically mediated disease [1]. There are high-prevalence populations of IBD in North America and Europe [1]. In India and Japan, the incidence is increasing [1]. Ulcerative colitis is a lifelong, immunologically mediated disease and results from the inappropriate activation of the mucosal immune system by intestinal luminal antigens [2], although the progress in treatment of ulcerative colitis has been observed [2, 3].

The prevalences of hepatitis B virus (HBV) and hepatitis C virus (HCV) in patients with IBD are similar to those in the general population [4, 5], although these data are controversial [6, 7]. Because the prevalences of HBV and HCV are higher in Asian countries, including Japan, than those in non-Asian countries [8, 9], the management of these infectious diseases is still important in patients with IBD.

Interferon-α, which was previously the most common treatment for HCV, is a proinflammatory cytokine and can provoke a relapse of ulcerative colitis [10]. The synthetic guanosine analogue ribavirin (1-beta-D-ribofuranosyl-1,2,4-triazole-3-carboxamide) is also used for HCV eradication [11, 12]. The exacerbation of ulcerative colitis has also been reported during and/or after combination therapy with peginterferon plus ribavirin for chronic hepatitis C [13–15].

Recent advances in the treatment of patients infected with HCV make it possible to eradicate this virus with interferon-free regimens. Sofosbuvir is a potent nucleotide inhibitor for HCV RNA-dependent polymerase [16]. The combination of sofosbuvir and ribavirin led to higher sustained virologic response (SVR) rates in HCV genotype 2-infected individuals [16]. We report an ulcerative colitis-patient who was chronically infected

* Correspondence: kandat-cib@umin.ac.jp
[1]Department of Gastroenterology and Nephrology, Chiba University, Graduate School of Medicine, 1-8-1 Inohana, Chuo-ku, Chiba 260-8670, Japan
Full list of author information is available at the end of the article

with HCV genotype 2 and was successfully treated with sofosbuvir plus dose reduction of ribavirin for 12 weeks.

Case presentation

A 56-year-old man with a 31-year history of ulcerative colitis was diagnosed with HCV infection at age 46. The patient received a blood transfusion at age 4 when he had surgery for his jaw and denied other risk factors for HCV infection, including tattoos or intravenous drug use. The patient drank alcohol (21 g daily) for 20 years; had a medical history of hypertension, IgA nephropathy, type 2 diabetes mellitus and dilated cardiomyopathy; and took several medications for these diseases. His ulcerative colitis was relatively well-controlled with oral sarazopyridine (4500 mg daily) and a sarazopyridine suppository (300 mg daily). The HCV genotype was 2b, and the patient was interferon treatment-naïve because he had ulcerative colitis, an autoimmune disease.

The patient's height and body weight were 172 cm and 88.3 kg, respectively, and his body temperature was 35.2 °C. His laboratory findings before treatment are shown in Table 1. Abdominal ultrasound findings showed no masses in the liver and no ascites. Liver stiffness as measured by transient elastography was 7.6 kPa, indicating the absence of cirrhosis. Although he had chronic significant amount of alcohol intake, the ultrasound findings did not show the fatty change of the liver. He wanted to be treated for his chronic hepatitis C.

The patient was treated with sofosbuvir at 400 mg daily and ribavirin at 600 mg daily. One week after the initiation of this treatment, the patient felt general malaise without any adverse events [white blood cell count (WBC), 7900/μL; hemoglobin, 14.7 g/dL; C-reactive protein (CRP) 0.0 mg/dL; AST, 35 IU/L; and ALT, 49 IU/L]. By week 3, the patient was having up to 10 loose bowel movements per day, with small amounts of blood. As the patient's HCV RNA became negative and he improved to having 5 loose bowel movements per day by week 4 [WBC, 8600/μL; hemoglobin, 14.3 g/dL; AST, 19 IU/L; and ALT, 19 IU/L], the dose of ribavirin was increased to 800 mg daily. By week 7, however, the patient was having up to 20 loose bowel movements per day, with small amounts of blood, and the dose of ribavirin was decreased to 400 mg daily [WBC, 8200/μL; hemoglobin, 14.7 g/dL; CRP 0.1 mg/dL; AST, 19 IU/L; and ALT, 17 IU/L]. By week 8, the patient improved to having 10 loose bowel movements per day [WBC, 8600/μL; hemoglobin, 14.2 g/dL; CRP 0.1 mg/dL; AST, 20 IU/L; and ALT, 17 IU/L], and by week 11, his diarrhoea had resolved. Finally, the patient was treated with sofosbuvir plus ribavirin for 12 weeks. By week 12 after the initiation of this treatment, the patient's HCV RNA was negative, and he had achieved a SVR 12 weeks (SVR12) after the stoppage of treatment [WBC, 14400/μL; hemoglobin, 16.2 g/dL; CRP 0.2 mg/dL; AST, 22 IU/L; and ALT, 22 IU/L] (Fig. 1). Three weeks post-treatment, an endoscopic examination of the colon-rectum confirmed that the mucosa was oedematous from the colon transversum to the rectum, although mucosal vascular permeability was reduced from the sigmoid colon to the rectum. The patient did not complain of abdominal pain or fever during treatment.

Discussion

In the present report, we present a 56-year-old HCV genotype 2-infected patient who was diagnosed with ulcerative colitis and achieved a SVR12 after combination

Table 1 Laboratory findings before treatment

Item	Value	Item	Value	Item	Value
AST	51 IU/L	BUN	16 mg/dL	HBsAg	negative
ALT	66 IU/L	Creatinine	0.68 mg/dL	Anti-HCV	positive
LDH	256 IU/L	UA	4.3 mg/dL	HCV RNA	6.4 logIU/mL
ALP	96 IU/L	Na	136 mEq/L	HCV genotype	2b
γ-GTP	88 IU/L	K	3.9 mEq/L	Anti-HIV	negative
T. Bil	1.2 mg/dL	Cl	104 mEq/L	Hyaluronic acid	37 ng/mL
TP	7.1 g/dL	WBC	5900/μL	AFP	7.4 ng/mL
Albumin	3.9 g/dL	RBC	477×10^4/μL	PIVKA-II	32 mAU/mL
Amylase	83 IU/L	Hemoglobin	14.4 g/dL	NH_3	58 μg/dL
CPK	102 IU/L	Haematocrit	40.7 %	HbA1c	7.8 %
T.CHO	115 mg/dL	Platelets	15.6×10^4/μL	CRP	0.1 mg/dL
TG	103 mg/dL	PT	100 %		

AFP α-Fetoprotein, *ALP* alkaline phosphatase, *BUN* blood urea nitrogen, *CPK* creatine phosphokinase, *CRP* C-reactive protein, *HbA1c* haemoglobin A1c, *LDH* lactate dehydrogenase, *PIVKA-II* protein induced by vitamin K absence or antagonists-II, *PT* prothrombin time, *RBC* red blood cell count, *T.Bil* total bilirubin, *T.CHO* total cholesterol, *TG* triglyceride, *TP* total protein, *UA* uric acid, *WBC* white blood cell count

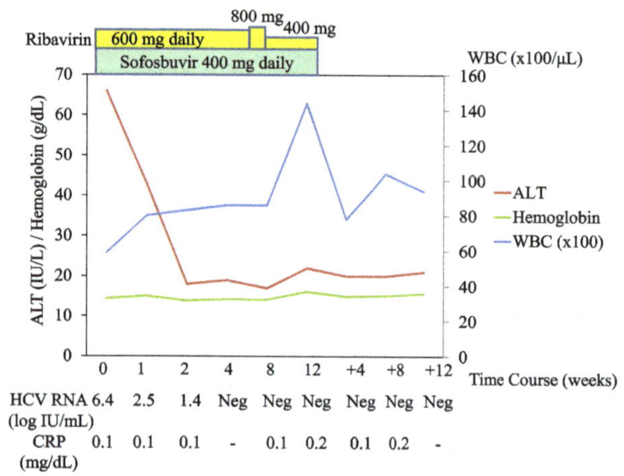

Fig. 1 Clinical course of the patient. *ALT* alanine transaminase, *WBC* white blood cells, *w* weeks, *Neg* negative

treatment with sofosbuvir plus ribavirin for 12 weeks. In Japanese multicentre, open-label phase 3 trial, HCV genotype 2-infected patients received 12 weeks of treatment with 400 mg of sofosbuvir, administered orally once daily, and ribavirin, administered orally twice daily, with doses determined according to body weight (1000 mg daily in patients with a body weight of >80 kg) [17]. But initial dose of the present case was 600 mg daily because we are afraid of adverse events of ribavirin. During treatment, the patient's diarrhoea worsened, and the reduction of ribavirin with no reduction of sofosbuvir led to improvement in this symptom and the completion of therapy.

The mechanism of the inhibition of HCV replication by ribavirin is as follows: (1) ribavirin induces mutagenesis in HCV RNA; (2) ribavirin inhibits HCV RNA-dependent polymerase; (3) ribavirin inhibits the inosine monophosphate dehydrogenase enzyme and reduces intracellular guanosine pools, which are essential for HCV replication; and (4) ribavirin stimulates the T helper 1 (Th1) antiviral response, which leads to HCV eradication [8, 11, 12]. Ulcerative colitis is vaguely associated with abnormal Th2 immunity [18]. Although we do not know the exact effects of ribavirin on mucosal immunity, ribavirin worsened the symptoms of the present case with ulcerative colitis.

Although 12-week-treatment with sofosbuvir and ribavirin could lead to diarrhoea in 9 % of HCV genotype 2/3-infected patients [16], of interest, 12-week-treatment with sofosbuvir and ledipasvir could lead to diarrhoea in only 4 % of HCV genotype 1-infected patients [19]. We could not completely rule out the possibility that the combination of sofosbuvir plus ribavirin might be responsible, compared the only ribavirin.

One year before treatment, an endoscopic examination of the colon-rectum demonstrated that mucosal vascular permeability was reduced from the sigmoid colon to the rectum with marked mucus exudates. We could not completely rule out the possibility that this patient had baseline active mucosal disease but asymptomatic and then developed diarrhoea due to the sofosbuvir and ribavirin treatment. Although one important differential diagnosis of flare of ulcerative colitis is infection, as this patient did not have a high fever, we did not perform stool culture or use any antibiotics other than sarazopyridine. So we excluded bacterial infection in this patient.

HCV infection is a current leading cause of HCC in Japan and the United States [12]. This patient should be followed up for the occurrence of HCC [12]. Coexistence of IBD and chronic liver diseases, including chronic hepatitis C, leads to higher mortality rates than IBD alone [20]. Interferon-free therapy with or without ribavirin could increase treatment efficacy and shorten treatment duration compared with previous standards of care, such as peginterferon plus ribavirin treatment. However, the clinician should pay special attention to the use of ribavirin in the management of HCV-infected patients with IBD.

Conclusion

We studied a HCV genotype 2b-infected patient with an ulcerative colitis exacerbation during sofosbuvir plus ribavirin treatment. The reduction of ribavirin improved this symptom, and the patient finally achieved a SVR12. Clinicians should pay careful attention to the ribavirin dose in the treatment of certain HCV patients with inflammatory bowel diseases, such as ulcerative colitis, in sofosbuvir plus ribavirin treatment.

Abbreviations

HBV, hepatitis B virus; HCV, hepatitis C virus; IBD, inflammatory bowel disease; SVR, sustained virologic response; SVR12, SVR at 12 weeks; Th, T helper

Acknowledgements

Authors thank all Chiba University Hospital's staff for patient's care.

Funding

Not applicable.

Authors' contributions

YO, TK and TK saw the patient and drafted the manuscript. All authors revised manuscript and approved the final manuscript.

Competing interests

TK and OY received lecture fees from Gilead Sciences. The other authors have no competing interest to disclose.

Author details

[1]Department of Gastroenterology and Nephrology, Chiba University, Graduate School of Medicine, 1-8-1 Inohana, Chuo-ku, Chiba 260-8670, Japan. [2]Department of Molecular Virology, Chiba University, Graduate School of Medicine, 1-8-1 Inohana, Chuo-ku, Chiba 260-8670, Japan.

References

1. Ananthakrishnan AN. Epidemiology and risk factors for IBD. Nat Rev Gastroenterol Hepatol. 2015;12(4):205–17.
2. Lawrance IC. Early investigational TNF receptor antagonists for the treatment of ulcerative colitis. Expert Opin Investig Drugs. 2015;24(6):761–8.
3. Seo GS, Chae SC. Biological therapy for ulcerative colitis: an update. World J Gastroenterol. 2014;20(37):13234–8.
4. Papa A, Felice C, Marzo M, Andrisani G, Armuzzi A, Covino M, et al. Prevalence and natural history of hepatitis B and C infections in a large population of IBD patients treated with anti-tumor necrosis factor-α agents. J Crohns Colitis. 2013;7(2):113–9.
5. Chevaux JB, Nani A, Oussalah A, Venard V, Bensenane M, Belle A, et al. Prevalence of hepatitis B and C and risk factors for nonvaccination in inflammatory bowel disease patients in Northeast France. Inflamm Bowel Dis. 2010;16(6):916–24.
6. Loras C, Saro C, Gonzalez-Huix F, Mínguez M, Merino O, Gisbert JP, et al. Prevalence and factors related to hepatitis B and C in inflammatory bowel disease patients in Spain: a nationwide, multicenter study. Am J Gastroenterol. 2009;104(1):57–63.
7. Lidar M, Langevitz P, Barzilai O, Ram M, Porat-Katz BS, Bizzaro N, et al. Infectious serologies and autoantibodies in inflammatory bowel disease: insinuations at a true pathogenic role. Ann N Y Acad Sci. 2009;1173:640–8.
8. Omata M, Kanda T, Yu ML, Yokosuka O, Lim SG, Jafri W, et al. APASL consensus statements and management algorithms for hepatitis C virus infection. Hepatol Int. 2012;6(2):409–35.
9. Sarin SK, Kumar M, Lau GK, Abbas Z, Chan HL, Chen CJ, et al. Asian-Pacific clinical practice guidelines on the management of hepatitis B: a 2015 update. Hepatol Int. 2016;10(1):1–98.
10. Sawada K, Ohnishi K, Fukunaga K, Shimoyama T. A new treatment for HCV-ulcerative colitis comorbidity intolerant to INF-alpha. Am J Gastroenterol. 2003;98(1):228–9.
11. Kanda T, Yokosuka O, Imazeki F, Tanaka M, Shino Y, Shimada H, et al. Inhibition of subgenomic hepatitis C virus RNA in Huh-7 cells: ribavirin induces mutagenesis in HCV RNA. J Viral Hepat. 2004;11(6):479–87.
12. Kanda T, Imazeki F, Yokosuka O. New antiviral therapies for chronic hepatitis C. Hepatol Int. 2010;4(3):548–61.
13. Sprenger R, Sagmeister M, Offner F. Acute ulcerative colitis during successful interferon/ribavirin treatment for chronic hepatitis. Gut. 2005;54(3):438–9.
14. Tursi A. Rapid onset of ulcerative colitis after treatment with PEG-interferon plus ribavirin for chronic hepatitis C. Inflamm Bowel Dis. 2007;13(9):1189–90.
15. Morimoto K, Yamagami H, Hosomi S, Ohira M, Suekane T, Kamata N, et al. Development of pouchitis with combination therapy with peg-interferon alpha-2b and ribavirin for chronic hepatitis C in a patient with ulcerative colitis who underwent pouch surgery. Am J Gastroenterol. 2009;104(6):1609–10.
16. Jacobson IM, Gordon SC, Kowdley KV, Yoshida EM, Rodriguez-Torres M, Sulkowski MS, et al. Sofosbuvir for hepatitis C genotype 2 or 3 in patients without treatment options. N Engl J Med. 2013;368(20):1867–77.
17. Omata M, Nishiguchi S, Ueno Y, Mochizuki H, Izumi N, Ikeda F, et al. Sofosbuvir plus ribavirin in Japanese patients with chronic genotype 2 HCV infection: an open-label, phase 3 trial. J Viral Hepat. 2014;21(11):762–8.
18. Neurath MF, Finotto S, Glimcher LH. The role of Th1/Th2 polarization in mucosal immunity. Nat Med. 2002;8(6):567–73.
19. Kowdley KV, Gordon SC, Reddy KR, Rossaro L, Bernstein DE, Lawitz E, et al. Ledipasvir and sofosbuvir for 8 or 12 weeks for chronic HCV without cirrhosis. N Engl J Med. 2014;370:1879–88.
20. Bargiggia S, Thorburn D, Anderloni A, Ardizzone S, Giorgi A, Bianchi Porro G, et al. Is interferon-alpha therapy safe and effective for patients with chronic hepatitis C and inflammatory bowel disease? A case-control study. Aliment Pharmacol Ther. 2005;22(3):209–15.

15

Therapeutic effects of different doses of polyethylene glycosylated porcine glucagon-like peptide-2 on ulcerative colitis in male rats

Ke-ke Qi, Jia-jia Lv, Jie Wu and Zi-wei Xu*

Abstract

Background: Polyethylene glycosylated (PEGylated) porcine glucagon-like peptide-2 (pGLP-2) considerably increases half-life and stability compared with the native pGLP-2, but the effective dose for intestinal damage is still unclear. This study aims to evaluate the available dose of polyethylene glycosylated porcine glucagon-like peptide-2 (PEG-pGLP-2), a modified, long-acting form of pGLP-2 in an experimental rat model of ulcerative colitis.

Methods: Thirty-five male rats were randomly assigned into five groups: control, dextran sodium sulphate (DSS), DSS + PEG–pGLP-2(L), DSS + PEG–pGLP-2(M) and DSS + PEG–pGLP-2(H). Rats in control group received only water; other rats were fed with 5% (w/v) DSS and intraperitoneally administered with 12.5, 25 and 100 nmol/kg PEG–pGLP-2 daily for 6 days.

Results: Compared with the control treatment, DSS treatment significantly ($p < 0.05$) decreased body weight change, colonic length, duodenal villus height and expression of zonula occludens-1, whereas significantly ($p < 0.05$) increased colonic damage score and expression of claudin-1, interleukin (IL)-1, IL-7, IL-10, interferon-γ and tumour necrosis factor (TNF)-α in colon. However, the three doses of PEG–pGLP-2 all reduced these effects; these treatments significantly ($p < 0.05$) increased body weight change and duodenal villus height, whereas significantly ($p < 0.05$) decreased colonic damage score and expression of IL-1, IL-7 and TNF-α in colon. Specifically, low-dose (12.5 nmol/kg/d) PEG–pGLP-2 was effective.

Conclusions: These results indicated that PEG–pGLP-2 is a novel and potentially effective therapy for intestinal healing in a relatively low dose.

Keywords: Porcine glucagon-like peptide-2, Ulcerative colitis, Tight junction, Inflammation cytokines

Background

Frequent injection of porcine glucagon-like peptide-2 (pGLP-2) because of the rapid degradation of pGLP-2 by the enzyme dipeptidyl peptidase-IV (DPP-IV) is the main impediment of pGLP-2 as a potential therapeutic agent for intestinal dysfunction and damage in weaning piglets [1]. For the first time, our team designed and purified polyethylene glycosylated (PEGylated) pGLP-2 (PEG-pGLP-2), whose half-life ($t_{1/2}$) is 16-fold longer than that of pGLP-2 in DPP-IV in vitro [2]. PEG-pGLP-2 infusion could alleviate the severity of intestinal injury in weaning piglets [3, 4]. The $t_{1/2}$ of teduglutide, a GLP-2 analogue, which is a candidate for the treatment of short bowel syndrome (SBS) in two phase III clinical studies [5], is 2.99 h in male patient [6]. Recently, our team proved that the $t_{1/2}$ of PEG-pGLP-2 is 3.38 h in male rats [7]. These findings provide a new perspective to the potential therapeutic use of PEG-pGLP-2 for weaning and diarrhoeal diseases in young pigs.

However, no reports about the therapeutic effect of PEG-pGLP-2, except that of our team, are available. Little information is also known about the dose and frequency of administration with PEG-pGLP-2. Thymann

* Correspondence: zjsnkyxzw@163.com
Institute of Animal Science, Zhejiang Academy of Agricultural Sciences, 198 Shiqiao Road, Jianggan, Hangzhou 310021, China

et al. [8] found that injection of acylated GLP-2 analogue 25 μg/(kg BW · 12 h) for 5 days increases intestinal weight and activity of brush border enzymes in weaned pigs when only using long-acting analogues or under diarrhoeal conditions. Kaji et al. [9] demonstrated high doses (240 μg/kg/day for 5 days) of continuous infusion result in the largest increases in microscopic and gross intestinal morphologic parameters in parenterally maintained rats. Similarly, Nakame et al. [10] found that high dose of GLP-2 (800 μg/kg BW every 6 h before stress) administration improves the incidence and survival rate of necrotising enterocolitis (NEC) in rats. Nevertheless, Sigalet et al. [11] found the effects of subcutaneous injection of weaning pigs with GLP-2 at a dose of 40 μg/kg/day for 42 days are limited to the gastrointestinal tract; GLP-2 could increase crypt cell proliferation rates and decrease in apoptosis; no effects were observed on activity, appetite, behaviour or food intake. Deng et al. [12] found that both low and high doses of exogenous GLP-2 (2 or 10 nmol/kg BW per day for 7 consecutive days) improve the growth of weaned piglets and protect them against LPS-induced intestinal damage. The various results of therapeutic methods of GLP-2 may be caused by the different agents, experimental animals and test environments. However, the substantially long $t_{1/2}$ of PEG-pGLP-2 provides us confidence to utilise it for post-weaning diarrhoea syndrome.

The present study was designed to examine the effect of different doses of long-acting pGLP-2, that is, PEG-p[Gly^2]GLP-2, on growth performance, intestinal morphology and expression levels of tight junction (TJ) proteins and inflammatory cytokines in an experimental rat model of ulcerative colitis. Results of this study may provide the dose reference for application of PEG-p[Gly^2]GLP-2 in post-weaning diarrhoea syndrome.

Methods

Materials

Porcine [Gly^2] GLP-2 (HGDGSFSDEMNTVLDNLATRDFINWLLHTKITDSL, > 98%) was synthesised by Chinese Peptide Company (Hangzhou, China). Monomethoxy PEG–succinimidyl propionate (mPEG–SPA; molecular weight (MW) = 5 kDa) was purchased from Beijing Kaizheng Biotech Development Co., Ltd. (Beijing, China). The ion-exchange chromatography (IEC) resin and column used were CM Sepharose Fast Flow (GE Healthcare Bio-Science AB, Uppsala, Sweden). Ultrafiltration membranes with a MW cutoff of 3000 were purchased from Millipore Corporation (Billerica, MA, USA). Dextran sodium sulphate (DSS) (MW = 36 000–50 000) was purchased from MP Biomedicals China (Shanghai, China). RNAiso Plus, PrimeScript®RT-reagent with gDNA Eraser Kit and SYBR® Premix Ex TaqTM were purchased from Takara Biotechnology Co., Ltd. (Dalian, China). RNA locker was purchased from TIANDZ (Beijing, China). Unless otherwise specified, all other chemicals and reagents were of analytical grade from Sigma–Aldrich and Fluka (Milan, Italy).

Preparation of PEG-p[Gly^2]GLP-2

The mono-PEGylated p[Gly^2]GLP-2 conjugates were prepared and purified as previously described [3]. Briefly, 1 mg/mL of p[Gly^2]GLP-2 in 50 mmol/L Tris-HCl buffer solution was reacted with 4 mole excess of mPEG$_{5k}$-SPA at room temperature for 30 min. The reaction was quenched by 1% trifluoroacetic acid/deionised water. The PEGylated p[Gly^2]GLP-2 mixtures were separated with IEC with C M Sepharose Fast Flow resin. The equilibration phase was 20 mmol/L of acetate buffer (pH 4.0), and the elution phase was 20 mmol/L acetate buffer (pH 4.0) + 1 mol/L NaCl. The PEGylated p[Gly^2]GLP-2 products were eluted in a linear gradient ranging from 0 to 60% for 60 min and to 100% for 30 min with 1 mL/min of elution buffer at 215 nm. The PEGylated products were collected, desalted, concentrated through 3 kDa cutoff, ultrafitrated and lyophilised to powder before the animal study.

Animal ethics statement and experimental protocol

Animal studies were conducted in accordance with the guidelines of the Zhejiang Farm Animal Welfare Council of China and approved by the ethics committee of Zhejiang Academy of Agricultural Sciences. Thirty-five male Sprague–Dawley rats were allocated into five treatments: control, DSS, DSS + PEG–pGLP-2(L), DSS + PEG–pGLP-2(M) and DSS + PEG–pGLP-2(H). Each treatment was performed in seven replicates on one rat. The rats were housed in a plastic bottom, wire-lid cages, maintained on a 12 h: 12 h light–dark cycle and allowed to acclimatise to the animal facility for 3 days. Rats in control group received only water; other rats were fed with 5% (w/v) DSS through their drinking water for 6 days from the first day of experiment, followed by 2 days of water consumption. The rats from the DSS + PEG–pGLP-2(L), DSS + PEG–pGLP-2(M) and DSS + PEG–pGLP-2(H) groups were intraperitoneally administered with 12.5, 25 and 100 nmol/kg PEG–pGLP-2, respectively, in 0.3 mL of saline solution daily from day 1 to day 6 of the trial. The rats in the control and DSS groups were administered with the same volume of saline solution. During the experimental period, behaviour and body weight were monitored daily. On day 8, all rats were anesthetised and sacrificed to collect their intestinal sample.

Collection samples

Samples collection was prepared as previously described [4]. The segment from the pylorus to the Trietz ligament and from the ileocecal valve to the rectum was considered the duodenum and colon, respectively; these segments were cut free from their mesentery and immediately placed on ice. The duodenum and colon were cleaned of luminal contents, weighed and measured with a balance and a ruler. The middle segments (1 cm) of duodenum and colon were fixed in 10% formalin for 48 h and embedded in paraffin using standard techniques for histology. One centimetre of the distal segment of colon was collected for RNA isolation, which was immediately placed in 1 mL of RNA locker.

Histology

Histology was prepared as previously described [3]. The paraffin-embedded sections were cut at 4 μm thickness and stained with haematoxylin and eosin. Duodenum villus-plus-crypt height was imaged using an Olympus DP-71 digital camera, and quantification was performed using an image processing system. Approximately 12 longitudinally oriented villi were measured from each H&E-stained section to make $n = 1$. All measurements were performed in a blinded manner. Colonic damage score (CDS), was evaluated in a blinded manner in tissue sections based on a grade scale ranging from 0 to 3 to measure the amount and depth of inflammation. The amount of crypt damage or regeneration was measured in a scale of 0–4, as indicated in Dieleman et al. [13]. These changes were also quantified in terms of the percentage involvement of the disease process: (1) 1–25%, (2) 26–50%, (3) 51–75% and (4) 76–100%. Each section was separately scored for each feature by establishing the product of the grade for that feature and the percentage involvement. The sum of the products of the four scores was the CDS for each rat.

Real-time PCR

Total RNA was isolated using RNAiso Plus kits following the manufacturers' instructions [4]. A 2 μL aliquot of the total RNA was used for first-strand cDNA synthesis using PrimeScript® RT-reagent Kit with gDNA Eraser. Real-time PCR was carried out with ABI plus one (Life Technologies, Carlsbad, CA, USA) using SYBR Premix Ex TaqTM. The primers used were in Table 1. RT-PCR analysis was performed with an ABI Step One Plus Real-Time PCR System (Applied Biosystems, Inc.) using SYBR® Premix Ex TaqTM. PCR reactions were performed in triplicate under the following conditions: 95 °C for 30 s; 40 cycles of 95 °C for 5 s and 60 °C for 30 s. Fluorescent data for quantification were collected at the end of each cycle. Melting curve analysis was performed at 55–95 °C to verify the single product generation at the end of the assay. Standard curves were generated based on the data obtained from the standards of the $2–2^{-6}$ dilution series template. Standard curve analysis was performed by using Step One Software (v2.2, Applied Biosystems, Inc.). Data were normalised to GADPH using the $2^{-\Delta\Delta Ct}$ quantitation method.

Statistical analysis

Data are expressed as the mean ± SD. Statistical differences between groups were compared through ANOVA with Duncan's multiple comparison tests at an alpha value of 0.05.

Results

Growth performance

As shown in Table 2, compared with the control treatment, the rats treated with 5% DSS for 6 days exhibited significantly decreased body weight change and colonic length ($p < 0.05$). Compared with the DSS group, body weight change and ratio between colonic weight and body weight of rats in DSS + PEG–pGLP-2(L) and DSS + PEG–pGLP-2(M) groups significantly ($p < 0.05$) increased, and the colonic length of rats in DSS + PEG–pGLP-2(L) group significantly ($p < 0.05$) increased; the body weight change in DSS + PEG–pGLP-2(H) also significantly ($p < 0.05$) increased. No significant differences in intestinal length and ratio of intestinal weight/body weight were observed among the five groups.

Table 1 Primer sequences (5′ to 3′) used for the quantitative polymerase chain reaction

Gene	Forward primer	Reverse primer
ZO-1	CCATCTTTGGACCGATTGCTG	TAATGCCCGAGCTCCGATG
Occludin	ACGGTGCCATAGAATGAGATGTTG	CAGCTAGTTGTTCATTTCTGCACCA
Claudin-1	CATCGCAGCTACTTGCCAGT	TTTTTTTTTTTTTTTTGCAAAAACGA
IL-1	TCAGGAAGGCAGTGTCACTCATTG	ACACACTAGCAGGTCGTCATCATC
IL-6	TAGAGTCACAGAAGGAGTGG	GCCAGTTCTTCGTAGAGA
IL-7	AACCTCCAAGAAACTACTGCC	CACCGATGCATGGTTGCTAAC
IL-10	CTCAGCACTGCTATGCTGCCTGCT	TCTTCACCTGCTCCACTGCCTTGC
INF-γ	TGTCATCGAATCGCACCT	TCAGCACCGACTCCTTTT
TNF-α	ACCCCCAACCTATGAAGAAA	TCCACGCAAAACGGAATGAA
GADPH	CCGAGGGCCCACTAAAGG	GCTGTTGAAGTCACAGGAGACAA

Table 2 Effects of polyethylene glycosylated (PEGylated) porcine glucagon-like peptide-2 (pGLP-2) on growth performance of colitis rats

Groups	Body weight change, %	Intestinal length, cm	Colonic length, cm	Intestinal weight (mg)/body weight (g)	Colonic weight (mg)/body weight (g)
Control	30.48 ± 3.44^{a}	94.72 ± 4.93	15.69 ± 1.90^{a}	30.61 ± 2.22	11.19 ± 1.90^{b}
Dextran sodium sulphate (DSS)	11.90 ± 5.04^{c}	92.88 ± 9.78	12.40 ± 1.94^{b}	35.19 ± 1.22	9.15 ± 1.79^{b}
DSS + PEG–pGLP-2(L)	21.45 ± 2.00^{b}	94.50 ± 7.07	14.74 ± 1.90^{a}	34.51 ± 3.09	14.13 ± 2.77^{a}
DSS + PEG–pGLP-2(M)	21.46 ± 4.65^{b}	99.10 ± 8.03	14.48 ± 1.42^{ab}	38.91 ± 4.23	14.22 ± 0.38^{a}
DSS + PEG–pGLP-2(H)	20.63 ± 3.4^{b}	99.56 ± 6.82	13.42 ± 0.80^{ab}	35.87 ± 1.73	11.52 ± 0.64^{b}

Data are expressed as means ± SD; no significant difference exists in that with no letter or the same letters ($p > 0.05$), and different letters ($p < 0.05$) indicate statistically significant difference

CDS of colon

The colonic morphology and CDS of the rats from the five treatments are shown in Fig. 1a–f. Compared with the control treatment, the CDS (Fig. 1f) of colon in rats of DSS group significantly ($p < 0.05$) increased, which was characterised as induced oedema of the intestinal wall, mucous epithelium destruction and multifocal dropouts of entire crypts in a large part of the colon (Fig. 1b). Compared with DSS group, the CDS (Fig. 1f) of colon in rats of DSS + PEG–pGLP-2(L) (Fig. 1c), DSS +

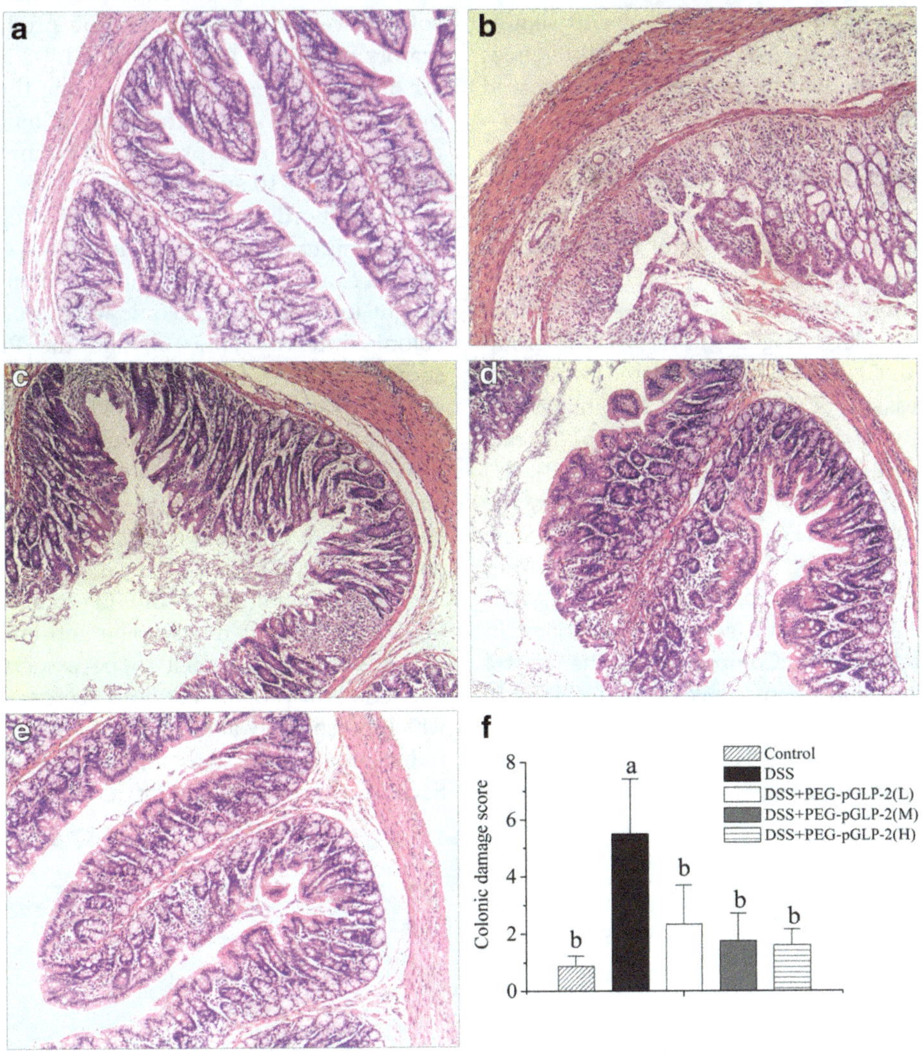

Fig. 1 Effects of PEG-pGLP-2 on the morphology and inflammation score of colon. **a**, **b**, **c**, **d**, **e** is the morphology of colon in group of Control, DSS, DSS + PEG–pGLP-2(L), DSS + PEG–pGLP-2(M), DSS + PEG–pGLP-2(H). Data of the colonic inflammation score (**f**) are expressed as means ± SD and different letters ($p < 0.05$) indicate statistically significant difference

PEG–pGLP-2(M) (Fig. 1d) and DSS + PEG–pGLP-2(H) (Fig. 1e) groups significantly ($p < 0.05$) decreased; such change was characterised as slight oedema of the intestinal wall, reconstruction of the mucous epithelium, increased goblet cells and decreased multifocal dropouts and focal lesions inflammatory cells; particularly, the colon morphological structures of DSS + PEG–pGLP-2(M) (Fig. 1d) and DSS + PEG–pGLP-2(H) (Fig. 1e) group were almost normal with no damage.

Morphology of duodenum

As shown in Table 3, compared with the control treatment, the villi height of duodenum in rats of DSS group significantly ($p < 0.05$) decreased. Compared with DSS group, the villi height of duodenum in rats of DSS + PEG–pGLP-2(L), DSS + PEG–pGLP-2(M) and DSS + PEG–pGLP-2(H) groups significantly ($p < 0.05$) increased, and the ratio of villi height/crypt depth in rats of DSS + PEG–pGLP-2(M) group significantly ($p < 0.05$) increased. No significant differences in crypt depth of duodenum in rats were observed among the five groups.

Expression of TJ and inflammation cytokines in colon

The expression levels of TJ proteins in colon are shown in Fig. 2a–c. Compared with the control treatment, the expression of zonula occludens-1(ZO-1) (Fig. 2a) in rats of DSS group significantly ($p < 0.05$) decreased, whereas the expression of claudin-1 (Fig. 2c) in rats of DSS group significantly ($p < 0.05$) increased. Compared with DSS group, the expression of ZO-1 (Fig. 2a) in rats of DSS + PEG–pGLP-2(H) and occludin (Fig. 2b) in rats of DSS + PEG–pGLP-2(M) and DSS + PEG–pGLP-2(H) groups significantly ($p < 0.05$) increased; moreover, the expression of claudin-1 (Fig. 2c) in rats of DSS + PEG–pGLP-2(M) and DSS + PEG–pGLP-2(H) group significantly ($p < 0.05$) decreased.

The expression levels of inflammatory cytokines in colon are shown in Fig. 2d–i. Compared with the control treatment, the expression of interleukin (IL)-1 (Fig. 2d), IL-7 (Fig. 2f), IL-10 (Fig. 2g), interferon-γ (IFN-γ) (Fig. 2h) and tumour necrosis factor-α (TNF-α) (Fig. 2i) in rats of DSS group significantly ($p < 0.05$) increased. Compared with DSS group, the expression of IL-1 (Fig. 2d), IL-7 (Fig. 2f) and TNF-α (Fig. 2i) in rats of DSS + PEG–pGLP-2(L), DSS + PEG–pGLP-2(M) and DSS + PEG–pGLP-2(H) groups significantly ($p < 0.05$) decreased; the expression of IL-10 (Fig. 2g) in rats of DSS + PEG–pGLP-2(L) and DSS + PEG–pGLP-2(M) groups significantly ($p < 0.05$) decreased; the expression of IFN-γ (Fig. 2h) in rats of DSS + PEG–pGLP-2(M) group significantly ($p < 0.05$) decreased. No significant differences in the expression of IL-6 (Fig. 2e) in colon of rats were observed among the five groups.

Discussion

This study is the first about the therapeutic effects of different doses of PEGylated pGLP-2 on DSS-induced colitis in rats. In this experiment, administration of 12.5, 25 or 100 nmol/kg/d PEG–pGLP-2 for 6 days could reduce the severity of colitis, improve the body weight and colonic weight, and decrease the production of inflammatory cytokines. PEG–p[Gly2]GLP-2 at 12.5 nmol/kg/d for 6 days is effective for recovering the colonic damage by DSS, which is indicated by colonic weight, length, damage score and expression of inflammatory cytokines (IL-1, IL-7, IL-10 and TNF-α).

DSS-induced ulcerative colitis is a reproducible model with symptoms of weight loss and colon shortening. GLP-2 can prevent DSS damage in mice, reverse body weight loss, decrease colonic inflammation and increase colonic integrity [14, 15], and the PEG-pGLP-2 here showed similar effects. There were some intreasting results in this study. First, PEG-pGLP-2 reduced the expression of both inflammation cytokines (IL-1, IL-7, TNF-α) and anti-inflammation cytokines (IL-10). Which was similar to previous reports regarding dextran sulphate-induced colitis [14, 16] and weaning piglets challenged with LPS [4]. Ivory et al. [17] demonstrated the anti-inflammation effects of GLP-2 are IL-10 independent in IL-10 knockout mouse. The anti-inflammatory effects of GLP-2 were assumed to be associated with the increased crypt proliferation and decreased crypt apoptosis, which presumably aid healing of lesions and subsequently reduce the production of inflammatory cytokines [18]. Second, expression of tight junction protein ZO-1 and

Table 3 Effects of PEG-pGLP-2 on morphology of duodenum in colitis rats

Groups	Villus height, μm	Crypt depth, μm	Villus height/Crypt depth
Control	1016.37 ± 49.60^{a}	401.79 ± 57.00	2.22 ± 0.12^{b}
DSS	777.99 ± 104.34^{b}	337.15 ± 30.19	2.28 ± 0.16^{b}
DSS + PEG–pGLP-2(L)	981.46 ± 136.04^{a}	400.76 ± 62.04	2.66 ± 0.49^{ab}
DSS + PEG–pGLP-2(M)	1006.42 ± 98.11^{a}	357.43 ± 52.21	2.98 ± 0.49^{a}
DSS + PEG–pGLP-2(H)	1003.03 ± 96.41^{a}	419.63 ± 51.00	2.39 ± 0.30^{b}

Data are expressed as means ± SD; no significant difference exists in that with no letter or the same letters ($p > 0.05$), and different letters ($p < 0.05$) indicate statistically significant difference

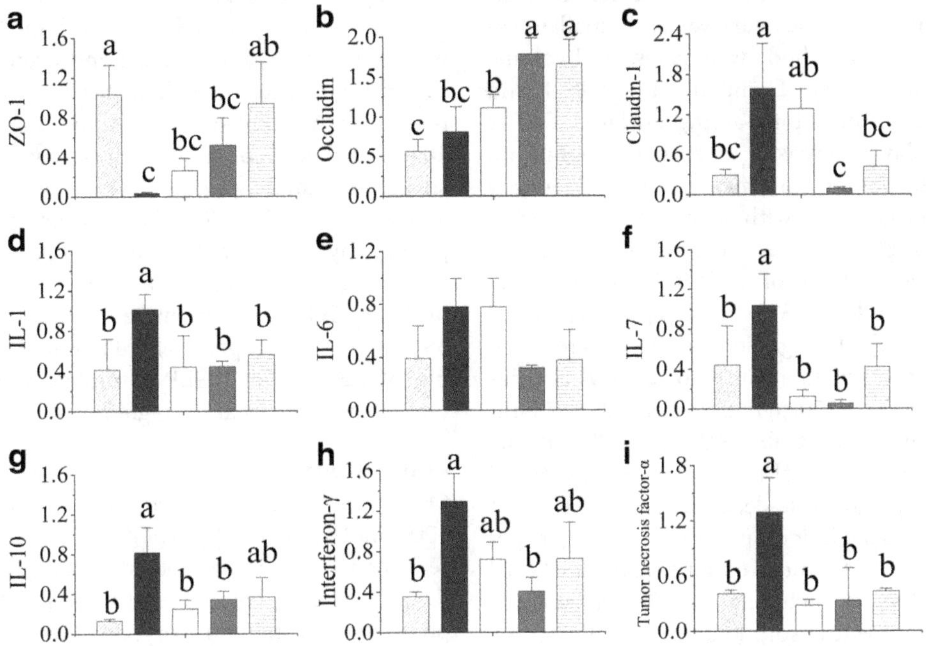

Fig. 2 Effects of PEG-pGLP-2 on the expression levels of tight junction proteins and inflammatory cytokines in colon of colitis rats. **a**, **b**, **c** is the expression levels of ZO-1, Occludin and Claudin-1. **d**, **e**, **f**, **g**, **h**, **i** is the expression levels of IL-1, IL-6, IL-7, IL-10, IFN-γ andTNF-α. Data are expressed as means ± SD; no significant difference exists in that with no letter or the same letters ($p > 0.05$), and different letters ($p < 0.05$) indicate statistically significant difference

Occludin increased while the tight junction protein Claudin-1 decreased. Tight junctions is an important junctional complex in epithelial cells, and contains several unique proteins, namely, claudins, the trans-membrane protein occludin and ZOs [19]. The impact of GLP-2 on the TJ proteins (ZO-1 and occludin) of the jejunum epithelia was confirmed by immunofluorescence staining in ob/ob mice injected with GLP-2 [20]. The different changes of Claudin-1 in tight junction protein could be explained by a possible compensatory role for claudin-1 in the damaged TJ of Poritz et al. [21], which found in dextran sulfate sodium (DSS) model of colonic inflammation, a decrease in ZO-1 but also a counterintuitive increase in claudin-1.

Effects of exogenous GLP-2 or its long-acting analogues on intestinal growth and healing have been studied in different animal models. Early time, the effective dose of GLP-2 is considerably high; Kato et al. [22] demonstrated that GLP-2 can enhance normal rat small intestine mucosal mass and absorption at 50 mg/kg/d for 14 days. The findings of Thymann et al. [8] may explain the above result; they found that animal living environment (normal animal or with disease) and modified GLP-2 are important for the intestinal therapeutic effects for piglets. Thymann et al. [8] also found that the significant effects of GLP-2 improve gut structure and function in weanling pigs only under diarrhoeal conditions and when using long-acting GLP-2 analogues. Thus, the dose of native GLP-2 shows relatively high effect. Nakame et al. [10] found subcutaneous administration of 800 μg/kg/day (224 nmol/kg/d) GLP-2 for 4 days could reduce the severity of NEC and improve the survival rate in rats. In the study of Kaji et al. [9], the continuous infusion of 240 μg/kg/day (67 nmol/kg/d) GLP-2 for 5 days induces intestinal growth and increases weight gain using a total parenteral nutrition (TPN) supported model in the rat. Thymann et al. [8] found that 200 μg/ kg · 12 h (56 nmol/kg · 12 h) GLP-2 for 7 days only increases goblet cell density, but shows limited effects on diarrhoea. No differences exist between two regimens (continuous GLP-2 infusion versus three daily GLP-2 injections) of 1 mg/day GLP-2 for 21 days on intestinal absorption in SBS patients [23]. Infusion of 100 μg/kg/d GLP-2 for 7 days augments adaptive growth and digestive capacity of the residual small intestine in a rat model of mid–small bowel resection [24]. Injection duration is also a major factor influencing the therapeutic effects. Sigalet et al. showed that chronic treatment of weaning pigs with GLP-2 at 40 μg/kg/day given by s.c. injection twice daily for 42 days increases the overall villus height and crypt depth; no effects were observed on activity, appetite, behaviour or food intake in weaning pigs [11].

However, when the peptide chain is changed or modified, the effective dose of GLP-2 is considerably low. L'Heureux and Brubaker (2003) used 40 μg/kg · q12 h

(11.5 nmol/kg · 12 h) human [Gly^2] GLP-2 for 10 consecutive days, which increases survival and small intestinal weight, and decreases body weight loss and colonic damage in DSS-mice [18]. Thymann et al. [8] found that 25 μg/ kg · 12 h of a long-acting acylated GLP-2 analogue for 5 days increases intestinal weight and activity of brush border enzymes in a low-sanitary environment. Pretreatment with a long-acting DPPIV inhibitor K579 (1 mg/kg, ig) for 1 day prevents the formation and promotes healing of IND-induced intestinal ulcers, although high-dose K579 (3 mg/kg) reverses the preventive effect [25]. Teduglutide, a DPP-IV-resistant GLP-2 analogue given subcutaneously for 21 days at three dose levels (30, 100 and 150 μg/kg/day), significantly increases intestinal wet weight absorption in SBS patients [26]. In the study of a neonatal piglet jejunostomy model by Thymann et al. [27], a dose-dependent (0.01, 0.02, 0.1 or 0.2 mg/kg/day teduglutide) increase in weight per length of the remnant intestine is obtained, but functional and structural endpoints, including digestive enzyme activity and enteral nutrient absorption, are not affected by treatments. XTEN is a long, unstructured, non-repetitive, hydrophilic sequence of amino acids. With the fusion of XTEN to the C-terminus of GLP2-2G, the serum half-life of GLP2-2G-XTEN in rats is 38 h, and 25 nmol/kg/day GLP2-2G-XTEN for 12 days significantly increases the length, reduces the number of trans-ulcerations and adhesions, and reduces the TNF-α content of the small intestine in rat indomethacin-induced disease model [28].

PEGylated pGLP-2, a site-specific mono-PEGylated derivative, was designed and purified by our team. This derivative exhibits longer half-life than native pGLP-2 in vitro and can reduce the severity of colonic injury in murine colitis [2]. We demonstrated that 10 nmol/kg/d PEG–pGLP-2 infusion alleviates the severity of intestinal injury in weaning piglets challenged with LPS by reducing the secretion of inflammatory cytokines and increasing the villus height/crypt depth ratio [3]. To provide references for the intestinal injury of weaned pigs by PEG–p[Gly^2]GLP-2, the pharmacokinetics of PEG–p[Gly^2]GLP-2 was conducted. The results showed that the half-life of p[Gly^2]GLP-2 and PEG–p[Gly^2]GLP-2 is 49 and 202 min in rat, respectively, which is longer than the half-life of intact pGLP-2 (8.4 min) [1]. PEGylated p[Gly^2]GLP-2 significantly improves the pharmacological profiles; increases half-time, peak time and mean residence time; decreases reduce clearance rate; and improves bioavailability [7]. Lee et al. [29] used a similar methodology to project the half-life of the GLP-1fusion; PEG(2 k)-Lys-GLP-1 improves the half-life with a 16- and 3.2-fold increase for intravenous and subcutaneous administrations, respectively.

The present study mainly aims to provide the dose reference for application of PEG-pGLP-2 in weaned pig. The effective dose of GLP-2 in pig is relatively low. Both low (2 nmol/kg BW/day) or high (10 nmol/kg BW/day) dose of human [Gly2]GLP-2_{1-34} 2 for 7 days improves the growth of weaned piglets and protects them against LPS-induced intestinal damage [12]. TPN-fed neonatal piglets with infused iv at three rates (2.5, 5.0 and 10.0 nmol/kg/d) of GLP-2 for 7 days exhibit increased small intestinal weight, DNA and protein content, and villus height [30]. This observation may be explained by the long half-life in different animals. Alters et al. [28] demonstrated that the serum half-life of GLP2-2G-XTEN in mice, rats and monkeys is 34, 38 and 120 h, respectively. Therefore, the longer half-life of PEG–p[Gly2]GLP-2 implies a lower total dose requirement in weaned piglet.

Conclusions

Our results demonstrated three doses (12.5, 25 or 100 nmol/kg/d) of PEG–pGLP-2, a long-acting pGLP-2, reduces the ulcerative colitis in male rats by recovering the body weight, colonic length, colonic damage score and production of inflammatory cytokines. PEG–pGLP-2 is a novel and potentially effective therapy for intestinal healing in a relatively low molar dose (12.5 nmol/kg/d).

Abbreviations

CDS: Colonic damage score; DPP-IV: Dipeptidyl peptidase-IV; DSS: Dextran sodium sulphate; IL: Interleukin; PEG–pGLP-2: Polyethylene glycosylated porcine glucagon-like peptide-2; $t_{1/2}$: Half-life; TJ: Tight junction; ZO-1: Zonula occludens-1

Acknowledgements

None.

Funding

This work was supported by a grant from the earmarked fund for the Modern Agro-Industry Technology Research System (Grant no. CARS-36) and Natural Science Funds of Zhejiang Province (Grant no. LY15C170002).

Authors' contributions

KKQ, JJL and JW performed the research; KKQ designed the research, analyzed the data, and wrote the paper; ZWX revised the manuscript critically. All authors read and approved the final manuscript.

Competing interests

The authors declare that they have no competing interests.

References

1. Pedersen NB, Hjollund KR, Johnsen AH, Orskov C, Rosenkilde MM, et al. Porcine glucagon-like peptide-2: structure, signaling, metabolism and effects. Regul Pept. 2008;146:310–20.
2. Qi KK, Wu J, Wan J, Men XM, Xu ZW. Purified PEGylated porcine glucagon-like peptide-2 reduces the severity of colonic injury in a murine model of experimental colitis. Peptides. 2014;52:11–8.
3. Qi KK, Wu J, Xu ZW. Effects of PEGylated porcine glucagon-like peptide-2 therapy in weaning piglets challenged with lipopolysaccharide. Peptides. 2014;58:7–13.
4. Qi KK, Wu J, Deng B, Li YM, Xu ZW. PEGylated porcine glucagon-like

peptide-2 improved the intestinal digestive function and prevented inflammation of weaning piglets challenged with LPS. Animal. 2015;9:481–9.
5. Seidner DL, Joly F, Youssef NN. Effect of teduglutide, a glucagon-like peptide 2 analog, on citrulline levels in patients with short bowel syndrome in two phase III randomized trials. Clin Transl Gastroenterol. 2015;6:e93.
6. Marier JF, Mouksassi MS, Gosselin NH, Beliveau M, Cyran J, et al. Population pharmacokinetics of teduglutide following repeated subcutaneous administrations in healthy participants and in patients with short bowel syndrome and Crohn's disease. J Clin Pharmacol. 2010;50:36–49.
7. Lv JJ, Wu J, Qi KK, Xu ZW. Pharmacokinetics studies in rats of porcine glucagon-like peptide-2 and its long-acting forms. Chin J Anim Nutr. 2016; 28:2650–6.
8. Thymann T, Le Huerou-Luron I, Petersen YM, Hedemann MS, Elinf J, et al. Glucagon-like peptide 2 treatment may improve intestinal adaptation during weaning. J Anim Sci. 2014;92:2070–9.
9. Kaji T, Tanaka H, Holst JJ, Redstone H, Wallace L, et al. The effects of variations in dose and method of administration on glucagon like peptide-2 activity in the rat. Eur J Pharmacol. 2008;596:138–45.
10. Nakame K, Kaji T, Mukai M, Shinyama S, Matsufuji H. The protective and anti-inflammatory effects of glucagon-like peptide-2 in an experimental rat model of necrotizing enterocolitis. Peptides. 2016;75:1–7.
11. Sigalet DL, de Heuvel E, Wallace L, Bulloch E, Turner J, et al. Effects of chronic glucagon-like peptide-2 therapy during weaning in neonatal pigs. Regul Pept. 2014;188:70–80.
12. Deng QH, Jia G, Zhao H, Chen ZL, Chen XL, et al. The prolonged effect of glucagon-like peptide 2 pretreatment on growth performance and intestinal development of weaned piglets. J Anim Sci Biotechnol. 2016;7:28.
13. Dieleman LA, Palmen MJ, Akol H, Bloemena E, Peña AS, Meuwissen SG, Van Rees EP. Chronic experimental colitis induced by dextran sulphate sodium (DSS) is characterized by Th1 and Th2 cytokines. Clin Exp Immunol. 1998; 114:385–91.
14. Drucker DJ, Yusta B, Boushey RP, Deforest L, Brubaker PL. Human [gly2]glp-2 reduces the severity of colonic injury in a murine model of experimental colitis. Am J Physiol. 1999;276(1):79–91.
15. Sigalet DL, Wallace LE, Holst JJ, Martin GR, Kaji T, Tanaka H, Sharkey KA. Enteric neuralpathways mediate the anti-inflammatory actions of glucagon-like peptide 2. Am J Physiol Gastrointest Liver Physiol. 2007;293:G211–21.
16. Wu J, Qi KK, Xu ZW, Wan J. Glucagon-like peptide-2-loaded microspheres as treatment for ulcerative colitis in the murine model. J Microencapsul. 2015; 32(6):598–607.
17. Ivory CP, Wallace LE, Mccafferty DM, Sigalet DL. Interleukin-10-independent anti-inflammatory actions of glucagon-like peptide 2. Am J Physiol Gastrointest Liver Physiol. 2008;295(6):1202–10.
18. L'Heureux MC, Brubaker PL. GLP-2 and DSS glucagon-like peptide-2 and common therapeutics in a murine model of ulcerative colitis. J Pharmacol Exp Ther. 2003;306:347–54.
19. Yu CS, Jia G, Jiang Y, Deng QH, Chen ZL, Xu ZW. Effect of glucagon-like peptide 2 on tight junction in jejunal epithelium of weaned pigs though MAPK signaling pathway. Asian Australas J Anim. 2014;27(5):733–42.
20. Cani PD, Possemiers S, Van de Wiele T, Guiot Y, Everard A, Rottier O, Geurts L, Naslain D, Neyrinck A, Lambert DM, Muccioli GG, Delzenne NM. Changes in gut microbiota control inflammation in obese mice through a mechanism involving GLP-2-driven improvement of gut permeability. Gut. 2009;58(8):1091–103.
21. Poritz LS, Garver KI, Green C, Fitzpatrick L, Ruggiero F, Koltun WA. Loss of the tight junction protein ZO-1 in dextran sulfate sodium induced colitis. J Surg Res. 2007;140:12–9.
22. Kato Y, Yu D, Schwartz MZ. GLP-2 Glucagonlike peptide-2 enhances small intestinal absorptive function and mucosal mass in vivo. J Pediatr Surg. 1999;34:18–20.
23. Naimi RM, Madsen KB, Askov-Hansen C, Brandt CF, Hartmann B, et al. A dose-equivalent comparison of the effects of continuous subcutaneous glucagon-like peptide 2 (GLP-2) infusions versus meal related GLP-2 injections in the treatment of short bowel syndrome (SBS) patients. Regul Pept. 2013;184:47–53.
24. Koopmann MC, Nelson DW, Murali SG, Liu X, Brownfield MS, et al. Exogenous glucagon-like peptide-2 (GLP-2) augments GLP-2 receptor mRNA and maintains proglucagon mRNA levels in resected rats. J Parenter Enteral Nutr. 2008;32:254–65.
25. Inoue T, Higashiyama M, Kaji I, Rudenkyy S, Higuchi K, et al. Dipeptidyl peptidase IV inhibition prevents the formation and promotes the healing of indomethacin-induced intestinal ulcers in rats. Dig Dis Sci. 2014;59:1286–95.
26. Jeppesen PB, Sanguinetti EL, Buchman A, Howard L, Scolapio JS, et al. Teduglutide(ALX-0600), a dipeptidyl peptidase IV resistant glucagon-like peptide 2 analogue, improves intestinal function in short bowel syndrome patients. Gut. 2005;54:1224–31.
27. Thymann T, Stoll B, Mecklenburg L, Burrin DG, Vegge A, et al. Acute effects of the glucagon-like peptide 2 analogue, teduglutide, on intestinal adaptation in short bowel syndrome. J Pediatr Gastroenterol Nutr. 2014;58: 694–702.
28. Alters SE, McLaughlin B, Spink B, Lachinyan T, Wang CW, et al. GLP2-2G-XTEN: a pharmaceutical protein with improved serum half-life and efficacy in a rat Crohn's. PLoS One. 2013;7(11):e50630.
29. Lee SH, Lee S, Youn YS, Na DH, Chae SY, et al. Synthesis, characterization, and pharmacokinetic studies of PEGylated glucagon-like peptide-1. Bioconjug Chem. 2005;16:377–82.
30. Burrin DG, Stoll B, Guan X, Cui L, Chang X, et al. Glucagon-like peptide 2 dose-dependently activates intestinal cell survival and proliferation in neonatal piglets. Endocrinology. 2005;146:22–32.

16

Prevalence of overlap syndromes and symptoms in pediatric functional dyspepsia

Craig A. Friesen[1*], John M. Rosen[1] and Jennifer V. Schurman[2]

Abstract

Background: The purpose was to evaluate the overlap frequency of irritable bowel syndrome (IBS), gastroesophageal reflux disease (GERD), and overactive bladder syndrome (OBS), as well as other gastrointestinal and systemic symptoms, in functional dyspepsia (FD). Additionally, we sought to determine whether adult Rome III FD subtypes were uniquely related to overlap syndromes or symptoms.

Methods: The study was a retrospective review of 100 consecutive pediatric patients, age 8–17 years, diagnosed with FD. All had completed a standardized medical history including gastrointestinal and systemic symptoms as well as specific symptoms related to GERD and OBS. The frequency of overlap with IBS, GERD, and OBS were determined for the whole group and for those fulfilling adult FD subtype criteria. Individual symptoms were also compared by FD subtype.

Results: Overlap IBS was present in 33 % of the FD patients. At least one GERD symptom was present in 74 % of patients with 41 % reporting heartburn. At least one OBS symptom was present in 44 % of patients with 29 % reporting urinary urgency. Other than pain, the most common reported gastrointestinal symptom was nausea (86 %). Systemic symptoms were common. Overlap syndromes/symptoms did not vary by FD subtype. Postprandial distress syndrome was associated with pain with eating, weight loss, and waking at night to have a stool.

Conclusions: FD is a heterogeneous condition in children and adolescents with significant variability in the presence of gastrointestinal and non-gastrointestinal symptoms and overlap syndromes. Varying symptom profiles need to be accounted for and analyzed in studies involving subjects with FD.

Keywords: Functional dyspepsia, Irritable bowel syndrome, Gastroesophageal reflux, Overactive bladder syndrome

Background

There are a number of pain-associated functional gastrointestinal disorders (FGIDs) defined by Rome III for children/adolescents, namely irritable bowel syndrome (IBS), functional dyspepsia (FD), abdominal migraines, functional abdominal pain, and functional abdominal pain syndrome [1]. In adults, there are two recognized FD subtypes, postprandial distress syndrome (PDS; defined by the presence of early satiety preventing completing a normal size meal or fullness following a normal sized meal) and epigastric pain syndrome (EPS; defined by the presence of pain or burning localized to the epigastrium) [2] These subtypes are not recognized in the pediatric Rome III criteria, although there is some evidence of their existence and indication that the distinction may be clinically meaningful in youth as well [3, 4]. For example, PDS-related symptoms (i.e., early satiety and/or bloating following a meal) have been associated with increased mucosal mast cells, anxiety, and depression in pediatric FD [4].

Most children and adolescents with chronic abdominal pain fulfill criteria for an FGID with FD and IBS being the two most common [1, 5, 6]. These diagnoses form the entry criteria for most abdominal pain studies and therapeutic trials. Utilization of these criteria for research (or clinical practice) presents challenges given some inherent ambiguity in the criteria, inconsistent application of the criteria, and differences in symptom reports between the patients and their parents or guardians [7]. Additionally, there may be overlap between FGIDs or overlap between FGIDs and other

* Correspondence: cfriesen@cmh.edu
[1]Division of Gastroenterology, Hepatology, and Nutrition, Children's Mercy Kansas City, 2401 Gillham Road, Kansas City, MO 64108, USA
Full list of author information is available at the end of the article

symptoms or conditions which may influence study results or therapeutic response. For adults, FD is well known to overlap with IBS, as well as other conditions such as gastroesophageal reflux disease (GERD) and overactive bladder syndrome (OBS) [8–11]. Overlap syndromes may be associated with greater psychopathology and electromechanical dysfunction [12, 13]. We have previously found that FD/IBS overlap accounts for 30 % of youth presenting for initial evaluation of chronic abdominal pain [6]. This represents another area of variability in utilization of Rome criteria as some investigators diagnose overlap FD/IBS while others presumably default to IBS when symptoms of both are present [7]. Overlap with GERD and OBS has been largely unstudied in a pediatric population. It is important to determine to what degree, if any, individual FGIDs overlap with other syndromes or symptoms in order to understand variability within a diagnostic category which may affect study results or patient outcomes.

The purpose of the current study was to evaluate the frequency of overlap IBS, potential GERD-related symptoms, and OBS-related symptoms, as well as other gastrointestinal and systemic symptoms, in a clinical sample of youth with FD. Additionally, we sought to determine the frequency of PDS and EPS in youth with FD, and whether these subtypes were uniquely related to overlap syndromes or other symptoms.

Methods

Study design

The current study was a retrospective chart review of pediatric patients who were identified as being diagnosed with FD after being seen for initial evaluation of chronic abdominal pain in a subspecialty abdominal pain clinic housed within a large Midwestern children's hospital between September, 2014 and June, 2015. All data described below were collected as part of standard care and were abstracted from the medical record and entered into a research database for analysis in the current study. The study was approved by the institutional review board at Children's Mercy Kansas City.

Study cohort and exclusion criteria

All patients selected for inclusion had been evaluated in a single subspecialty abdominal pain clinic. Patients were 8–17 years, inclusive, and reported pain at least weekly for a minimum of 8 weeks per standard entry criteria for the clinic. The diagnosis of FD was determined according to Rome III criteria by a single board-certified pediatric gastroenterologist based on an extensive history and physical examination conducted with each child and family during the initial clinic visit [1]. All patients had undergone upper endoscopy with biopsy after failing to respond to acid reduction therapy of at least 2 weeks duration. All were without gross pathology (including nodularity, erosions, and ulceration. Per standard protocol at the participating hospital, all patients had at least 2 biopsies obtained from each of the lower one-third of the esophagus and the gastric antrum and at least four biopsies from the duodenum for histologic evaluation. All patients were negative for *Helicobacter pylori* on antral biopsy. Mild histologic esophagitis (peak eosinophils < 5/hpf) and/or mild chronic gastritis did not exclude the patient from selection. Patients diagnosed with other pathology, including eosinophilic gastroenteritis, celiac disease, inflammatory bowel disease, or giardiasis, were excluded from the study cohort. Eosinophilic gastritis and duodenitis were diagnosed at the discretion of the evaluating board-certified pathologist as no widely accepted criteria exist regarding eosinophil density.

Data sources

Pathology

As a prerequisite for inclusion in the study cohort, patients had to have previous biopsies to evaluate for the presence of histologic esophagitis as assessed by a board certified pediatric pathologist as part of routine care. The pathology report provided the histologic data for analysis.

Gastrointestinal and systemic symptoms

All patients seen for initial evaluation in the abdominal pain clinic from which the sample was selected had completed a standardized medical history. This medical history included questions regarding the presence of upper abdominal pain or discomfort, as well as any relation to a change in stool frequency or consistency or a history of relief from stooling. In addition, specific locations of the pain were obtained by asking the patient to mark pain locations on a diagram of the abdomen. The nature of the pain (e.g. burning, crampy) was asked of each patient. Patients were specifically asked whether pain wakes them at night and whether pain increases after a meal. Patients also were asked about the presence of nausea and/or vomiting and whether nausea increases after a meal. Relevant to the issue of FD subtyping, patients were asked specifically about the presence of early satiety and postprandial bloating [2].

Patients also are asked about the presence of a number of other gastrointestinal and systemic symptoms. Gastrointestinal symptoms that are assessed include the presence of stool symptoms such as loose stools, hard stools, mucus in stools, blood in stools, and waking at night to have a stool, as well as the presence of excessive gas. Systemic symptoms that are assessed include hayfever, fatigue, headache, fainting, dizziness, chest pain, muscle pain, joint pain, mouth sores, weight loss, and fever. In addition to the above, patients are asked about the presence of 4 symptoms related to gastroesophageal reflux (bitter, salty, or sour taste in mouth; excessive belching or burping; regurgitation; heartburn) and 3 symptoms related to overactive bladder syndrome (increased frequency of urination; waking during the night to urinate; sudden urge to urinate).

Information from the medical history, once abstracted and entered into the research database, was used to evaluate dyspeptic symptoms and assign an FD subtype based on adult Rome III criteria. Patients were defined as having postprandial distress syndrome if they endorsed early satiety or postprandial bloating [2]. Patients were defined as having epigastric pain syndrome if they endorsed burning or pain localized only to the epigastric region [2]. Diagnoses of potentially overlapping symptoms and conditions (i.e., IBS, GERD, OBS) also were assigned based on symptom information abstracted from the patient's medical history.

Table 1 Frequency of specific gastrointestinal and systemic symptoms in FD patients

Symptom	% Reporting Symptom
Waking at night with pain	64
Pain increased with eating	68
Increased appetite	4
Decreased appetite	61
Nausea	86
Vomiting	32
Early satiety	74
Postprandial bloating	62
Fatigue	47
Headache	66
Dizziness	53
Weight loss	30
Muscle pain	28
Joint pain	26

Statistical analysis

Statistical analysis was performed using SPSS Version 20 (SPSS Inc, Chicago, IL). Frequencies were determined for individual symptoms and diagnoses. The frequencies of individual reflux symptoms were compared between patients with and without mild histologic esophagitis by chi-square analysis or Fisher's exact tests, as appropriate given cell frequencies. The frequencies of an IBS diagnosis, reflux symptoms, and overactive bladder symptoms, respectively, were compared between genders, between patients <13 years of age and those ≥13 years of age, and between patients with and without PDS by chi-square analysis or Fisher's exact tests, as appropriate given cell frequencies. A p value of <0.05 was considered statistically significant for all of the analyses. Given the exploratory nature of the current study, trends were reported for p values >0.05 but <0.07.

Results

Demographics of the study cohort

One hundred patients ranging in age from 8 to 17 years with a mean age of 13 years 9 months were evaluated. Seventy-six percent were female. Pain was reported to occur daily in 76 %, several times/week in 19 %, and weekly in 5 % of patients. Pain was described as intermittent by 60 % and continuous by 40 % of patients. For patients reporting nausea ($n = 86$), the nausea occurred daily in 36 % and at least weekly in 76 %. Sixty-three percent reported that nausea increased with eating. Frequencies of other selected gastrointestinal symptoms and systemic symptoms are shown in Table 1. All patients had failed to respond clinically to acid reduction therapy. Forty percent were treated with ranitidine (>6 mg/Kg/day up to 150 mg twice daily) and 72 % were treated with a proton pump inhibitor (PPI; >1 mg/Kg/day up to 40 mg twice daily for omeprazole, pantoprazole, and esomeprazole and up to 30 mg twice daily for lansoprazole). Twelve percent received courses of both ranitidine and a PPI. Of those treated with a PPI, 32 % received twice daily dosing and 21 % received multiple courses of different PPIs. As a requirement, all patients underwent upper endoscopy with biopsies. No patients had a previous upper gastrointestinal barium study, gastric emptying study, or pH-impedance study. No patients reported previous food allergy testing and while some patients were avoiding specific foods, none had been on a full elimination diet.

FD subtypes

Seventy-two percent of patients met criteria for PDS. Bloating was reported by 62 % and early satiety by 74 % of all FD patients. Of those endorsing early satiety, 85 % reported that it prevented finishing a regular meal. While 52 % of all patients reported epigastric pain or burning, only 3 % localized this pain and/or burning only to the epigastrium as required to fulfill criteria for EPS. Twenty-five percent of patients met criteria for FD but not PDS or EPS subtypes.

Overlap syndromes/symptoms in FD

One-third (33 %) of FD patients also fulfilled criteria for IBS. Frequencies for GERD-related symptoms are shown in Table 2. At least one symptom was reported by 74 %, 2 or more symptoms by 49 %, 3 or more symptoms by 29 %, and all 4 symptoms by 6 % of patients. Patients with mild histologic esophagitis reported higher frequencies compared to those with normal histology for bitter/

Table 2 Frequency of overlap syndromes and symptoms in FD patients

Syndrome/Symptom	% of patients
IBS	33
GERD: bitter, salty, or sour taste	35
GERD: excessive belching or burping	30
GERD: regurgitation	57
GERD: heartburn	41
OBS: increased frequency of urination	13
OBS: waking at night to urinate	33
OBS: sudden urge to urinate	29

salty taste (52 vs. 29 %; $p = .046$), belching/burping (62 vs. 22 %; $p = .001$), regurgitation (64 vs. 54 %; $p = .042$), and heartburn (71 vs. 32 %; $p = .001$). Frequencies for OBS-related symptoms are shown in Table 2. Of the patients reporting night time urination, 67 % reported that this occurred at least weekly. At least one symptom was reported by 44 %, 2 or more symptoms by 23 %, and all 3 symptoms by 8 %. No differences were found in the frequencies of overlap relative to age or gender with one exception. Specifically, IBS overlap was more common in females 13 years of age and older as compared to younger females (36 vs. 13 %; $p = .037$).

Overlap syndromes/symptoms by FD subtype

Patients fulfilling criteria for PDS (as compared to those who did not) were more likely to report pain with eating (79 vs. 43 %; $p = .001$), weight loss (36 vs. 14 %; $p = .026$), and waking at night to have a stool (27 vs. 7 %; $p = .025$). There also were trends for patients with PDS to be more likely to report nausea with eating (70 vs. 50 %; $p = .052$), pain relief with a stool (39 vs. 21 %; $p = .069$), mucus in the stool (17 vs. 4 %; $p = .067$), and increased gas (44 vs. 25 %; $p = .066$). Although other gastrointestinal and systemic symptoms were found to be relatively common in the broader group of patients with FD, no other correlations emerged between these symptoms and the PDS subtype. PDS also did not have any significant associations with any GERD-related or OBS-related symptoms. Associations with overlap syndromes/symptoms were not examined for EPS given the low base rate (3 %) in the study cohort.

Discussion

The current study indicates that FD is a heterogeneous condition in children and adolescents. There is significant variability in the presence of gastrointestinal, as well as non-gastrointestinal, symptoms. It is important to understand this variability within diagnostic categories, and also within individual patients as each patient appears to have a somewhat unique symptom profile within the broad category of FD.

Overlap IBS was present in 33 % of the FD patients in the current study. Previously we found IBS overlap in 54 % of patients fulfilling FD criteria [6]. Consistent with these pediatric findings, IBS overlap has been reported in 33–56 % of adults with FD [14–16]. In adults, IBS occurs more often in those with FD (37 %) as compared to those without FD (7 %) [12]. IBS has been found to be more common with the PDS subtype in some, but not all, studies in adults [12, 15]. We found no association between overlapping IBS and PDS; however, the PDS subtype patients were more likely to report the individual symptom of waking at night to have a stool. There was also a trend towards increased reporting of pain improvement with a stool in the PDS subgroup. Associations with EPS could not be assessed given the low EPS frequency. In adults, FD/IBS overlap patients were more likely to be female. (13) We did not find any main effect of gender in our pediatric cohort, however, females 13 years of age and older were more likely to report overlap than were younger females (12 years of age and under).

Evaluating for the presence of GERD overlap in youth with FD presents a challenge, as there is no gold standard test for GERD. Symptoms and available tests lack high sensitivity or specificity. However, the North American Society for Pediatric Gastroenterology, Hepatology, and Nutrition guidelines concluded, based on expert opinion, that the diagnosis of GERD can be made in adolescents with typical heartburn symptoms [17]. Heartburn is considered to be a reasonably sensitive indicator of GERD in adults [18]. Heartburn was reported by 41 % of the patients in the current study. Although a definitive statement isn't possible, our data suggest that reflux-like symptoms are common in youth with FD. The correlation between reflux-like symptoms and mild histologic esophagitis adds some support for these symptoms being related to GERD in at least some patients. Reported prevalence of GERD in adults with FD has ranged from 13.3 to 56 %, with the prevalence being near 50 % in most studies [12]. This overlap appears to be greater in those patients with non-erosive GERD (NERD) and, within this group, overlap is greatest among those with heartburn [8, 9]. It has been suggested that heartburn should be considered an integral part of the dyspepsia complex in adults [19].

Overactive bladder symptoms were common in FD patients in the current study, with at least one symptom present in 44 %. In adults, OAB is defined as a symptom complex of urinary urgency usually with urinary frequency and nocturia [10]. The hallmark of OAB in children is urgency. (20) In the current study, urgency was reported by 29 % of the patients. This is similar to the

20.5 % prevalence of OAB in adults with FD [11]. Pathophysiologic processes implicated in OAB are similar to those that appear relevant to FD (and IBS) including nerve hypersensitivity and mucosal mast cells [20–22].

The FD subtypes, PDS and EPS, are well recognized in adults but were not included in the pediatric FD criteria [1]. In adults, some studies have shown good separation of PDS and EPS while others have reported significant overlap of the two subtypes [23]. It appears that separation is better in the general population than in patients who seek medical care [24]. In one pediatric study, Turco and colleagues evaluated 100 pediatric patients with FD and found EPS alone in 17 %, PDS alone in 47 %, and overlap in 36 %; however, many of these patients crossed over their diagnosis between PDS and EPS over time [3]. In the current study, 72 % of our pediatric cohort met criteria for PDS, while only 3 % met criteria for EPS. Similar to our previous findings regarding EPS, 52 % of the patients in the current study reported epigastric pain or burning, but only 3 % localized this pain exclusively to the epigastrium, a requirement for diagnosing EPS under the Rome III adult criteria [4].

Adult data suggests that meal-related symptoms, including pain and nausea, may be the norm in FD [25]. The PDS subtype did have some associations with other GI symptoms in our pediatric cohort, including increased pain with eating (79 %) and weight loss (36 %), as well as a trend toward increased nausea with eating (70 %). Thus, the consequences of eating may be more widespread than just early satiety. In adult studies, nausea has been reported by 39–65 % of FD patients [24]. Overall, nausea was reported by 86 % of pediatric patients in the current study with 70 % reporting an increase in nausea with eating. In another pediatric abdominal pain study, nausea was reported by 87 % of subjects who met adult criteria for FD [26]. Thus, nausea appears to be a common component of FD in both adults and youth. However, nausea may be more associated with PDS than EPS in children [3]. Nausea is important to consider as it is associated with poor school functioning and greater social disability [26]. These meal related symptoms may also be associated with nutritional consequences. As noted above, weight loss was common in the current study being reported by 36 % of PDS patients. This is similar to adults where weight loss correlates most strongly with early satiety [27].

The main strength of the current study is the relatively large population size with symptom reporting performed in a standardized fashion across a wide array of gastrointestinal and non-gastrointestinal symptoms. The main limitation is that the study design did not allow evaluation of the natural history of these symptoms. It is known that symptoms may evolve across time and patients may change FD subtype classification [3].

Conclusions

In sum, pediatric FD is a heterogeneous syndrome exhibiting variable symptoms from patient to patient with many, but not all, fulfilling criteria for PDS. The clinical presentation of FD also varies with regard to non-FD symptoms, exhibiting significant overlap with IBS as well as symptoms consistent with GERD and OBS. These varying symptom profiles need to be considered in providing care to FD patients. For example, an FD patient with overlap may have a different pathogenic process or respond differently to a treatment regimen than a patient with FD alone or FD with overlap GERD. Likewise, varying symptom profiles need to be accounted for and analyzed in studies involving subjects with FD. Clinical trials need to be designed to fit the patients that are actually encountered, rather than the clean diagnostic boxes we create.

Abbreviations

EPS, epigastric pain syndrome; FD, functional dyspepsia; FGID, functional gastrointestinal disorder; GERD, gastroesophageal reflux disease; hpf, high power field; IBS, irritable bowel syndrome; OBS, overactive bladder syndrome; PDS, postprandial distress syndrome

Funding

There was no funding for this study.

Authors' contributions

CAF contributed to study design, data collection and analysis, manuscript writing, and final editing. JMR contributed to study design, data analysis, manuscript writing, and final editing. JVS contributed to study design, data analysis, manuscript writing, and final editing. All authors have read and approved the final version of the manuscript.

Competing interests

The authors declare that they have no competing interests.

Author details

Division of Gastroenterology, Hepatology, and Nutrition, Children's Mercy Kansas City, 2401 Gillham Road, Kansas City, MO 64108, USA. [2]Division of Developmental and Behavioral Sciences, Children's Mercy Kansas City, 2401 Gillham Road, Kansas City, MO 64108, USA.

References

1. Rasquin A, Di Lorenzo C, Forbes D, Guiraldes E, Hyams JS, Staiano A, Walker LS. Childhood functional gastrointestinal disorders: child/adolescent. Gastroenterology. 2006;130:1527–37.
2. Tack J, Talley NJ, Camilleri M, Holtmann G, Hu P, Malagelada JR, Stanghellini V. Functional gastroduodenal disorders. Gastroenterology. 2006;130:1466–79.
3. Turco R, Russo M, Martinelli M, Castiello R, Coppola V, Miele E, Staiano A. Do distinct functional dyspepsia subtypes exist in children? J Pediatr Gastroenterol Nutr 2015; doi: 10.1098/MPG.0000000000000944.
4. Schurman JV, Singh M, Singh V, Neilan N, Friesen CA. Symptoms and subtypes in pediatric functional dyspepsia: relation to mucosal inflammation and psychological functioning. J Pediatr Gastroenterol Nutr. 2010;51:298–303.
5. Walker L, Lipani TA, Greene JW, Caines K, Stutts J, Polk DB, Caplan A, Rasquin-Weber A. Recurrent abdominal pain: symptom subtypes based on the Rome II criteria for pediatric functional gastrointestinal disorders. J Pediatr Gastroenterol Nutr. 2004;38:187–91.

6. Schurman JV, Friesen CA, Danda CE, Andre L, Welchert E, Lavenbarg T, Cocjin JT, Hyman PE. Diagnosing functional abdominal pain with Rome III criteria: parent, child, and clinician agreement. J Pediatr Gastroenterol Nutr. 2005;41:291–5.
7. Friesen CA, Schurman JV, Abdel-Rahman SM. Present state and future challenges in pediatric abdominal pain therapeutics research: Looking beyond the forest. World J Gastrointest Pharmacol Ther. 2015;6:96–104.
8. Quigley EM, Lacy BE. Overlap of functional dyspepsia and GERD- diagnostic and treatment implications. Nat Rev Gastroenterol Hepatol. 2013;10:175–86.
9. Yarandi SS, Christie J. Functional dyspepsia in review: Pathophysiology and challenges in the diagnosis and management due to coexisting gastroesophageal reflux disease and irritable bowel syndrome. Gastroenterol Res Pract. 2013;2013:351086.
10. Homma Y, Yoshida M, Seki N, Yokoyama O, Kakizaki H, Gotoh M, Yamanishi T, Yamaguchi O, Takeda M, Nishizawa O. Symptom assessment tool for overactive bladder syndrome- overactive bladder symptom score. Urology. 2006;68:318–23.
11. Matsuzaki J, Suzuki H, Fukushima Y, Hirata K, Fukuhara S, Okada S, Hibi T. High frequency of overlap between functional dyspepsia and overactive bladder. Neurogastroenterol Motil. 2012;24:821–7.
12. Fujiwara Y, Arakawa T. Overlap in patients with dyspepsia/functional dyspepsia. J Neurogastroenterol Motil. 2014;20:447–57.
13. Corsetti M, Caenepeel P, Fischler B, Janssens J, Tack J. Impact of coexisting irritable bowel syndrome on symptoms and pathophysiological mechanisms in functional dyspepsia. Am J Gastroenterol. 2004;99:1152–9.
14. Wang AJ, Liao XH, Xiong LS, Peng S, Xiao YL, Liu SC, Hu PJ, Chen MH. The clinical overlap between functional dyspepsia and irritable bowel syndrome based on Rome III criteria. BMC Gastroenterol. 2008;8:43.
15. Xiong LS, Shi Q, Gong XR, Cui Y, Chen MH. The spectra, symptom profiles and overlap of Rome III functional gastrointestinal disorders in a tertiary center in South China. J Dig Dis. 2014;15:538–44.
16. Van Oudenhove L, Vandenberghe J, Vos R, Holvoet L, Tack J. Factors associated with co-morbid irritable bowel syndrome and chronic fatigue-like symptoms in functional dyspepsia. Neurogastroenterol Motil. 2011;23:524–e202.
17. Vandenplas Y, Rudolph CD, Di Lorenzo C, Hassall E, Liptak G, Mazur L, Sondheimer J, Staiano A, Thomson M, Veereman-Wauters G, Wenzl TG. Pediatric gastroesophageal reflux clinical practice guidelines: Joint recommendations of the North American Society for Pediatric Gastroenterology, Hepatology, and Nutrition (NASPGHAN) and the European Society for Pediatric Gastroenterology, Hepatology, and Nutrition (ESPGHAN). J Pediatr Gastroenterol Nutr. 2009;49:498–547.
18. Lacy BE, Weiser K, Chertoff J, Fass R, Pandolfino JE, Richter JE, Rothstein RI, Spangler C, Vaezi MF. The diagnosis of gastroesophageal reflux disease. Am J Med. 2010;123:583–92.
19. Talley NJ. Functional (non-ulcer) dyspepsia and gastroesophageal reflux disease: one not two diseases? Am J Gastroenterol. 2013;108:775–7.
20. Franco I. Functional bladder problems in children: pathophysiology, diagnosis, and treatment. Pediatr Clin North Am. 2012;59:783–817.
21. Gamper M, Regauer S, Welter J, Eberhard J, Viereck V. Are mast cells still good biomarkers for bladder pain syndrome/interstitial cystitis? J Urol. 2015;193:1994–2000.
22. Liu HT, Shie JH, Chen SH, Wang YS, Kuo HC. Differences in mast cell infiltration, E-cahedrin, and zonula occludens-1 expression between patients with overactive bladder and interstitial cystitis/bladder pain syndrome. Urology. 2012;80:225.e13–18.
23. Shin CM. Overlap between postprandial distress and epigastric pain syndromes in functional dyspepsia: its implications for research and clinical practice. Am J Gastroenterol. 2013;108:767–74.
24. Tack J, Talley NJ. Functional dyspepsia- symptoms, definitions and validity of Rome III criteria. Nat Rev Gastroenterol Hepatol. 2013;10:134–41.
25. Talley NJ. Functional dyspepsia and the Rome criteria: a success story. Neurogastroenterol Motil. 2015;27:1052–6.
26. Kovacic K, Williams S, Li BU, Chelimsky G, Miranda A. High prevalence of nausea in children with pain-associated functional gastrointestinal disorders: are Rome criteria applicable? J Pediatr Gastroenterol Nutr. 2013;57:311–5.
27. Tack J, Jones MP, Karamanolis G, Coulie B, Dubois D. Symptom pattern and pathophysiologic correlates of weight loss in tertiary-referred functional dyspepsia. Neurogastroenterol Motil. 2010;22:29–e5.

17

Primary tumor location predicts poor clinical outcome with cetuximab in *RAS* wild-type metastatic colorectal cancer

Dalyong Kim[1,4†], Sun Young Kim[1†], Ji Sung Lee[2], Yong Sang Hong[1], Jeong Eun Kim[1], Kyu-pyo Kim[1], Jihun Kim[3], Se Jin Jang[3], Young-Kwang Yoon[2] and Tae Won Kim[1,2*]

Abstract

Background: In metastatic colorectal cancer, the location of the primary tumor has been suggested to have biological significance. In this study, we investigated whether primary tumor location affects cetuximab efficacy in patients with *RAS* wild-type metastatic colorectal cancer.

Methods: Genotyping by the SequenomMassARRAY technology platform (OncoMap) targeting *KRAS*, *NRAS*, *PIK3CA*, and *BRAF* was performed in tumors from 307 patients who had been given cetuximab as salvage treatment. Tumors with mutated *RAS* (*KRAS* or *NRAS*; $n = 127$) and those with multiple primary location ($n = 10$) were excluded. Right colon cancer was defined as a tumor located in the proximal part to splenic flexure.

Results: A total of 170 patients were included in the study (right versus left, 23 and 147, respectively). Patients with right colon cancer showed more mutated *BRAF* (39.1% vs. 5.4%), mutated *PIK3CA* (13% vs. 1.4%), poorly differentiated tumor (17.4% vs. 3.4%), and peritoneal involvement (26.1% vs. 8.8%) than those with left colon and rectal cancer. Right colon cancer showed poorer progression-free survival (2.0 vs.5.0 months, $P = 0.002$) and overall survival (4.1 months and 13.0 months, $P < 0.001$) than the left colon and rectal cancer. By multivariable analysis, *BRAF* mutation, right colon primary, poorly differentiated histology, and peritoneal involvement were associated with risk of death.

Conclusions: In *RAS* wild-type colon cancer treated with cetuximab as salvage treatment, right colon primary was associated with poorer survival outcomes than left colon and rectal cancer.

Keywords: Primary tumor location, Metastatic colorectal cancer, Cetuximab, *RAS* wild-type, EGFR

Background

Colorectal cancer (CRC) represents 10% of cancer incidence globally, and it is the fourth leading cause of cancer-related deaths worldwide. South Korea has one of the highest incidences of CRC in the world [1]. The survival of metastatic CRC has gradually been improved with advancements in medical therapy, which include not only the development of new drugs but also the discovery of predictive biomarkers.

Previous studies have suggested that primary tumor location (PTL) may be a surrogate for tumor biology that may affect treatment outcomes [2, 3]. In terms of embryology and molecular carcinogenesis, CRC can be divided into distinct disease entities according to the PTL; the right side of the colon, including the cecum, the ascending colon, and the transverse colon is derived from the midgut, while the remaining parts of the colon and rectum come from the hindgut [2]. Tumors of the right colon (RC) tend to more frequently exhibit a poorly differentiated histology, *BRAF* mutation, a hypermethylated phenotype, and microsatellite instability (MSI), while *c-MYC* expression occurs more commonly

* Correspondence: twkimmd@amc.seoul.kr
†Equal contributors
[1]Department of Oncology, Asan Medical Center, University of Ulsan College of Medicine, 88, Olympic-ro 43-gil, Songpa-gu, Seoul 05505, Republic of Korea
[2]Clinical Research Center, Asan Institute for Life Sciences, Asan Medical Center, University of Ulsan College of Medicine, Seoul, South Korea
Full list of author information is available at the end of the article

in tumors of left colon and rectum(LC) than in those in the RC [2, 4, 5].

The prognostic and predictive implications of PTL have been addressed in numerous studies, but there is no clear consensus on the role of PTL in treatment decisions. Generally, RC cancer is associated with poorer survival compared to LC cancer [6, 7], and recent evidences have shown that patients with RC cancer may respond poorly to anti-epidermal growth factor receptor (EGFR) antibodies, such as cetuximab or panitumumab, which are the backbone of treatment for metastatic CRC [8, 9]. However, the predictive value of PTL should be analyzed in consideration of *RAS* mutation,the most powerful predictor of response of anti-EGFR antibodies [10, 11].

In our current study, we investigated the association between PTL and clinical outcomes in *RAS* wild-type metastatic CRC patients who received cetuximab as a salvage treatment.

Methods

Patients

We retrospectively reviewed the medical records of 307 metastatic CRC patients treated with cetuximab with or without irinotecan as a salvage treatment between December 2003 and June 2013 at Asan Medical Center, Seoul, Republic of Korea. All of them were given cetuximab as a third or later line of treatment for metastatic CRC and had sufficient tissue to conduct extended *RAS* analyses. After extended *RAS* testing, 127 *RAS* mutant patients were excluded from the analysis, and additional 10 patients with synchronous multiple colon cancers were excluded due to an inability to define PTL. Finally, 170 patients were analyzed and assigned to either RC or LC group (Fig. 1). Clinicopathologic variables, including age, gender, initial stage, histologic differentiation, metastatic sites, MSI status (determined as previously described [12] by the Bethesda panel), and details of treatment given before cetuximab were extracted from medical records. This study was conducted in accordance with the declaration of Helsinki and was approved by the Institutional Review Board of Asan Medical Center. Informed consent was obtained in all participants except patients who were dead at the time of this study. Institutional Review Board of Asan Medical Center approved to waive the requirement to obtain informed consent from the dead according to Bioethics and Biosafety Act in Korea.

Genotyping

Mutational analysis was done using the Sequenom-MassARRAY technology platform (OncoMap version 4.0), as previously described [13, 14]. A pathologist (JK) reviewed formalin-fixed paraffin-embedded tissue and marked tumor portions, where DNA was extracted from using the QIAamp DNA Tissue kit (Qiagen, Hilden, Germany) according to the manufacturer's instructions. Multiplex polymerase chain reaction amplification using iPLEXchemistry (#10134–2; Sequenom, San Diego, CA), and homogenous mass extension validation of mutation were implemented. Single-base extension was done and a MALDI-TOF mass spectrometer was used to determine the unique mass value according to the mutation site. Target genes were *KRAS* (exon 2, 3, and 4), *NRAS* (exon 2, 3, and 4), *PIK3CA* (exon 9 and 20), and *BRAF* (exon 15).

Tumor locations

The tumor location was determined based on operation records and colonoscopy findings. The RC group consisted of cancers occurring in the cecum, the ascending colon, hepatic flexure, and the transverse colon, while the LC group included primary tumors from the splenic flexure to the rectum.

Statistical analysis

The statistical tests were exploratory in nature. Demographic and baseline clinical characteristics were compared according to the PTL. Fisher's exact test and the Mann–Whitney U-test were used for categorical variables and continuous variables, respectively. The Kaplan–Meier method was used to estimate progression-free survival (PFS) and overall survival (OS), and the survival outcomes were compared according to PTL by the log-rank test. PFS was defined as the time from the date of the first administration of cetuximab to the date of documented disease progression or the date of death from any cause, if progression was not documented before death. OS was defined as the time from the date of first cetuximab dose to the date of death from any cause. To evaluate clinical outcomes by PTL, the Cox proportional hazards regression model was used for multivariable analysis. In these analyses, we selected statistically significant or clinically meaningful variables as predictors for the final model. Thus, PFS and OS were adjusted for age, sex, presence of peritoneal seeding, histologic grade, and *BRAF* mutational status. Hazard ratio (HR) associated with each variable was suggested with 95% confidence interval (CI). All statistical analyses were two-sided, with a level of significance established at $p < 0.05$, and performed using the Statistical Package for Social Sciences version 21.0 (IBM Corp., Armonk, NY). The Kaplan–Meier curves were drawn using STATA software (StataCorp. 2015. *Stata Statistical Software: Release 14*. College Station, TX: StataCorp LP).

Role of the funding source

The study funders had no role in the design, analysis, interpretation or manuscript preparation. All authors prepared the drafts of this report and approved the

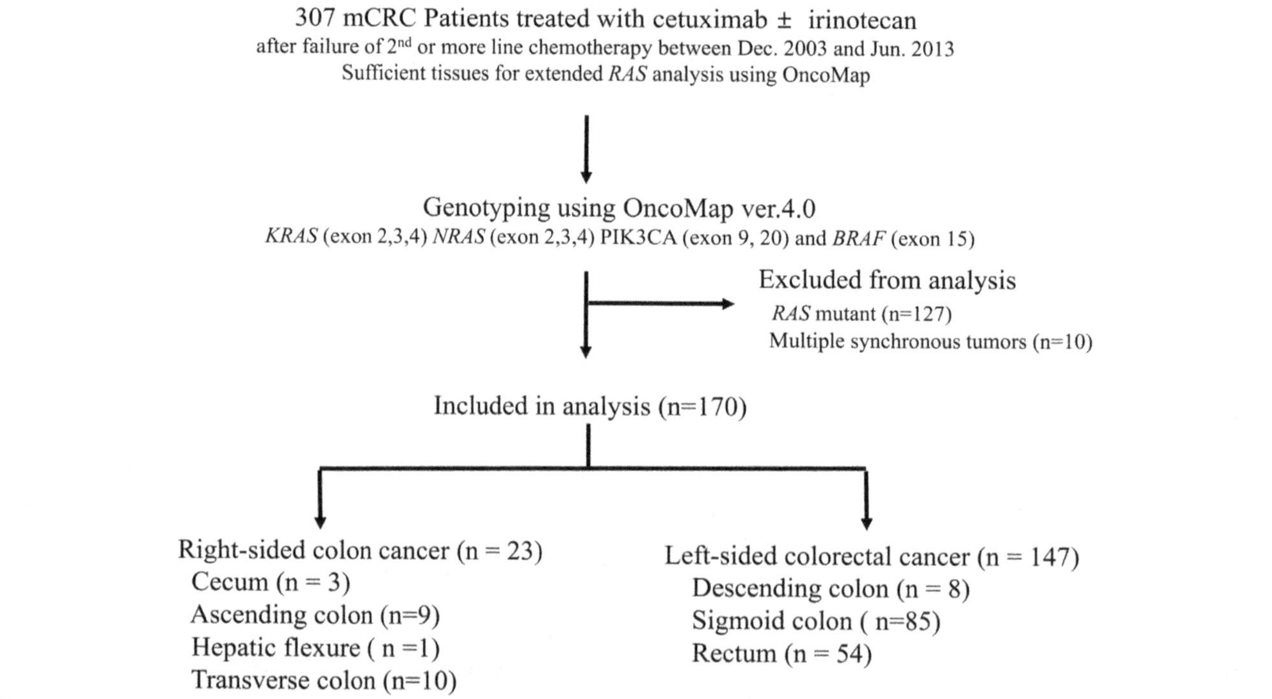

Fig. 1 Flow diagram for the patient selection process. mCRC, metastatic colorectal cancer

submission. The corresponding author had full access to all the data and final responsibility to submit for publication.

Results

Patient characteristics

Among a total of 170 *RAS* wild-type patients, 23 were classified as belonging to the RC group and 147 as belonging to the LC group (Fig. 1). The baseline characteristics of the study patients are presented in Table 1. All patients were treated with cetuximab as third or later-line therapy, and half of them received it in combination with irinotecan. All patients were treated with irinotecan before cetuximab; no significant difference was seen in previously exposed chemotherapeutic agents (oxaliplatin, fluoropyrimidine, and bevacizumab). The median age was similar between the groups, while the proportion of female patients was higher in the RC group, without statistical significance. The most common metastatic organ was liver in both groups, while peritoneal metastasis was more common in RC cancer than in LC cancer (26.1% vs. 8.8%, $p = 0.026$). The proportion of unfavorable histology, including poorly differentiated adenocarcinoma and signet ring cell carcinoma, was 20.0% in RC and 5.0% in LC ($p = 0.031$). The interval between first-line chemotherapy and cetuximab treatment was slightly shorter in the RC group than the LC group, without statistical significance (16.4 vs. 18.2 months, $p = 0.552$).

Molecular information according to PTL

The results of genotyping are summarized in Table 1. The *BRAF* V600E mutation was detected in nine (39.1%) patients in the RC group and eight (5.4%) in the LC group. The *PIK3CA* mutation was also more frequently detected in the RC group (13% vs. 1.4%, $p = 0.018$). The MSI test is not routinely performed for metastatic CRC in our institution, so information for MSI status was only available for 108 patients (63.5%), among whom only 1 patient, in the LC group, had an MSI-high tumor.

Clinical outcomes by primary tumor location

A profound difference in OS according to PTL was observed: 4.1 months (95% CI, 2.1 to 8.1) in the RC group and 13.0 months (95% CI 11.5 to 14.0) in the LC group ($p < 0.001$) (Fig. 2a). The PFS was also poorer in the RC group (2.0 months, 95% CI 0.9 to 4.0) than in the LC group (5.0 months, 95% CI 4.5 to 6.3, $p = 0.002$) (Fig. 2b).

BRAF mutation was significantly associated with poor clinical outcome: OS in *BRAF* wild-type and mutants were 13.0 months and 4.1 months ($p < 0.0001$), respectively. PFS was 5.1 months in *BRAF* wild-type, and 1.2 months in *BRAF* mutants ($p < 0.0001$).

Within the *RAS* and *BRAF* wild-type population (n = 153, 14 in RC group and 139 in LC group), OS was still poorer in the RC group than in the LC group (5.7 months vs. 13.2 months, respectively), with marginal significance ($p = 0.055$, Fig. 2c). PFS did not significantly

Table 1 Baseline characteristics according to primary tumor location

Characteristics	Right colon (*n* = 23)	Left colon and rectum (*n* = 147)	*P*-value*
Age (years)			0.546
Median (range)	57 (36–72)	55 (24–74)	
Gender			0.154
Female	10 (43.5%)	42 (28.6%)	
Male	13 (56.5%)	105 (71.4%)	
Stage at presentation			0.292
Stage IV	20 (87.0%)	110 (74.8%)	
Stage I-III	3 (13.0%)	37 (25.2%)	
Histology			0.031
W/D or M/D	16 (80.0%)	136 (95.0%)	
P/D or SRCC	4 (20.0%)	7 (5.0%)	
Number of metastasized organs			>0.999
1	13 (56.5%)	81 (55.1%)	
≥ 2	10 (43.5%)	66 (44.9%)	
Metastasized organ			
Liver	12 (52.2%)	106 (72.1%)	0.086
Lung	7 (30.4%)	65 (44.2%)	0.260
Peritoneum	6 (26.1%)	13 (8.8%)	0.026
Treatment lines			0.921
3	16 (69.6%)	104 (70.7%)	
4	6 (26.1%)	35 (23.8%)	
≥5	1 (4.3%)	8 (5.4%)	
Prior treatment			
Oxaliplatin	23 (100%)	144 (98.0%)	1.00
Bevacizumab	7 (30.4%)	25 (17.0%)	0.151
5-fluoropyrimidine	20 (87.0%)	136 (92.5%)	0.408
Regimen			0.482
Cetuximab + irinotecan	13 (56.5%)	97 (66.0%)	
Cetuximab monotherapy	10 (43.5%)	50 (34.0%)	
BRAF			<0.001
Wild-type	14 (60.9%)	139 (94.6%)	
Mutant	9 (39.1%)	8 (5.4%)	
PIK3CA			0.018
Wild-type	20 (87.0%)	145 (98.6%)	
Mutant	3 (13.0%)	2 (1.4%)	
MSI status			0.156
MSS	19 (82.6%)	85 (57.8%)	
MSI-low	0 (0%)	3 (2.0%)	
MSI-high	0 (0%)	1 (0.7%)	
Not checked	4 (17.4%)	58 (39.5%)	

Abbreviations: *W/D* well-differentiated, *M/D* moderately differentiated, *P/D* poorly differentiated, *SRCC* signet ring cell carcinoma, *MSI* microsatellite instability, *MSS* microsatellite stable

**P*-value by Fisher's exact test or Mann-Whitney U-test as appropriate

differ between the two groups when *BRAF* mutants were excluded (3.7 months in RC group vs. 5.3 months in LC group, $p = 0.219$; Fig. 2d).

The presence of peritoneal metastasis, *BRAF* mutation, unfavorable histology (poorly differentiated adenocarcinoma or signet ring cell carcinoma), and PTL were statistically meaningful parameters in bivariate analysis for OS and PFS using the Cox proportional hazard model (Tables 2 and 3). By multivariable analysis, RC was associated with a poorer OS (hazards ratio 1.84, 95% CI 1.10 to 3.09, $p = 0.021$, Table 2), and there was a trend toward a lower PFS (HR 1.55, 95% CI 0.92 to 2.61, $p = 0.099$, Table 3).

Discussion

We observed in our current analysis that RC was associated with poor OS and PFS outcomes in *RAS* wild-type metastatic CRC patients treated with cetuximab as salvage therapy. OS was still poorer in the RC group when *BRAF* mutants were excluded. These findings suggest that PTL may be a factor in deciding on salvage chemotherapy with cetuximab in *RAS* wild-type patients.

Several studies have suggested that clinical benefits from anti-EGFR treatment may differ according to PTL. In data from a phase II trial of cetuximab-based chemotherapy, LC cancer was found to be associated with significantly longer PFS and OS than RC cancer in *KRAS* exon 2 wild-type patients [9]. Similarly, the NCIC CO.17 trial, a phase III study that compared cetuximab with the best supportive care in refractory metastatic CRC, showed that patients with LC cancer had benefit from cetuximab in terms of PFS, but those with RC cancer did not in *KRAS* exon 2 wild-type population [8]. Post-hoc analysis of the CALGB 80405 trial, a phase III trial that compared cetuximab and bevacizumab in front-line settings, also showed that cetuximab-treated *KRAS* exon 2 wild-type patients with RC cancer had markedly poorer survival than those with LC cancer (16.7 months in RC and 36.0 in LC, $p < 0.0001$) [15]. All of these analyses were performed in *KRAS* exon 2 wild-type patients, so the possibility that *RAS* mutations other than *KRAS* exon 2 may have contributed to the relatively poorer outcome in RC cancer in these studies could not be excluded. Recent studies for *RAS* wild-type subgroup of randomized trials which compared anti-EGFR treatment with chemotherapy +/− bevacizumab addressed this issue, by showing OS, PFS and objective response rate with anti-EGFR treatment was poorer in RC cancer than in LC cancer [16, 17].

A strength of our present study is that we excluded all *RAS* mutants from our analysis using a highly sensitive high-throughput method, the SequenomMassARRAY system. Our previous study showed that this method was more helpful for selecting candidates for cetuximab

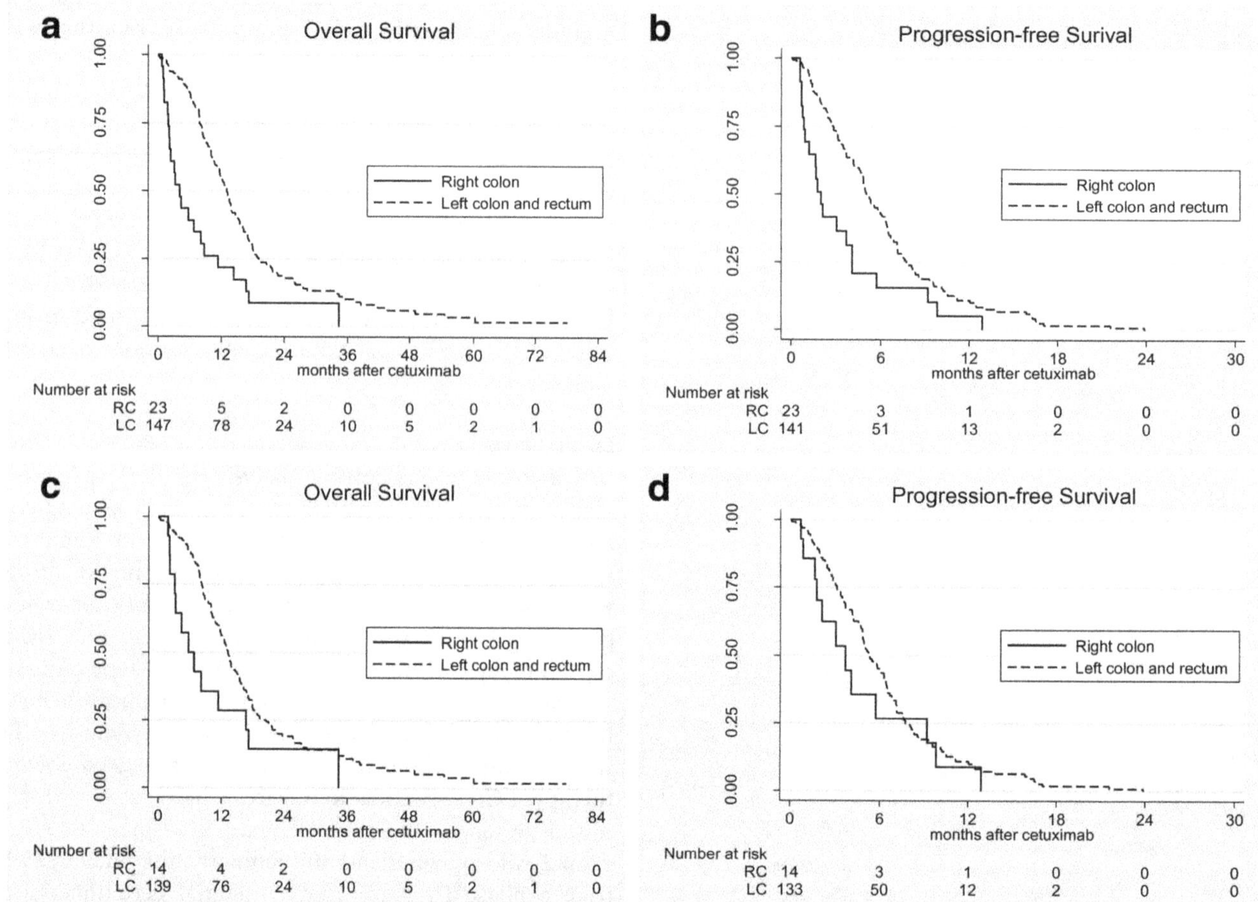

Fig. 2 Kaplan–Meier estimates of (**a**) overall survival and (**b**) progression-free survival according to primary tumor location in *RAS* wild-type metastatic colorectal cancer patients ($n = 170$), and (**c**) overall survival and (**d**) progression-free survival in *RAS* and *BRAF* wild-type patients ($n = 153$)

treatment than less-sensitive Sanger sequencing [14]. This means that the poorer outcomes with anti-EGFR treatment in RC cancer than in LC cancer were maintained even after all *RAS* mutants with low-allele frequency were excluded.

We further found in our analysis that *BRAF* and *PIK3CA* mutants were enriched in RC cancer, as shown in previous studies [5], which may partly explain the different therapeutic effects of anti-EGFR according to the PTL. However, the difference in OS was still retained, even after excluding *BRAF* mutants. Although we should be careful interpreting this subset analysis due to small sample size and relatively low proportion of RC (in *RAS* and *BRAF* wild-type subgroup, $n = 14$ for RC compared to $n = 139$ in LC), PTL may be associated with poor prognostic biological features other than *RAS* or *BRAF* mutation. The prognostic impact of PTL irrespective of *RAS* and *BRAF* mutation was also suggested by subgroup analyses of 3 randomized trials on anti-EGFR vs. chemotherapy +/− bevacizumab (FIRE3, PRIME, and PEAK), which showed poor prognosis of RC in patients with *RAS/BRAF* wild-type metastatic CRC [18, 19].

Recent studies have suggested that biologic features of RC cancer that may explain the poor prognosis or resistance to anti-EGFR treatment. A translational study in PETACC-3 trial reported that *BRAF*-mutant-like tumors, which were *BRAF* wild-type but shared similar gene expression profile with *BRAF* mutant tumors, were enriched in RC and had poor prognosis [20]. The abundant expression of epiregulin and amphiregulin, which are known to be predictors of good response to anti-EGFR treatment, was shown to be more prevalent in LC cancer than in RC cancer [21]. On the other hand, MiR-31-3p, a poor predictor for anti-EGFR response, was shown to be overexpressed more frequently in RC cancer than in LC cancer [22]. In addition, Consensus Molecular Subtype (CMS)1, which is associated with a poorer survival rate after relapse, is more common in RC [23]. However, there might be more unknown features of biologic relevance of PTL, since recent translational study

Table 2 Bivariate and multivariable analysis for overall survival

Characteristic	Crude HR (95% CI)	*P*-value* (bivariate[a])	Adjusted HR (95% CI)	*P*-value* (multivariable[a])
Primary tumor location				
Right vs. Left	2.29 (1.46–3.62)	<0.001	1.84 (1.10–3.09)	0.021
Age				
>60 years vs. ≤ 60	1.06 (0.76–1.47)	0.750	1.07 (0.75–1.51)	0.720
Gender				
Female vs. Male	0.92(0.65–1.30)	0.623	0.97 (0.66–1.40)	0.852
Stage at presentation				
Stage IV vs. Stage I-III	1.12 (0.77–1.63)	0.554		
Histologic grade				
P/D or SRC vs. W/D or M/D	4.35 (2.21–8.57)	<0.001	3.08 (1.49–6.34)	0.002
Presence of liver metastasis				
Yes vs. No	1.29 (0.91–1.82)	0.156		
Presence of lung metastasis				
Yes vs. No	0.84 (0.61–1.15)	0.279		
Presence of peritoneal metastasis				
Yes vs. No	2.91 (1.79–4.75)	<0.001	2.05 (1.17–3.60)	0.013
Number of metastasized organs				
≥ 2 vs. 1	1.10 (0.80–1.52)	0.540		
BRAF				
Mutant vs. Wild-type	3.24 (1.94–5.43)	<0.001	2.84 (1.60–5.03)	<0.001
PIK3CA				
Mutant vs. Wild-type	1.97 (0.80–4.84)	0.138		

Abbreviations: *HR* hazard ratio, *CI* confidence interval, *P/D* poorly differentiated, *SRCC* signet ring cell carcinoma, *W/D* well-differentiated, *M/D* moderately differentiated
[*]*P*-value by Cox's proportional hazards regression
[a]Clinically meaningful variables and those with $p < 0.05$ by bivariate analysis were entered into the multivariable analysis model

from CALGB 80405 showed PTL was independent prognostic factor when adjusted to *BRAF* mutation, MSI and CMS [24].

It is uncertain whether PTL is just a negative prognostic indicator reflecting tumor biology irrespective of treatment or is a genuine predictive marker of the response to anti-EGFR treatment. In CALGB 80405 trial, the OS was better in LC than in RC cancer in bevacizumab-treated patients, although the interaction between the PTL and the treatment (cetuximab versus bevacizumab) was significant ($p = 0.005$) [15]. This prognostic as well as predictive impact of PTL was consistently shown by the pooled analysis of 6 randomized trials (5 in first-line and 1 in second-line setting) on anti-EGFR in terms of OS and PFS although the interaction between sidedness and treatment effect was not always significant in all of the trials [16]. However, in NCIC CO.17 study, a randomized study in chemo-refractory setting, PFS and OS in the best supportive care arm was not affected by PTL, implying that it was not prognostic, but only predictive of PFS benefit from cetuximab (interaction $p = 0.002$) [8]. To date, collective evidences are suggesting high likelihood of no clinical benefit from anti-EGFR in RC cancer, at least in first-line setting, and possibly in later-line treatment. PTL seems to be also prognostic for metastatic CRC in first-line setting, but unclear in chemo-refractory patients.

In our current study, PTL showed a significant relationship with OS in multivariable analysis, but not in PFS; the prognostic impact of PTL seems to be more prominent than the predictive role in these results. However, the limitations of our present analysis hamper such an interpretation; the sample size of our patients with RC cancer was too small and we did not include a control group without cetuximab. Thus, it was difficult to conclude whether PTL is purely prognostic or predictive from our present study.

The characteristics of our study patients were comparable to those of previous reports, namely frequent poorly differentiated histology and peritoneal seeding, as well as the mutation profile previously mentioned [2, 6, 25]. However, the proportion of RC patients in our study population was relatively too small (13.5%, 23/170) to have adequate power of comparison according to PTL.

Table 3 Bivariate and multivariable analysis for progression-free survival

Characteristic	Crude HR (95% CI)	*P*-value* (bivariate[a])	Adjusted HR (95% CI)	*P*-value* (multivariable[a])
Primary tumor location				
Right vs. Left	2.09 (1.31–3.33)	0.002	1.55 (0.92–2.61)	0.099
Age				
>60 years vs. ≤ 60	0.77 (0.54–1.08)	0.133	0.77 (0.53–1.13)	0.180
Gender				
Female vs. Male	1.15 (0.80–1.64)	0.449	1.11 (0.75–1.64)	0.616
Stage at presentation				
Stage IV vs. Stage I-III	0.99 (0.66–1.49)	0.965		
Histologic grade				
P/D or SRC vs. W/D or M/D	5.37(2.24–12.87)	<0.001	3.06 (1.22–7.67)	0.017
Presence of liver metastasis				
Yes vs. No	1.04 (0.73–1.50)	0.816		
Presence of lung metastasis				
Yes vs. No	0.87 (0.63–1.21)	0.419		
Presence of peritoneal metastasis				
Yes vs. No	2.53 (1.53–4.19)	<0.001	2.08 (1.19–3.63)	0.010
Number of metastasized organs				
≥ 2 vs. 1	1.11 (0.80–1.53)	0.543		
BRAF				
Mutant vs. Wild-type	3.56 (2.11–6.01)	<0.001	3.07 (1.73–5.46)	<0.001
PIK3CA				
Mutant vs. Wild-type	2.60 (0.95–7.11)	0.062		

Abbreviations: *HR* hazard ratio, *CI* confidence interval, *P/D* poorly differentiated, *SRCC* signet ring cell carcinoma, *W/D* well-differentiated, *M/D* moderately differentiated
*P-value by Cox's proportional hazards regression
[a]Clinically meaningful variables and those with $p < 0.05$ by bivariate analysis were entered into the multivariable analysis model

This probably resides in the low proportion of proximal colon cancer in Korean populations: 18.6% in male and 24.2% in female according to 2009 statistics from national registry [26]. This is consistent with the racial difference in subsite-specific CRC incidence in United States; Asia-Pacific islanders had lowest proportion of proximal colon cancer (28% in male, 34% in female) compared to other racial groups (usually ≥40%) [27]. The association of racial difference in subsite distribution and prognosis according to treatment warrants further investigation.

Our current study had other limitations, including its retrospective nature, the heterogeneous regimen of cetuximab, insufficient information on MSI, and the lack of biological information other than hotspot mutation profiles, such as gene expression or the CpG island methylation profile.

Conclusions

PTL in RC might be associated with a poor OS outcome in patients with *RAS* wild-type metastatic CRC being treated with cetuximab as salvage treatment. Despite of the limitations from the retrospective study of small sample size, this finding supports the conclusions of previous studies that PTL may be a surrogate for tumor biology and should be considered as a biomarker and as a stratification factor in conducting clinical trials. Further studies are needed to validate the impact of PTL on treatment outcomes in various clinical settings.

Abbreviations

CI: Confidence interval; CRC: Colorectal cancer; EGFR: Epidermal growth factor receptor; HR: Hazard ratio; LC: Left colon and rectum; MSI: Microsatellite instability; OS: Overall survival; PFS: Progression-free survival; PTL: Primary tumor location; RC: Right colon

Acknowledgments

Not applicable.

Funding

This study was funded by the National R&D Program for Cancer Control, Ministry of Health and Welfare, Republic of Korea (1420030), and the Asan Institute for Life Sciences, Seoul, Republic of Korea (2016–0735), and was supported in part by CJ HealthCare, Corp, Seoul, Korea.

Authors' contributions

DK, SYK, YSH, JEK, KK, YY and TWK contributed conception and design of this study. DK and SYK contributed to clinical data acquisition and manuscript drafting. DK, SYK and JSL contributed to statistical analysis. JK and SJJ contributed to genomic data acquisition. All the authors have read and approved the manuscript.

Competing interests

The authors declare that they have no competing interests.

Author details

[1]Department of Oncology, Asan Medical Center, University of Ulsan College of Medicine, 88, Olympic-ro 43-gil, Songpa-gu, Seoul 05505, Republic of Korea. [2]Clinical Research Center, Asan Institute for Life Sciences, Asan Medical Center, University of Ulsan College of Medicine, Seoul, South Korea. [3]Department of Pathology, Asan Medical Center, University of Ulsan College of Medicine, Seoul, South Korea. [4]Department of Hematology/Oncology, Yuseong Sun Hospital, 93, Bugyuseong-daero, Yuseong-gu, Daejeon 34084, South Korea.

References

1. GLOBOCAN. 2012: estimated cancer incidence, mortality and prevalence worldwide in 2012. International Agency for Research on Cancer: Lyon; 2015.
2. Lee GH, Malietzis G, Askari A, Bernardo D, Al-Hassi HO, Clark SK. Is right-sided colon cancer different to left-sided colorectal cancer? - a systematic review. Eur J Surg Oncol. 2015;41(3):300–8.
3. Yahagi M, Okabayashi K, Hasegawa H, Tsuruta M, Kitagawa Y. The worse prognosis of right-sided compared with left-sided colon cancers: a systematic review and meta-analysis. J Gastrointest Surg. 2016;20(3):648–55.
4. Rothberg PG, Spandorfer JM, Erisman MD, Staroscik RN, Sears HF, Petersen RO, Astrin SM. Evidence that c-myc expression defines two genetically distinct forms of colorectal adenocarcinoma. Br J Cancer. 1985;52(4):629–32.
5. Shen H, Yang J, Huang Q, Jiang MJ, Tan YN, JF F, Zhu LZ, Fang XF, Yuan Y. Different treatment strategies and molecular features between right-sided and left-sided colon cancers. World J Gastroenterol. 2015;21(21):6470–8.
6. Benedix F, Kube R, Meyer F, Schmidt U, Gastinger I, Lippert H. Comparison of 17,641 patients with right- and left-sided colon cancer: differences in epidemiology, perioperative course, histology, and survival. Dis Colon rectum. 2010;53(1):57–64.
7. Meguid RA, Slidell MB, Wolfgang CL, Chang DC, Ahuja N. Is there a difference in survival between right- versus left-sided colon cancers? Ann Surg Oncol. 2008;15(9):2388–94.
8. Brule SY, Jonker DJ, Karapetis CS, O'Callaghan CJ, Moore MJ, Wong R, Tebbutt NC, Underhill C, Yip D, Zalcberg JR, et al. Location of colon cancer (right-sided versus left-sided) as a prognostic factor and a predictor of benefit from cetuximab in NCIC CO.17. European journal of cancer (Oxford, England : 1990). 2015;51(11):1405–14.
9. von Einem JC, Heinemann V, von Weikersthal LF, Vehling-Kaiser U, Stauch M, Hass HG, Decker T, Klein S, Held S, Jung A, et al. Left-sided primary tumors are associated with favorable prognosis in patients with KRAS codon 12/13 wild-type metastatic colorectal cancer treated with cetuximab plus chemotherapy: an analysis of the AIO KRK-0104 trial. J Cancer Res Clin Oncol. 2014;140(9):1607–14.
10. Douillard JY, Oliner KS, Siena S, Tabernero J, Burkes R, Barugel M, Humblet Y, Bodoky G, Cunningham D, Jassem J, et al. Panitumumab-FOLFOX4 treatment and RAS mutations in colorectal cancer. N Engl J Med. 2013;369(11):1023–34.
11. Sorich MJ, Wiese MD, Rowland A, Kichenadasse G, McKinnon RA, Karapetis CS, Extended RAS. Mutations and anti-EGFR monoclonal antibody survival benefit in metastatic colorectal cancer: a meta-analysis of randomized, controlled trials. Ann Oncol. 2015;26(1):13–21.
12. Kim JE, Hong YS, Ryu MH, Lee JL, Chang HM, Lim SB, Kim JH, Jang SJ, Kim MJ, CS Y, et al. Association between deficient mismatch repair system and efficacy to irinotecan-containing chemotherapy in metastatic colon cancer. Cancer Sci. 2011;102(9):1706–11.
13. Kim YM, Lee SW, Chun SM, Kim DY, Kim JH, Kim KR, Kim YT, Nam JH, van Hummelen P, MacConaill LE, et al. Analysis and comparison of somatic mutations in paired primary and recurrent epithelial ovarian cancer samples. PLoS One. 2014;9(6):e99451.
14. Kim D, Hong YS, Kim JE, Kim KP, Lee JL, Chun SM, Kim J, Jang SJ, Kim TW. Use of a high-throughput genotyping platform (OncoMap) for RAS mutational analysis to predict Cetuximab efficacy in patients with metastatic colorectal cancer. Cancer Res Treat. 2016;49(1):37–43.
15. Venook AP, Niedzwiecki D, Innocenti F, Fruth B, Greene C, O'Neil BH, Shaw JE, Atkins JN, Horvath LE, Polite BN, et al. Impact of primary tumor location on overall survival (OS) and progression-free survival (PFS) in patients (pts) with metastatic colorectal cancer (mCRC): Analysis of CALGB/SWOG 80405 (Alliance). J Clin Oncol. 2016;34 Suppl:3504-3504.
16. Arnold D, Lueza B, Douillard JY, Peeters M, Lenz HJ, Venook A, Heinemann V, Van Cutsem E, Pignon JP, Tabernero J, et al. Prognostic and predictive value of primary tumour side in patients with RAS wild-type metastatic colorectal cancer treated with chemotherapy and EGFR directed antibodies in six randomised trials. Ann Oncol. 2017;28(8):1713–29.
17. Tejpar S, Stintzing S, Ciardiello F, et al. Prognostic and predictive relevance of primary tumor location in patients with ras wild-type metastatic colorectal cancer: retrospective analyses of the crystal and fire-3 trials. JAMA oncology. 2017;3(2):194–201.
18. Peeters M: Outcome according to Left vs. Right side in the Panitumumab studies. In: *ESMO 2016 Congress*.
19. Heinemann V: Outcome according to Left vs. Right side in the FOLFIRI Cetuximab and FIRE 3 study. In: *ESMO 2016 Congress*.
20. Popovici V, Budinska E, Tejpar S, Weinrich S, Estrella H, Hodgson G, Van Cutsem E, Xie T, Bosman FT, Roth AD, et al. Identification of a poor-prognosis BRAF-mutant-like population of patients with colon cancer. J Clin Oncol. 2012;30(12):1288–95.
21. Seligmann JF, Elliott F, Richman SD, Jacobs B, Hemmings G, Brown S, Barrett JH, Tejpar S, Quirke P, Seymour MT. Combined Epiregulin and Amphiregulin expression levels as a predictive biomarker for Panitumumab therapy benefit or lack of benefit in patients with RAS wild-type advanced colorectal cancer. JAMA Oncol. 2016;2(5):633–42.
22. Laurent-Puig P, Grisoni ML, Heinemann V, Fontaine K, Vazart C, Decaulne V, Rousseau F, Courtieu B, Lieabert F, Jung A et al.: MiR-31-3p is a predictive biomarker of cetuximab response in FIRE3 clinical trial. Ann Oncol 2016, 27(suppl_6):457O-457O.
23. Guinney J, Dienstmann R, Wang X, de Reynies A, Schlicker A, Soneson C, Marisa L, Roepman P, Nyamundanda G, Angelino P, et al. The consensus molecular subtypes of colorectal cancer. Nat Med. 2015;21(11):1350–6.
24. Venook AP, Ou F-S, Lenz H-J, Kabbarah O, Qu X, Niedzwiecki D, Zemla T, Goldberg RM, Hochster HS, O'Neil BH. Primary (1°) tumor location as an independent prognostic marker from molecular features for overall survival (OS) in patients (pts) with metastatic colorectal cancer (mCRC): Analysis of CALGB/SWOG 80405 (Alliance). J Clin Oncol. 2017;35 Suppl:3503-3503.
25. Yamauchi M, Morikawa T, Kuchiba A, Imamura Y, Qian ZR, Nishihara R, Liao X, Waldron L, Hoshida Y, Huttenhower C, et al. Assessment of colorectal cancer molecular features along bowel subsites challenges the conception of distinct dichotomy of proximal versus distal colorectum. Gut. 2012;61(6):847–54.
26. Shin A, Kim KZ, Jung KW, Park S, Won YJ, Kim J, Kim DY, JH O. Increasing trend of colorectal cancer incidence in Korea, 1999-2009. Cancer research and treatment : official journal of Korean Cancer Association. 2012;44(4):219–26.
27. Wu X, Chen VW, Martin J, Roffers S, Groves FD, Correa CN, Hamilton-Byrd E, Jemal A. Subsite-specific colorectal cancer incidence rates and stage distributions among Asians and Pacific islanders in the United States, 1995 to 1999. Cancer Epidemiol Biomarkers Prev. 2004;13(7):1215–22.

Secreted protein acidic and rich in cysteine-like 1 suppresses metastasis in gastric stromal tumors

Chaoyong Shen[1†], Yuan Yin[1†], Huijiao Chen[2], Ruixue Wang[3], Xiaonan Yin[1], Zhaolun Cai[1], Bo Zhang[1*], Zhixin Chen[1] and Zongguang Zhou[4*]

Abstract

Background: Malignant growth and metastasis of gastrointestinal stromal tumors (GIST) occur in some patients even during the course of treatment, but their mechanisms remains poorly understand at the molecular level so far.

Methods: Profiles of protein expression in gastric GIST tissues were explored using protein microarray analysis, down-regulation of SPARCL1 (secreted protein acidic and rich in cysteine-like protein 1) was validated by RT-qPCR, western blot and immunohistochemistry. The effect of specific shRNA-induced SPARCL1 downregulation on the biological traits of GIST 882 cell was investigated. We then employed a mouse xenograft model to investigate whether the low-expression of SPARCL1 impact the metastasis ability of GIST cells in vivo.

Results: SPARCL1 was significantly downregulated in the gastric GIST with high-grade malignance as compared with low-grade malignance, its expression was closely correlated with tumor size, mitotic index, distant metastasis at the time of initial diagnosis and tumor progression of GIST ($P < 0.05$). Moreover, results of the Cox analysis showed that expression of SPARCL1 is an independent prognostic predictors for gastric GIST ($P = 0.008$; HR 0.157, 95% CI 0.040~ 0.612). Downregulation of SPARCL1 promoted cell migration and invasion, but did not affect proliferation, cell cycle and apoptosis of GIST 882 cells. In mouse xenograft model, GIST cells with the decreased expression of SPARCL1 presented an enhanced ability of liver metastasis ($P < 0.05$).

Conclusions: Taken together, our present study demonstrated that SPARCL1 have a certain degree of malignancy-suppressing potential through inhibiting the metastasis of gastric GIST.

Keywords: Gastrointestinal stromal tumors, Microarray, SPARCL1, Malignization, Metastasis

Background

Gastrointestinal stromal tumors (GIST) is by far the most common mesenchymal neoplasm in the human digestive tract, which originating from the interstitial cells of Cajal or their progenitor cells [1, 2]. In the past few decades, despite tremendous efforts such as radical resection, targeted therapy and immunotherapy, have been made to improve the long-term outcome of GIST patients, the prognosis of advanced GIST patients is still unfavorable [3, 4]. The gain-of-function mutations of *c-KIT* or platelet-derived growth factor receptor alpha (*PDGFRα*) has been reported as the main cause of GIST instead of the primary promoter of the malignant potential of GIST [5]. Therefore, in addition to the *c-kit/PDGFRa* gene, other mechanisms must be involved in and ultimately determined the development and outcome of GIST.

Several risk-stratification schemes for defining malignant potential of GIST have been already proposed by researchers, which mainly comprise prognostic parameters such as tumor size, mitosis and tumor location, but these criteria are established merely rely on clinicopathological features and also do not clarify the biology mechanism

* Correspondence: hxwcwk@126.com; zhou767@163.com
†Chaoyong Shen and Yuan Yin contributed equally to this work.
[1]Department of Gastrointestinal Surgery, West China Hospital, Sichuan University, Chengdu 610041, Sichuan, China
[4]Institute of Digestive Surgery and State Key Laboratory of Biotherapy, West China Hospital, Sichuan University, Chengdu 610041, Sichuan, China
Full list of author information is available at the end of the article

underlying the clinical aggressiveness [6–9]. Undoubtedly, the mitotic rate and tumor size, which are powerful prognostic indicators for the risk assessment of GIST, are still key factors to distinguish different degrees of malignancy for those tumors with same locations. Additionally, as reported in previous study, gastric GIST have become malignant progression from preexisting less aggressive tumors, namely a stepwise progression from low- to high-grade malignancy [10]. The metastasis rate or tumor-related mortality for gastric GIST with tumor size ≤2 cm and mitotic rate ≤ 5 mitoses/50 HPFs and those with tumor size > 10 cm and mitotic rate > 5 mitoses/50 HPFs are 0.0 and 86.0%, respectively, according to the NCCN guidelines (Version 2. 2017). In other words, the former is more likely to be benign or low-grade malignancy while the latter is thought to be high-grade malignancy and may behave in an aggressive manner. However, the molecular events involved in GIST malignization remains unclear by far. As such, a better understanding of the molecular mechanism responsible for GIST metastasis is of critical significance, and would eventually result in new anticancer drug targets and greatly contribute to advances in diagnostic approaches.

To identify the candidate proteins which are closely related to the malignant biological potential of GIST, a common and straightforward microarray analysis was performed to clarify a list of differentially expressed proteins between low- and high-grade malignant gastric GISTs. Based on this approach, we found a potential novel candidate protein which was markedly down-regulated in high-grade malignant gastric GIST when compared to those with low-grade malignancy. We hypothesized that this protein might be mechanistically involved with the metastasis of GIST. Thus, we tested this idea for this candidate protein (secreted protein acidic and rich in cysteine-like protein 1, SPARCL1) and explored the relationship between SPARCL1 and gastric GIST progression. SPARCL1, which is also known as Hevin, MAST9, and SC1, is an extracellular matrix glycoprotein encoded by a conserved gene localized at chromosome 4q22 [11]. There is a wealth of evidences indicating that SPARCL1 participates in many physiological functions such as de-adhesive activity, cell proliferation, and facilitates lymphocyte transendothelial migration [12, 13]. SPARCL1 is expressed in a wide range of normal tissues and organs, such as lung, placenta, muscle, heart, lymphatic gland, colon, gastric mucosa and brain neurons. However, in contrast to its widespread expressed in normal tissues, downregulation of SPARCL1 has been reported as a putative tumor-suppressor factor in a wide variety of human malignancies including breast, colorectal, prostate and pancreatic cancers [13–19]. Furthermore, a few reports have shown that SPARCL1 inhibited prostate, colorectal and pancreatic cancer cell migration and invasion in vitro/vivo, suggesting that SPARCL1 may be a potential suppressor of metastatic progression in many cancers [13, 16, 17]. However, there is little known about the expressive characteristics of SPARCL1 as well as its potential role in the initiation and progression of GIST, particularly whether SPARCL1 can suppress the metastasis of GIST has not been addressed to date.

In this study, we aim to explore the expression pattern and clinicopathological significance of SPARCL1 in a Chinese gastric GIST cohort, as well as to investigate whether the downregulation of SPARCL1 can enhance the invasion/migration ability of GIST cells in vitro or facilitate liver metastasis of GIST cells in vivo.

Methods

Specimens and patients collection

To construct the protein expression profiles in gastric GIST, tumor and corresponding adjacent normal tissues were sampled from 4 primary gastric GIST patients (Table 1) during the surgical procedure. Moreover, additional 8 pairs of fresh gastric GIST and corresponding adjacent normal tissues were obtained from the Biological Specimen Banks (West China Hospital, Sichuan University, China.) to confirm the reliability of microarray results (Table 1). GIST tissues were categorized into low-grade malignancy (LGM, tumor size ≤2 cm and mitotic rate ≤ 5

Table 1 Clinicopathological characteristics of the 20 gastric GIST (No. 1~ 4 were used for microarray analysis and No. 5~ 20 were utilized to western blot/RT-qPCR analysis)

No.	Gender	Age (years)	Size (cm)	Mitoses (/50HPF)
1	Female	47	2 × 2	3
2	Male	62	2 × 1.8	2
3	Female	51	12 × 10	14
4	Male	35	15 × 12	16
5	Male	48	1.5 × 1	3
6	Male	35	2 × 1	2
7	Female	62	1.8 × 1.5	1
8	Male	52	2 × 1.5	2
9	Female	49	2 × 2	2
10	Female	58	1.5 × 1	3
11	Male	49	1 × 1	1
12	Female	61	2 × 1.8	2
13	Male	57	12 × 10	14
14	Female	46	15 × 12	16
15	Male	53	20 × 18	57
16	Male	51	15 × 13	12
17	Male	48	10 × 10	17
18	Male	63	11 × 10	> 20
19	Male	68	16 × 8	11
20	Female	42	15 × 10	18

mitoses/50 HPFs) and high-grade malignancy (HGM, tumor size > 10 cm and mitotic rate > 5 mitoses/50 HPFs), according to the NCCN guidelines. Additionally, formalin-fixed paraffin-embedded GIST specimens ($n = 98$) gathered from the Department of Pathology (West China Hospital, Sichuan University, from January 2010 to December 2013) were included in immunohistochemical analysis. In the present study, all samples were collected from patients without pre-treatment of radiotherapy and/or chemotherapy preoperatively as well as the history of other associated malignant tumors. The clinicopathological characteristics and follow-up data, including age at diagnosis, gender, hospital stay, tumor size, mitotic count, clinical symptom, tumor rupture, distant metastasis, risk classifications and so on, were collected from the patients' medical records. Informed consents were provided by each patient before surgery, and the protocol of this study was approved by the Research Ethics Board of West China Hospital, Sichuan University, China.

Protein microarray analysis

Human Cytokine Antibody Array (Raybiotech, Norcoss, GA, USA), which comprising 1000 cytokines, was utilized according to the manufacture's instruction. Briefly, the arrays were blocked and incubated at room temperature for 30 min, incubated with biotin-conjugated antibodies for 1–2 h and with HRP-conjugated streptavidin for 2 h at room temperature. The membranes were incubated with chemiluminescent substrate and then exposed to x-ray film, signals were directly detected from membranes using chemiluminescene imaging system. The intensities of signals can be quantified by densitometry. Quantitative array analysis was performed using Array Vision Evaluation 8.0 (GE Healthcare Life Science, Little Chalfont, Buckinghamshire, UK). Proteins with significantly differential expression were selected with Fold change-value > 2.0 or < 0.5 and P-value < 0.05.

Real-time quantitative PCR

Total RNA was extracted from the cultured cells and fresh-frozen gastric GIST tissues using the Trizol reagent (Invitrogen, CA, USA), according to the protocol of manufacturer. A NanoDrop ND-1000 spectrophotometer was utilized to determine the concentration and purity of isolated RNA. Real-time quantitative RCR reaction was performed using SYBR® Premix Ex Taq™ kit (Takara, Kyoto, Japan) as described by the manufacture. β-actin was used as an endogenous control. Primers were obtained from Invitrogen. The primers used for detection of SPARCL1 mRNA were 5′-ATG AAG CCA ACT CTG AAC ACG C-3′ (Forward) and 5′-ATG GTC CCC AGC CAA AAG C-3′ (Reverse), and for β-actin the primers were 5′-GTG GCC GAG GAC TTT GAT TG-3′ (Forward) and 5'-CCT GTA ACA ACG CAT CTC ATA TT-3′ (Forward). The PCR reactions were performed as follows: 95 °C for 10 min, then 40 cycles of 10 s at 95 °C and 30 s at 60 °C. All samples were run in triplicate, and the quantification of SPARCL1 was normalized to β-actin expression using the 2-ΔΔCt method.

Protein extraction and western blot

Total cellular protein was extracted from fresh-frozen tumor tissues and cultured cells with a RIPA Lysis Buffer (Beyotime, Beijing, China) containing protease inhibitor, phenylmethylsulfonyl fluoride and phosphatase, protein concentration was measured using a BCA protein assay kit (Pierce, Rockford, IL, USA) in accordance with manufacturer's instruction. Equal amounts of tissue or cell lysate per lane were loaded onto 20% sodium dodecyl sulfate polyacrylamide gels (SDS-PAGE). Proteins were then transferred to PVDF membranes (Millipore, Bedford, USA), and blocked with 5% skimmed milk under ambient temperature for 1 h. Membranes were incubated with rabbit polyclonal antibody specific for human SPARCL1 (1:1000 dilution, Abcam, Cambridge, United Kingdom) at 4 °C overnight, after washing three times with TBST, membranes were subsequently incubated with the horseradish peroxidase-conjugated goat anti-rabbit second antibody (Invitrogen) at a dilution of 1:5000 for 2 h at room temperature. Imaging was performed with a ChemiDoc™ XRS+ System (BIO-RAD, Hercules, CA, USA), and quantification was conducted using the pre-installed software. β-actin was used as loading control for normalization.

Immunohistochemistry (IHC) and scoring of IHC

Briefly, paraffin-embedded samples were sliced into sections with thickness of 3–4 μm, which were then deparaffinized in xylene and rehydrated in gradually decreasing concentrations of alcohol to water. The tissue sections were heated in citrate buffer (pH 6.0) in a high-pressure cooker under the temperature of 95 °C for 5 min to retrieve antigen. Thereafter, the activity of endogenous peroxidase was blocked using 3% hydrogen peroxide, sections were incubated with primary rabbit polyclonal antibody against human SPARCL1 (1:100 dilution, Abcam) at 4 °C overnight, washed 3 times using phosphate-buffered saline (PBS) and then incubated with a secondary biotin-labeled antibody (ZSGB-BIO, Beijing, China) at 37 °C for 1.5 h. After washing again, sections were incubated with DAB-chromogen substrate mixture (DAKO, Glostrup, Denmark). Finally, sections were counterstained with hematoxylin, dehydrated in graded alcohol and xylene, mounted and coversliped. Immunostaining was evaluated individually and independently by two experienced pathologists using an Olympus CX31 microscope (Olympus, Tokyo, Japan) who were blinded to each other's findings. The scoring was conducted according to ratio and intensity of positive-staining cells [20]. The mean percentage of positive tumor cells was assigned from 0 to 100% (< 10%, 0; 10~ 25%, 1; 26~ 50%, 2;

51~ 75%, 3; ≥76%, 4), staining intensity was scored as follows: (negative)% × 0 + (weak)% × 1 + (moderate)% × 2 + (intensive)% × 3. Finally, an IHC expressing score was generated for each case (staining ratio + intensity of staining). Low-expression of SPARCL1 was defined as score ≤ 3, whereas the slides with scored 4~ 7 were defined as SPARCL1 over-expression.

GIST cell line and cell culture

Human GIST 882 line cells was obtained from Shanghai Cancer Institute (Shanghai, China). Cells were cultured in RPMI 1640 medium containing 20% fetal bovine serum (FBS) and 1% penicillin/streptomycin and incubated at 37 °C in a humidified atmosphere containing 95% air and 5% CO_2.

Construction of plasmids and cell transfection

GIST 882 cells were seeded into 6-well plates at a density of 5×10^5 cells per well. SPARCL1-targeting double-stranded short hairpin RNA (shRNA) was cloned into the lentiviral vector (GV248, hU6-MCS-Ubiquitin-EGFP-IRES-puromycin). The scrambled sequences (shRNA 1: AGAGAAATAAAGTCAAGAA; shRNA 2: ACCC AATCTGATGATATTT; shRNA 3: ACCTATGCA CCAGGTATTT) were synthesized by Genechem Corporation (Shanghai, China). All vectors were verified through sequencing. Lentiviral particles were produced as followings: transfected the lentiviral vectors into 293 T cells according to the manufacture's instruction, collected supernatants after 48-h incubation, filtrated by 0.45 μm filters (Merck Millipore, Billerica, MA, USA), condensed by ultracentrifugation (Beckman Coulter TL-100, Miami, FL, USA). The harvested lentiviral particles were transfect GIST 882 cells based on manufacturer's protocol using Lipofectamine 2000 (Invitrogen). The mRNA and protein levels of SPARCL1 in the transfected GIST 882 cells were evaluated by RT-qPCR and western blotting, respectively. Meanwhile, GIST 882 cells transfected with empty vectors in the same way were used as a negative control (Lv-shNC group). All transfecting experiments were conducted for three times. Subsequently, stable SPARCL1-knockdown GIST 882 cell line was established (Lv-shSPARCL1 group).

Cell proliferation assay

After transfection, cells were harvested and reseeded in a 96-well plate under regular conditions with an initial density of 3×10^3/well. A cell counting kit-8 cell proliferation assay (Dojindo, Kumamoto, Japan) was performed. The absorbing data at 450 nm were measured over next 3 days. All experiments were performed three times independently.

Flow cytometry analysis of cell cycle and apoptosis

Flow cytometry was utilized to analyzed cell cycle and apoptosis. Cells were inoculated in 6-well culture plates at a density of 1×10^6 cells per well. Following the pretreatments, the harvested cells were fixed with 70% ethanol at 4 °C overnight. Whereafter, cells were washed with PBS and then stained with propidium iodide (PI, 1 mg/mL). Flow cytometry (BD Biosciences, San Diego, CA, USA) was used to analyze the DNA content and comparing cells in G0/G1, S as well as G2/M stage.

For the additional analysis of cell apoptosis, an Annexin V-FITC apoptosis detection kit was used according to the manufacturer's instruction. Cells were washed with ice-cold PBS, then 5 μL of PI (50 μg/mL), 5 μL of fluorescein isothiocyanate, and 100 μL of annexin V binding buffer were added to the cell suspensions and incubated in a dark condition at room temperature for 15 min. Flow cytometry was conducted to analyze the samples within 1 h. All assays were repeated in triplicate.

In vitro cell migration

Wound-healing assay was adopted to evaluate the ability of cell migration, 3×10^5 viable cells were seeded in 12-well plates and cultured with serum-free RPMI 1640 medium. After overnight incubation, the monolayer cells were scraped with a 1 mL sterilized pipette tip to form a linear wound. The plates were washed three times and cultured at 5% CO_2 and 37 °C for another 24 h. Images were taken at the time of point of 0 h and 24 h, the wound area in each plate were detected using Image-Pro Plus 6.0 (IPP 6.0, produced by Media Cybernetics Corporation, USA) software. Wound-healing rate = [(scratch width at 0 h) - (scratch width at 24 h)]/(scratch width at 0 h)*100%.

Transwell invasion assay

Assays were performed using 24-well plates with 8-μm polycarbonate filter membrane coated from bottom with Matrigel as an extracelluar matrix barrier. Cells (5×10^4 cells per well) were seeded in the upper chambers and incubated with serum-free medium. Cell culture medium containing 20% FBS was added to the bottom of 24-well plates as a chemoattractant. After 24 h incubation at 37 °C, the non-migratory cells were removed from the upper surface by gentle scrubbing with a cotton tip. Subsequently, invading cells were fixed in 90% ethanol, stained with crystal violet and counted under a light microscopy. Each well counted 5 random fields, the experiments were carried out in triplicate.

Construction of Xenografted nude mouse models

All animal experiments were conducted under an approved protocol from Sichuan University Institutional Animal Care and Use Committee. Experimental mice were housed and maintained in sterile environment. For subcutaneous Xenograft experiments, 5-week-old athymic nude mice (BALB/$c^{nu/nu}$, $n = 24$) were randomized into three groups (half male and half female): normal control group, GIST Lv-shSPARCL1 group, and Lv-shNC group. Eight mice in each group were injected subcutaneously with 1×10^7 cells into the costal region of naked mice. Animals were weighted at the initial of the experiment and the tumor size was measured every 3 days. Moreover, the volume of tumors (TV) was calculated as previously described [21]. Mice were sacrificed by cervical dislocation at day 32 postinjection to collect and weight the generated tumors. For hepatic metastasis mice model, thirty mice were kept at least 1 week before experiment manipulation and were grouped as mentioned above. After disinfection, mice were anesthetized with 1% pentobarbital sodium at a dosage of 75 mg/kg. The middle abdominal incision was carried out to expose the spleen. A total of 1×10^7 viable tumor cells were implanted into splenic subcapsular space carefully to avoid extravasations, and gently pressed spleen injection point for minutes. Then, spleen was excised completely and abdominal incision was stitched. The mice were euthanized on day 30 postinjection or when the body weight was lost in more than 20% mice. Abdominal autopsy were performed to confirm hepatic metastatic nodules. The fresh tumor specimen and metastases were fixed with 10% formalin for the following pathologic examination.

Statistical analysis and follow-up

All statistical analyses were determined using the Statistical Package for the Social Science (SPSS), version 21.0 for Windows (SPSS Inc., Chicago, IL, USA). Measurement data were expressed as mean ± standard deviation and enumeration data were described as percentage. Differences between groups were analyzed using analysis of variance for consecutive data and χ^2 test or Fisher's exact test for categorical variables. Cumulative survival was determined using the Kaplan-Meier method and log rank test. Progression-free survival (PFS) was defined from the start of any treatment until disease progression. Follow-ups were carried out by office visit, telephone call, or outpatient clinic visit from July 2016 to August 2016. The univariate and multivariate analyses were used to explore independent prognostic factors by Cox regression. Differences with two-sided $P < 0.05$ were considered as statistically significant.

Results

Microarray analysis of the gastric GIST patients with high- and low-grade malignancy

To investigate the underlying mechanisms for malignant transformation in GIST, protein expression profiles in four primary gastric GIST and corresponding adjacent normal tissues were analyzed using a protein microarray. After normalization, 64 out of 1000 proteins were significant differentially expressed in gastric GIST between low- and high-grade malignance. And 41 proteins were up-regulated, while 23 proteins were down-regulated in tumors with high-grade malignancy when compare with that of low-grade malignancy (fold change > 2 or < 0.5; $P < 0.05$). The top 10 up- and down-regulated proteins as compared to low-grade malignancy were shown in Tables 2 and 3, respectively. And then unsupervised hierarchical clustering classified them into two groups according to their protein expression (Fig. 1). The differentially expressed proteins were shown in the volcano plot (Additional file 1: Figure S1).

Validation for differentially expression protein

As mentioned above, SPARCL1 is expressed in many tissues and downregulated in a wide variety of human malignancies, which suggests that SPARCL1 might play a role as a tumor suppressor gene. Moreover, former microarray analysis showed that SPARCL1 was significantly downregulated in tumors with high-grade malignancy. Thus, to verify the microarray results and to evaluate the significance of the findings, SPARCL1 was chosen to examine the expression level by real-time quantitative PCR and Western blot in a larger cohort of 4 pairs of gastric GIST samples. Relative to a loading control β-actin, SPARCL1 mRNA levels were down-regulated in tumors of HGM in comparison to the samples with LGM ($P < 0.05$), which was in consistency with prior microarray data (Fig. 2a). In addition, high expression of SPARCL1 mRNA was observed in adjacent normal tissues in contrast to gastric GIST ($P < 0.05$). To determine whether SPARCL1 protein expression decreased in tumors of HGM, we also evaluated SPARCL1 expression by Western blot. SPARCL1 expression was decreased in tumors of HGM in accordance with microarray and PCR data (Fig. 2b, c). These data suggested that the downregulation of SPARCL1 in GIST might be responsible for the pathogenesis and progression, and then we further investigated the functional role of SPARCL1 in gastric GIST.

Associations of SPARCL1 expression with Clinicopathological parameters in gastric GIST

The entire cohort comprised 98 patients with gastric GIST and included 47 (47.96%) females and 51 (52.04%) males with a mean age of 57.28 ± 11.55 years and a median age of 58.8 years (range, 30~ 84 years). The mean tumor size was 7.37 ± 6.13 cm and with a median size of 6 cm (range, 1~ 35 cm). A total of 20 patients received adjuvant therapy with targeted drug (imatinib/sunitinib). Immunochemistry staining showed a significant SPARCL1 overexpression in normal gastric tissues, and SPARCL1 was mainly located in the cytoplasm. High expression of SPARCL1 was observed in a majority of cases (71/98), while lower expression of SPARCL1 was detected in 27 of 98 gastric GIST (Fig. 3).

Table 2 Proteins significantly up-regulated in gastric GIST with HGM as compared to tumors with LGM

Name	Fold change	Standardized value in LGM	Standardized value in HGM	*P* value
pro-MMP13	15.746	8.000	125.969	0.012
FAP	8.385	11.359	95.250	0.036
FABP2	6.553	14.094	92.359	0.005
Chymase	5.991	16.953	101.563	0.001
PSP	5.564	3.656	20.344	0.005
Vitamin K-dependent protein S	5.338	14.250	76.063	0.023
Calsyntenin-1	4.666	12.875	60.078	0.031
HAI-2	4.643	18.531	86.047	0.000
Fetuin A	4.409	12.797	56.422	0.035
E-Cadherin	4.316	17.344	74.859	0.022

GIST gastrointestinal stromal tumors, *HGM* high-grade malignancy, *LGM* low-grade malignancy

Table 4 indicates the association between SPARCL1 expression and clinicopathological characteristics in gastric GIST. Specifically, there was significantly correlation between SPARCL1 expression and tumor size, mitotic index (/50HPF), distant metastasis at the time of initial diagnosis ($P < 0.05$). In other words, the later clinical stage of tumor, the lower expressing of SPARCL1 would be. No significant differences, however, were noted between SPARCL1 expression and age, gender, and radical degree, etc.

Relationship between SPARCL1 expression and patient prognosis

A total of 6 patients died due to tumor progression or other causes for the entire cohort with a median follow-up of 49.5 months (range, 6~ 78 months). The 1, 2, 3 years progression-free survival rate of gastric GIST patients was 95.9, 89.8 and 86.5%, respectively. Factors associated with PFS by Kaplan-Meier univariate analysis were radical degree ($P < 0.001$), distant metastasis at the time of initial diagnosis ($P < 0.05$), tumor size ($P < 0.001$), mitotic count ($P < 0.001$), NIH risk classification ($P < 0.001$), and SPARCL1 expression ($P < 0.001$). We learned that low expression of SPARCL1 was related with poor prognosis for gastric GIST. The median survival was not achieved for patients with SPARCL1-high expression versus 36 months (range, 0~ 67 months) for patients with SPARCL1-low expression ($P < 0.001$, Fig. 4). By incorporating these factors, except the highly collinear variables, into the Cox multivariate regression proportional hazards model, we found that radical degree (HR 7.266, 95% CI 1.222~ 43.221; $P = 0.029$), tumor size (HR 4.518, 95% CI 1.172~ 17.410; $P = 0.028$), and SPARCL1 expression (HR 0.157, 95% CI 0.040~ 0.612; $P = 0.008$) were independent prognostic predictors in gastric GIST (Table 5). Above findings suggested that SPARCL1 may function as a tumor suppressor in gastric GIST.

Transfecting cells with shRNA for knocking down SPARCL1

The moderate abundance of SPARCL1 expression was detected in cultured GIST 882 cells (parental cell) by qPCR. So, to investigate the functional significance of SPARCL1 knockdown on GIST 882 cells, a lentivirus shRNA-based system was used, which resulting in Lv-shSPARCL1 and

Table 3 Proteins significantly down-regulated in gastric GIST with HGM as compared to tumors with LGM

Name	Fold change	Standardized value in LGM	Standardized value in HGM	*P* value
SPARCL1	25.099	134.906	5.375	0.002
INSL3	6.418	72.203	11.250	0.020
HSP27	6.051	216.141	35.719	0.031
NPTX1	5.722	118.469	20.703	0.003
PSA-Free	5.344	143.125	26.781	0.044
ROCK1	5.058	68.359	13.516	0.041
Ceruloplasmin	5.005	289.969	57.938	0.032
NR3C3	4.948	108.703	21.969	0.037
Hck	4.770	108.656	22.781	0.005
Lyn	4.165	117.016	28.094	0.001

GIST gastrointestinal stromal tumors, *HGM* high-grade malignancy, *LGM* low-grade malignancy

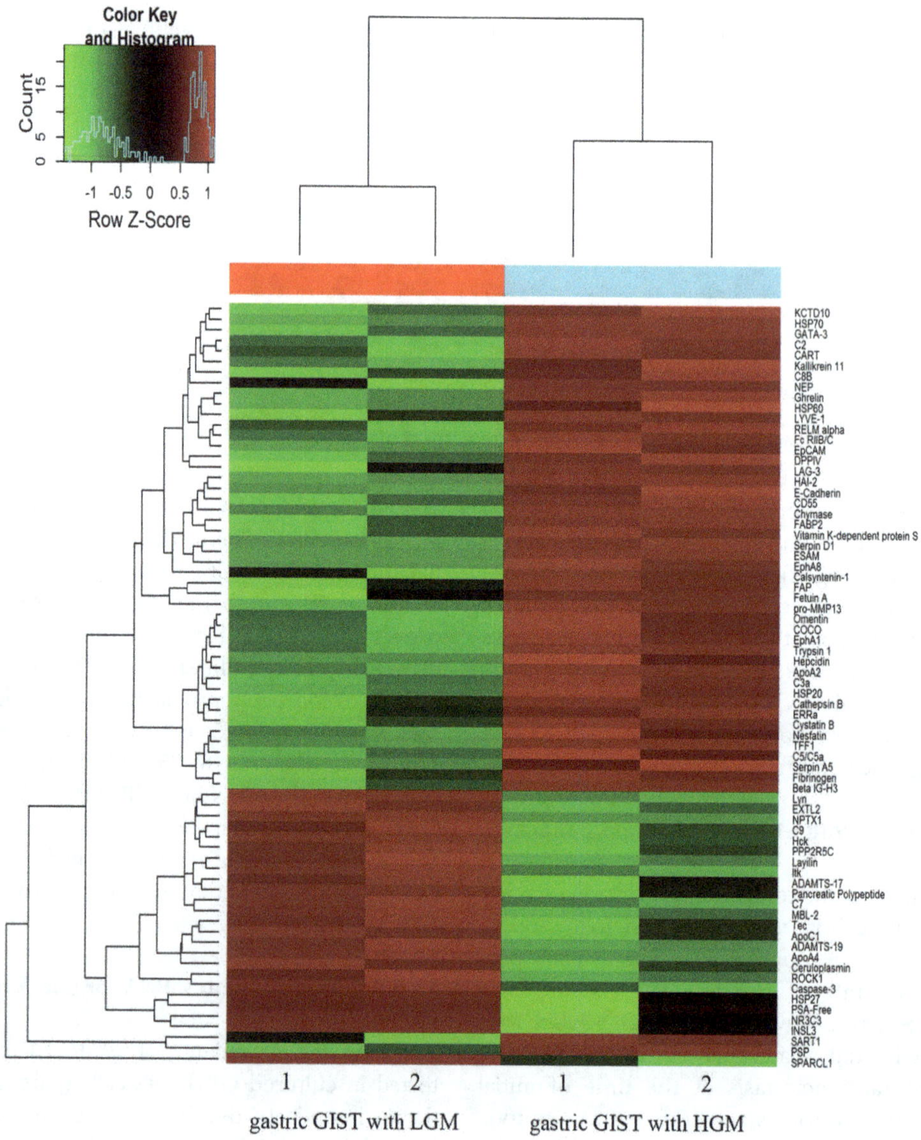

Fig. 1 Heatmap of the hierarchical cluster analysis of the differentially expressed proteins between LGM and HGM in gastric GIST. Each column represents a single tissue specimen and each row represents a protein. Pseudocolors indicate differential expression, with red indicating high expression, green for low expression and black indicating for the mean expression levels

Lv-shNC. The relative transcribing and expressing quantities of SPARCL1 in the group treated with shRNA were significantly lower to those in the normal control ($P < 0.05$) and Lv-shNC group ($P < 0.05$) after normalizing to β-actin (Fig. 5a, b). Because the interference efficiency of RNAi-3 was more efficient than the others, so a series of in vitro functional assays were performed by using this interference group.

Effects of SPARCL1 downregulation on GIST cell proliferation, cell cycle and apoptosis

CCK-8 cell proliferation assay was conducted to determine the changes of SPARCL1 knockdown on GIST cell growth. According to the Fig. 5, the proliferation rates of the Lv-shSPARCL1, Lv-shNC and normal control group were similar in 24-, 48- and 72-h measurements ($P > 0.05$), which demonstrating that downregulation of SPARCL1 had no significant effect on GIST 882 cell growth in vitro. The influence of SPARCL1 silencing on cell-cycle progression was determined by flow cytometry with the aim of observing the changes in cell cycles induced by knocking out SPARCL1. The ratio value of cells in the G0/G1 phase in the Lv-shSPARCL1 group was significantly higher than those in the Lv-shNC and normal control group ($P < 0.05$), while the percentages of cells in the G2/M phase decreased in the Lv-shSPARCL1 group, and which indicated that

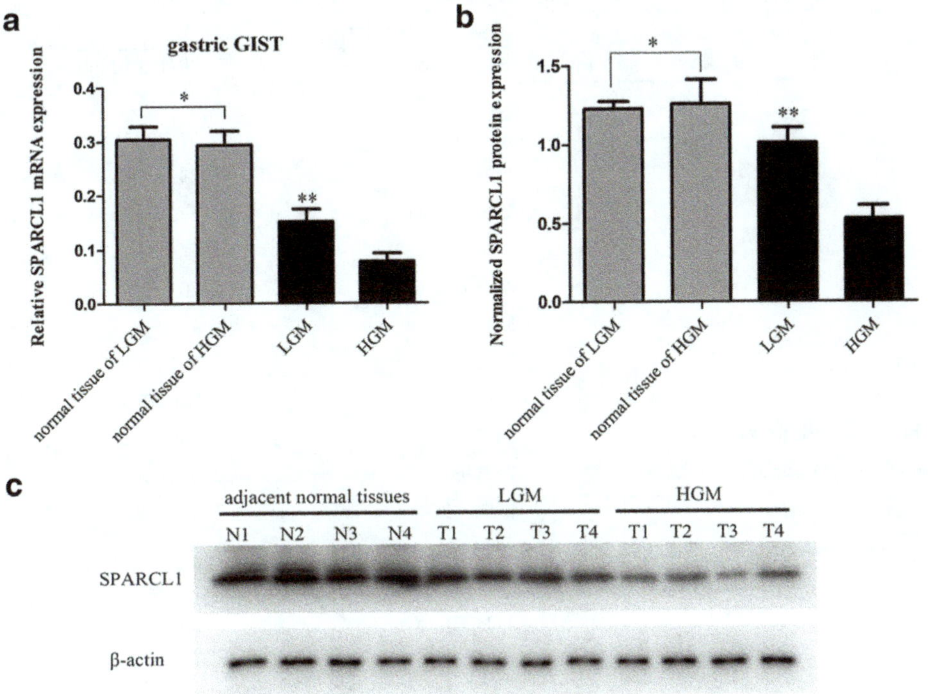

Fig. 2 SPARCL1 is downregulated in human gastric GIST. The protein expression of SPARCL1 was determined by RT-qPCR and western blot with β-actin as a loading control. **a** Relative SPARCL1 mRNA level was significantly decreased in gastric GSIT with HGM as compared with those with LGM (**$P < 0.05$), while no statistical significance was noted between matched normal tissues from HGM and LGM (*$P > 0.05$); **b**, **c** A significant reduced expression of SPARCL1 in gastric GIST with HGM compared to those with LGM was determined by western blot analysis (**$P < 0.05$). N1~N2 for adjacent normal tissue of LGM, while N3~N4 for adjacent tissue of HGM. The bars represent mean ± SD ($n = 4$)

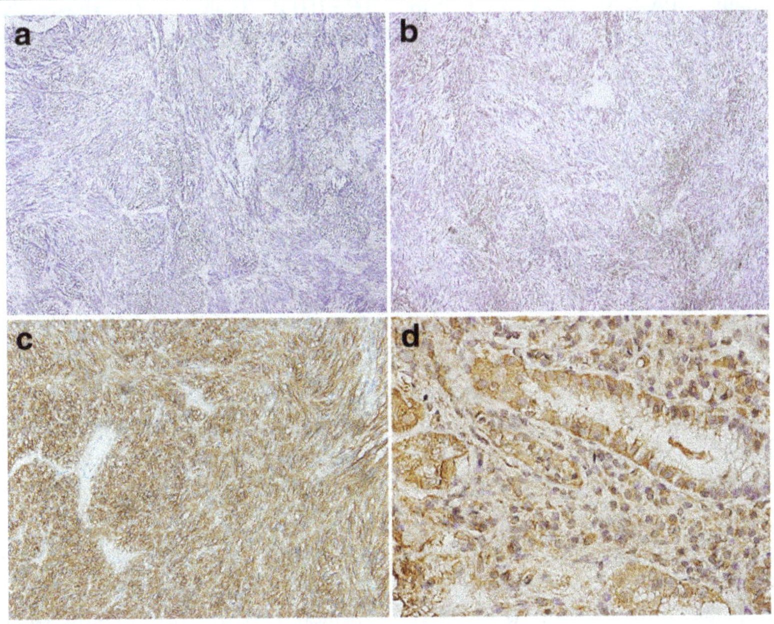

Fig. 3 Representative immunohistochemical staining of SPARCL1 in gastric GIST and normal gastric tissues. **a**, **b** Negative/low expression of SPARCL1 in gastric GIST; (**c**, **d**) Gastric GIST and normal gastric tissues showed high expression of SPARCL1, separately. Original magnification: × 200 for **a**, **b**, **c** and × 600 for **d**

Table 4 Association of SPARCL1 expression with clinicopathological factors of gastric GIST (*n* = 98)

Variables	SPARCL1 expression		*P* value
	SPARCL1-low	SPARCL1-high	
Gender			0.182
Male	10 (37.04)	37 (52.11)	
Female	17 (62.96)	34 (47.89)	
Age (years)	55.67 ± 14.11	57.89 ± 10.46	0.398
Surgical margins			0.062
R0	24 (88.89)	70 (98.59)	
Not R0	3 (11.11)	1 (1.41)	
Multivisceral resection (n, %)	7 (25.93)	2 (2.82)	0.002
Tumor rupture (n, %)	1 (3.70)	0 (0.00)	0.276
Hepatic metastasis at initial diagnosis (n, %)	5 (18.52)	0 (0.00)	0.001
Peritoneal metastasis at initial diagnosis (n, %)	7 (25.93)	0 (0.00)	< 0.001
Tumor size (cm)	11.94 ± 9.04	5.63 ± 3.24	< 0.001
Mitotic count (n, %)			< 0.001
≤5/50 HPF	3 (11.11)	35 (49.30)	
6~ 10/50 HPF	9 (33.33)	20 (28.17)	
> 10/50 HPF	15 (55.56)	16 (22.54)	
NIH risk classification (n, %)			0.127
Very low	0 (0.00)	4 (5.63)	
Low	1 (3.70)	20 (28.17)	
Intermediate	4 (14.81)	22 (30.99)	
High	22 (81.48)	25 (35.21)	

SPARCL1 secreted protein acidic and rich in cysteine-like protein 1, *GIST* gastrointestinal stromal tumors, *HPF* high power field, *NIH* National Institutes of Health, *"Not R0"* includes surgeries of R1 and R2 resections

SPARCL1 silencing could induce the arresting of cell cycles in G0/G1 phase. Additionally, SPARCL1 downregulation did not affect apoptosis of GIST 882 cell among three groups (Lv-shSPARCL1, Lv-shNC and normal control group, $P > 0.05$).

Downregulation of SPARCL1 suppresses migration and invasion of GIST 882 cells

The ability to migrate or invade was considered as the main malignant phenotype and prerequisite for tumor cell metastasis. To determine whether downregulation of SPARCL1 changed cell motility, an in vitro wound healing assay was utilized. In wound healing assay, it was shown that the cell migration abilities of GIST 882 was remarkably promoted after knocking out of SPARCL1 in comparison with those in the normal control and Lv-shNC group at 24 h ($P <$ 0.001). Moreover, we also investigated the SPARCL1 effect on invasive capability of GIST 882 cells. In a 24-h transwell cell invasion assay, there were more Lv-shSPARCL1 cells passing through membranes coated with Matrigel compared to Lv-shNC and normal control group ($P < 0.001$, Fig. 5). The SPARCL1 notably decreased the invasion ability of GIST 882 cells by 3.2-fold when compared with vector control cells ($P < 0.001$), while no statistical significance was observed between the Lv-shNC and normal control group ($P > 0.05$). Collectively, these data support a role for SPARCL1 in reducing abilities of migration and invasion in GIST 882 cell line.

Effect of SPARCL1 on GIST growth and liver metastasis in a mouse xenograft model

To gain insight into whether SPARCL1 impacts tumor growth and metastasis in vivo, mouse xenograft models were performed by means of implanting Lv-shSPARCL1, Lv-shNC and parental cells. The subcutaneous model in nude nice was successfully established, and the tumor volume was monitored every 3 days from 14 days after the injection of these cells. No tumorigenesis were observed in 1 and 3 nude mice for the normal control group and Lv-shSPARCL1 group, respectively. There was no statistical significance in terms of average tumor volume and tumor weight among three groups ($P > 0.05$). The SPARCL1 expression for xenograft groups was verified by RT-qPCR and IHC staining, and it was found that SPARCL1 was downregulated in the Lv-shSPARCL1 xenograft group as compared with that of the Lv-shNC and normal control group. Moreover, the representative images for the hematoxylin and eosin staining were shown in Fig. 6. Due to the liver

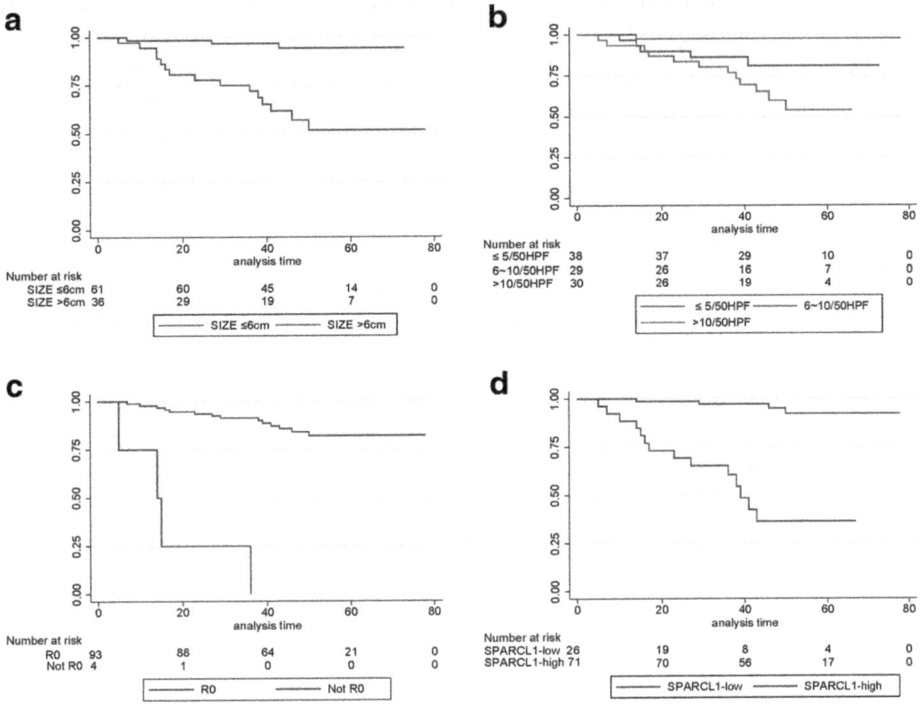

Fig. 4 Kaplan-Meier survival curves of progression-free survival in patients with primary gastric GIST ($n = 98$). **a** Comparison of progression-free survival between tumors with ≤6 cm and > 6 cm ($P < 0.001$); **b** The tumors with mitotic count ≤5/50HPF showed significant better PFS compared with those of 6~ 10/50HPF and > 10/50HPF ($P < 0.001$); **c** Patients with R0 resection showed better PFS than that who did not achieve R0 resection ($P < 0.001$); **d** A worse prognosis was noted in patients with SPARCL-low expression in comparison to those with SPARCL1-high expression ($P < 0.001$)

accounts for the most of the GIST metastases, the intrasplenic implantation was conducted to assess the influence of SPARCL1 on hepatic metastasis. There were 1, 1 and 6 nude mice occurred liver metastasis in the normal control group, Lv-shNC group and Lv-shSPARCL1 group, respectively. Review of metastasis from sacrificed mice indicated that the metastatic nodules formation was significantly higher in the Lv-shSPARCL1 group than those in the Lv-shNC and normal control group ($P < 0.05$). Furthermore, the expression of SPARCL1 in each tissue sample was determined by RT-qPCR and IHC staining (Fig. 6). These results demonstrated that SPARCL1 downregulation could inhibit the development of liver metastasis of GIST cells in vivo.

Discussion

SPARCL1 is a secreted matricellular glycoprotein belonging to SPARC family, which plays important roles in the regulation of cell adhesion, proliferation, cell cycle, and migration [13, 22]. In recent years, a multitude of studies have reported that SPARCL1 implicated in the initiation and progression of various cancer, including prostate, colorectal, gastric, liver, breast cancer [23, 24]. Here, we first explored the molecular basis of GIST malignization by studying the expression profile of proteins, and found that SPARCL1 was expressed at lower level in high-grade malignance gastric GIST compared with low-grade ones. The Kaplan-Meier and Cox proportional hazard analyses demonstrated that SPARCL1 can be considered as a protective factor in gastric GIST. In vitro and in vivo experiments suggested that downregulation of SPARCL1 significantly enhanced the invasion and liver metastasis ability of GIST 882 cell, but did not influence the GIST cell proliferation, cell cycle, and apoptosis. These studies validate that SPARCL1 may play a crucial role in gastric GIST progression.

According to the NCCN guidelines (Version 2. 2017), all GIST have potential malignancy-transforming ability even if the tumor is small and asymptomatic [25]. Several risk-stratification systems were proposed, which incorporated the prognostic factors such as tumor location, mitotic count and tumor size, to assess the malignant potential or risk level of GIST in clinics. However, the intrinsic mechanism in progression of GIST is not well defined to date. To this end, in the present work, we explored differential expression of proteins which might be involved in gastric GIST malignization, and further validation of selected candidate (SPARCL1) was performed. Identifying molecular biomarkers associated with the recurrence risk of GIST could contribute to novel treatment approaches, and also complement the existing risk evaluation criteria [26].

Table 5 Univariate and multivariate analysis of factors with PFS in gastric GIST using Cox proportional hazards regression modeling ($n = 98$)

Variables	*P* univariate	Multivariate analysis	
		HR (95% CI)	*P*
Surgical margins			
R0		Reference	
Not R0	< 0.001	7.266(1.222~ 43.221)	0.029
Multivisceral resection			
No		Reference	
Yes	< 0.001	1.553(0.439~ 5.489)	0.495
Peritoneal metastasis at initial diagnosis			
No		Reference	
Yes	< 0.001	2.201(0.512~ 9.466)	0.289
Hepatic metastasis at initial diagnosis			
No		Reference	
Yes	0.003	2.281(0.384~ 13.533)	0.364
Tumor size			
≤6 cm		Reference	
> 6 cm	< 0.001	4.518(1.172~ 17.410)	0.028
NIH risk classification			
Very low/low		Reference	
Intermediate/high	0.005	1.681(0.309~ 9.155)	0.548
Mitotic count			
≤5/50 HPF		Reference	
6~ 10/50 HPF		3.752(0.379~ 37.105)	0.258
> 10/50 HPF	< 0.001	8.924(0.908~ 87.698)	0.060
SPARCL1 expression			
Low		Reference	
High	< 0.001	0.157(0.040~ 0.612)	0.008

PFS progression-free survival, *GIST* gastrointestinal stromal tumors, *HR* hazard ratio, *CI* confidential interval, *HPF* high power field, *NIH* National Institutes of Health, *SPARCL1* secreted protein acidic and rich in cysteine-like protein 1, *"Not R0"* includes surgeries of R1 and R2 resections

Growing evidences show that SPARCL1 often presents a reduced or absent expression pattern in many human epithelial cancers, suggesting its role as tumor suppressor [16, 17]. In 2012, Li and colleagues reported that both SPARCL1 mRNA and protein levels were relevantly downregulated compared to normal tissues in a large series of patients harboring gastric cancer [27]. In agreement with their findings, data from both PCR and western blot analyses indicated that SPARCL1 was decreased in gastric GIST compared with normal gastric tissues; and its expression level was decreased with the increase of malignancy in gastric GIST. However, an increased expression of SPARCL1 was noted in a few of other types of human tumors which derived from liver, colon and rectum when compared to corresponding healthy tissues [15, 23]. These reports indicating that SPARCL1 exactly participates in cancer occurrence and development, but its expression pattern as well as functionary mechanisms in various tumor conditions may be different.

Pilot studies have analyzed the associations of SPARCL1 expression with the clinicopathological factors. As reported, Loss of SPARCL1 was more observed in N1/2-stage and high/moderate-differentiated tumors than in N0-stage and poor/un-differentiated hilar cholangiocarcinoma, respectively [28]. Additionally, expression of SPARCL1 was closely associated with tumor grade, tumor size, regional lymph nodes, and TNM stages in gastric cancer [27]. In the present study, an analysis of the clinicopathological features showed that low expression ratio of SPARCL1 markedly increased tumor size, mitotic index (/50HPF), and number of distant metastasis at the time of initial diagnosis and tumor progression. The aforementioned parameters are known to be factors for evaluating recurrence risk or malignant potential of GIST. Thus, our study indicates that SPARCL1 expression is negatively related to the malignant biological

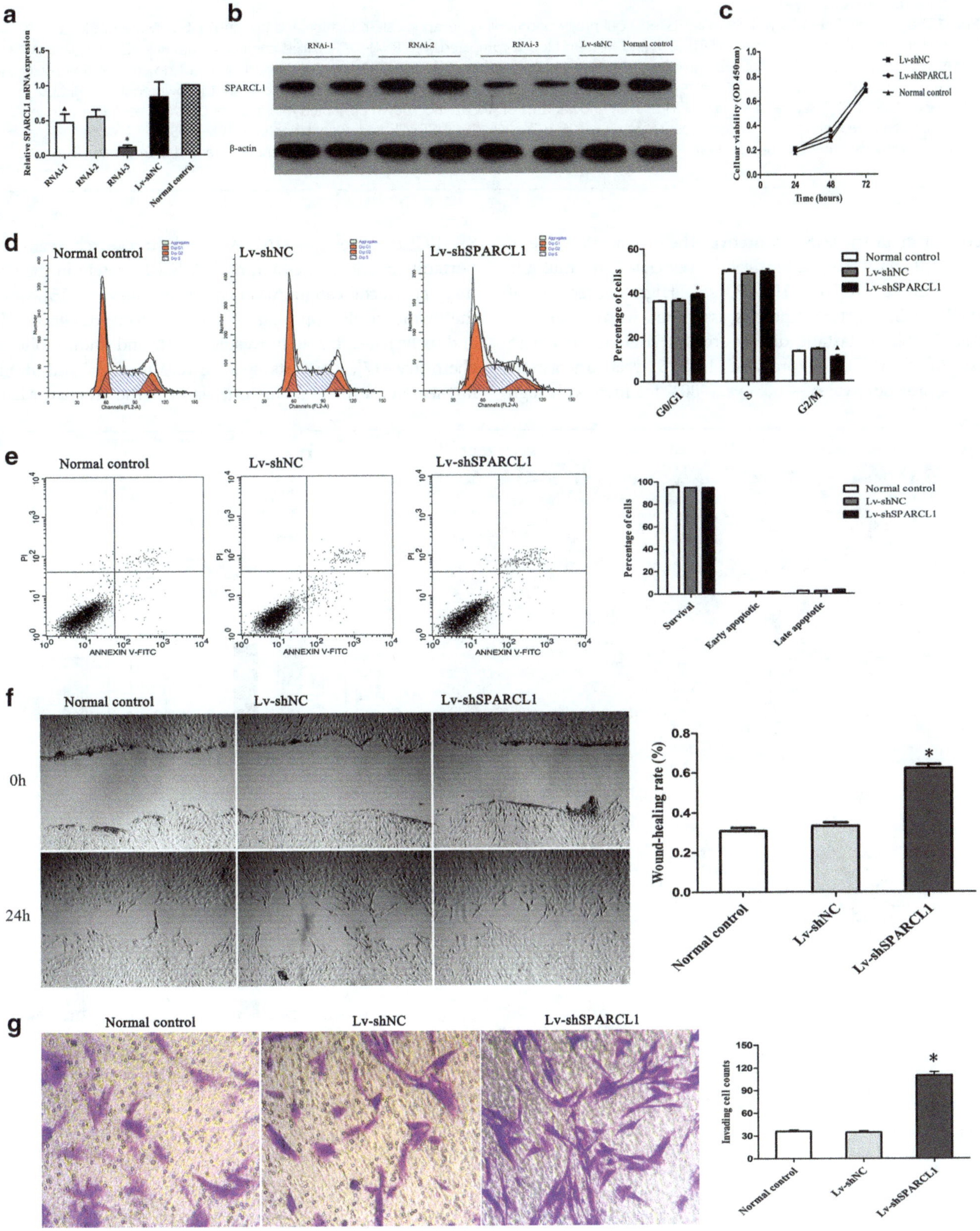

Fig. 5 (See legend on next page.)

(See figure on previous page.)

Fig. 5 The roles of SPARCL1 knockdown in GIST 882 cell proliferation, cell cycle, apoptosis, migration and invasion. **a**, **b** Downregulation of SPARCL1 in GIST cells was confirmed by RT-qPCR and western blot. ▲compared with RNAi-3, $P < 0.05$; * compared with RNAi-2, $P < 0.05$. **c**: A CCK-8 assay was performed to evaluate the influence of SPARCL1 knockdown on GIST 882 cell proliferation. **d**: SPARCL1 downregulation could induce the arrest of cell cycles in G0/G1 phase. ▲ * compared with the other two groups, both $P < 0.05$. **e** SPARCL1 downregulation did not affect apoptosis of GIST 882 cell. **f** Wound-healing assay showed that SPARCL1 knockdown promoted migration of GIST 882 cells after cultured for 24 h. * compared with the other two groups, both $P < 0.05$. **g** The invasive GIST cells and quantitation of invasive GIST cell counts. * compared with the other two groups, both $P < 0.05$. Data represent the mean of three independent experiments, and the error bars refer to SD from the mean

behavior in gastric GIST. Moreover, the prognostic value of SPARCL1 has been extensively investigated in multiple solid tumors [16, 17, 19, 27, 28]. High expression of SPARCL1 in prostate cancer is associated with better survival, 5 year metastatic disease-free survival of men with loss of SPARCL1 expression had 5 year metastatic disease-free survival of ~ 60% vs. ~ 80% for men with high SPARCL1 expression [16]. A Swedish research team reported that over-expression of SPARCL1 protein in the primary colorectal carcinomas had a short survival [15], while the diametrically opposing conclusions were drawn by Hu and colleagues through western blot and immunohistochemistry [17]. Thus, its specific role in GIST still awaits further confirmation. In our study, the Kaplan-Meier

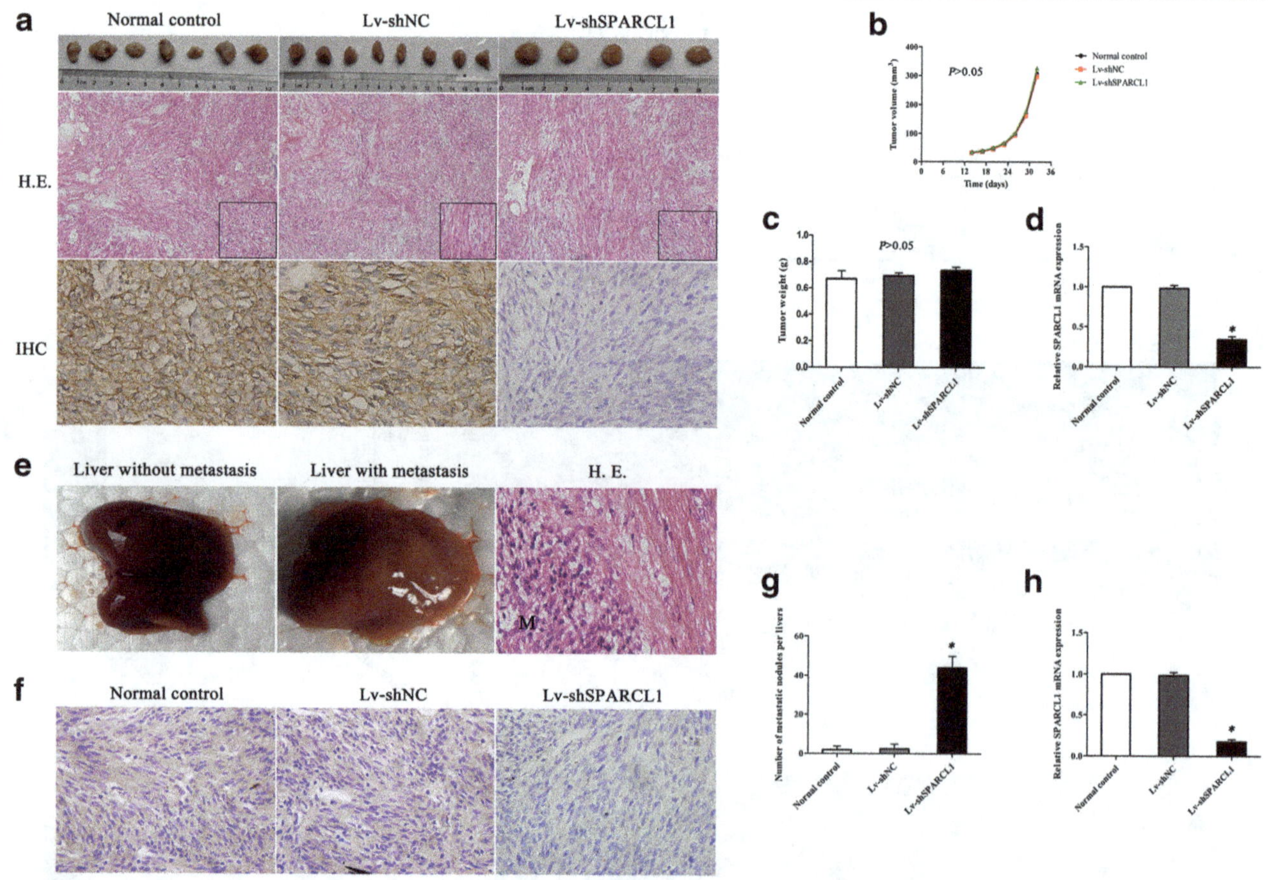

Fig. 6 Downregulation of SPARCL1 in GIST 882 cells promoted liver metastasis in xenograft mouse models. **a** Representative images of hematoxylin and eosin staining (HE ×100) and IHC staining (×600) of SPARCL1 in xenografted tumors; **b**, **c** Quantification of tumor volume and tumor weight for tumorigenesis among three groups in nude mice ($P > 0.05$). The error bars refer to SD ($n = 7$, 8, and 5 for normal control, Lv-shNC and Lv-shSPARCL1, respectively); **d** Expression level of SPARCL1 mRNA was significantly decreased in Lv-shSPARCL1 group as compared to other two groups ($^*P < 0.05$). The error bars present SD ($n = 7$, 8, and 5 for normal control, Lv-shNC and Lv-shSPARCL1, respectively); **e** Representative of gross view of liver without and with metastasis, and HE staining of liver metastatic tumor (M); **f** Low expression of SPARCL1 in liver metastatic nodules was observed in Lv-shSPARCL1 group as compared to other two groups; **g** The number of liver metastatic nodules was increased in Lv-shSPARCL1 group when compared to other two groups ($^*P < 0.05$); **h** The relative SPARCL1 mRNA level of liver metastatic nodules of nude mice ($^*P < 0.05$). The error bars refer to SD from the mean

analysis revealed that low expression of SPARCL1 was related with poor prognosis for gastric GIST, which was consistent with previous reports. The median survival was not achieved for patients with SPARCL1-high expression versus 36 months (range, 0~ 67 months) for patients with SPARCL1-low expression. Furthermore, in addition to the clinicopathological factors, we have introduced biomarker, SPARCL1, into the Cox regression model, and found that SPARCL1 expression functions as a protective factor (HR 0.157; 95%CI 0.040~ 0.612; $P = 0.008$).

Metastasis is the main cause of cancer-related death. The hallmarks of cancer comprise six biological capabilities: sustaining proliferative signaling, evading growth suppressors, evasion of apoptosis, limitless replicative potential, inducing angiogenesis, and ability to invade and metastasize [29]. It is worthy that the final hallmark of caner, invasion and metastasis, underlies its deadly progressive nature. Many tumors prefer certain organs, particularly the lungs, bone marrow, and liver, as metastatic sites. Specifically, cancerous cells preferentially metastasized to liver tissue, which caused the high recurrence (about 55~ 72%) and low survival rates to patients with GIST [30, 31]. Given the above findings, which showed the malignancy-suppressing ability of SPARCL1, we further examined whether downregulation of SPARCL1 affects GIST cell invasion and migration in vitro and in vivo. Our results suggested that SPARCL1 suppressed the invasion and migration of GIST cell in vitro, but did not inhibit cell proliferation and apoptosis. Results from in vivo study showed that downregulation of SPARCL1 significantly promoted the ability of liver metastasis, suggesting that SPARCL1 may participate in the progression of gastric GIST, which was consistent with previous reports [14, 16, 17]. Hurly et al. demonstrated that SPARCL1 blocks the activation of the Ras homolog gene family, member C, thereby inhibiting cellular movement [16]. In addition, SPARCL1 may also promote differentiation possibly via mesenchymal-epithelial transition, which inhibits the aggressiveness of colorectal cancer [17]. Besides, unlike the influence to colorectal and pancreatic cancer cells, SPARCL1 did not inhibit the proliferation of hilar cholangiocarcinoma cells and prostate cells in vitro [13, 14, 16, 17, 28]. Our study demonstrated a crucial role for SPARCL1 in facilitating GIST invasion and migration both in vitro and vivo, strongly suggested SPARCL1 functioning as a metastatic suppressor and may serve as a potential therapeutic target for patients with metastatic gastric GIST. However, the detail mechanism of SPARCL1 involving in GIST malignization should be explored in further study, which is also the major limitation of this study.

Downregulation of SPARCL1 in human tumors has not been well addressed yet. The possible mechanism of gene inactivation may result from gene mutations, loss of heterozygosity (LOH), and epigenetic alteration such as promoter methylation. Esposito and colleagues found that promoter demethylation slightly increased SPARCL1 mRNA, suggesting that hypermethylation is not the key mechanism accounting for low expression of SPARCL1 in pancreatic cancer cell [13]. Meanwhile, result from a previous study showed that no mutation or deletion that might be responsible for downregulation of SPARCL1 was noted in lung tumor [32]. In a recent study, Li et al. showed that no methylation variable positions and no mutation were observed in gastric cancer, but a possible mechanism involving the LOH of SPARCL1 gene was revealed [27].

Conclusions

Overall, the collective findings from our study show for the first time that SPARCL1 might have a certain degree of malignancy-suppressing potential, which suppresses metastasis of gastric GIST. Additionally, this study also sets the stage for further investigations on the basic mechanisms that underlie GIST metastasis.

Additional file

Additional file 1: Figure S1. Volcano plots of differential expression proteins. The vertical lines correspond to 2.0-fold up and down, respectively, and the horizontal line represents a *p*-value of 0.05. The red point in the plot represents the differentially protein with statistically significance. (A: gastric GIST with LGM; B: gastric GIST with HGM; C: corresponding adjacent normal tissues for LGM; D: corresponding adjacent normal tissues for HGM).

Abbreviations

GIST: Gastrointestinal stromal tumors; HGM: High-grade malignancy; HPFs: High power field; HR: Hazard ratio; IHC: Immunohistochemistry; LGM: Low-grade malignancy; NCCN: National Comprehensive Cancer Network; PCR: Polymerase chain reaction; PDGFRa: Platelet-derived growth factor receptor alpha; PFS: Progression-free survival; SPARCL1: Secreted protein acidic and rich in cysteine-like protein 1; TV: Volume of tumor

Acknowledgements

The authors gratefully acknowledge the whole staffs of Department of Gastrointestinal Surgery, West China Hospital, who generously provided assistance in the collection of data throughout the duration of the study.

Funding

This work was supported by the National Natural Science Foundation of China (no. 81572931).

Authors' contributions

ZB, CZX and ZZG conceived and designed the study. SCY, YY, CHJ and WRX performed the experiments. YXN and CZL analyzed the data. SCY and YY drafted the manuscript. All authors read and approved the final manuscript.

Competing interests

The authors declare that they have no competing interests.

Author details

[1]Department of Gastrointestinal Surgery, West China Hospital, Sichuan University, Chengdu 610041, Sichuan, China. [2]Department of Pathology, West

China Hospital, Sichuan University, Chengdu 610041, Sichuan, China. [3]State Key Laboratory of Biotherapy and Cancer Center/Collaborative Innovation Center for Biotherapy, West China Hospital, Sichuan University, Chengdu 610041, Sichuan, China. [4]Institute of Digestive Surgery and State Key Laboratory of Biotherapy, West China Hospital, Sichuan University, Chengdu 610041, Sichuan, China.

References

1. Wang X, Mori I, Tang W, Utsunomiya H, Nakamura M, Nakamura Y, Zhou G, Kakudo K. Gastrointestinal stromal tumors: are they of cajal cell origin? Exp Mol Pathol. 2002;72:172–7.
2. Miettinen M, Lasota J. Gastrointestinal stromal tumors–definition, clinical, histological, immunohistochemical, and molecular genetic features and differential diagnosis. Virchows Arch. 2001;438:1–12.
3. Lin JX, Chen QF, Zheng CH, Li P, Xie JW, Wang JB, Lu J, Chen QY, Cao LL, et al. Is 3-years duration of adjuvant imatinib mesylate treatment sufficient for patients with high-risk gastrointestinal stromal tumor? A study based on long-term follow-up. J Cancer Res Clin Oncol. 2017;143:727–34.
4. Joensuu H, Wardelmann E, Sihto H, Eriksson M, Sundby Hall K, Reichardt A, Hartmann JT, Pink D, Cameron S, et al. Effect of KIT and PDGFRA mutations on survival in patients with gastrointestinal stromal tumors treated with adjuvant Imatinib: an exploratory analysis of a randomized clinical trial. JAMA Oncol. 2017;3:602–9.
5. Baskin Y, Kocal GC, Kucukzeybek BB, Akbarpour M, Kayacik N, Sagol O, Ellidokuz H, Oztop I. PDGFRA and KIT mutation status and its association with Clinicopathological properties, including DOG1. Oncol Res. 2016;24:41–53.
6. Joensuu H. Risk stratification of patients diagnosed with gastrointestinal stromal tumor. Hum Pathol. 2008;39:1411–9.
7. Gold JS, Gönen M, Gutiérrez A, Broto JM, García-del-Muro X, Smyrk TC, Maki RG, Singer S, Brennan MF, et al. Development and validation of a prognostic nomogram for recurrence-free survival after complete surgical resection of localised primary gastrointestinal stromal tumour: a retrospective analysis. Lancet Oncol. 2009;10:1045–52.
8. Miettinen M, Sobin LH, Lasota J. Gastrointestinal stromal tumors of the stomach: a clinicopathologic immunohistochemical, and molecular genetic study of 1765 cases with long-term follow-up. Am J Surg Pathol. 2005;29:52–68.
9. Joensuu H, Vehtari A, Riihimäki J, Nishida T, Steigen SE, Brabec P, Plank L, Nilsson B, Cirilli C, et al. Risk of recurrence of gastrointestinal stromal tumour after surgery: an analysis of pooled population-based cohorts. Lancet Oncol. 2012;13:265–74.
10. Nakajima T, Ushijima T, Kihara A, Murata K, Sugiyama T, Tsuneyama K, Imura J, Fukushima J, Horiuchi H. A gastrointestinal stromal tumor of the stomach demonstrating a stepwise progression from low- to high-grade malignancy. Case Rep Gastrointest Med. 2012;2012:606832.
11. Girard JP, Springer TA. Cloning from purified high endothelial venule cells of hevin, a close relative of the antiadhesive extracellular matrix protein SPARC. Immunity. 1995;2:113–23.
12. Girard JP, Springer TA. Modulation of endothelial cell adhesion by hevin, an acidic protein associated with high endothelial venules. J Biol Chem. 1996;271:4511–7.
13. Esposito I, Kayed H, Keleg S, Giese T, Sage EH, Schirmacher P, Friess H, Kleeff J. Tumor-suppressor function of SPARC-like protein 1/Hevin in pancreatic cancer. Neoplasia. 2007;9:8–17.
14. Xiang Y, Qiu Q, Jiang M, Jin R, Lehmann BD, Strand DW, Jovanovic B, DeGraff DJ, Zheng Y, et al. SPARCL1 suppresses metastasis in prostate cancer. Mol Oncol. 2013;7:1019–30.
15. Zhang H, Widegren E, Wang DW, Sun XF. SPARCL1: a potential molecule associated with tumor diagnosis, progression and prognosis of colorectal cancer. Tumour Biol. 2011;32:1225–31.
16. Hurley PJ, Marchionni L, Simons BW, Ross AE, Peskoe SB, Miller RM, Erho N, Vergara IA, Ghadessi M, et al. Secreted protein, acidic and rich in cysteine-like 1 (SPARCL1) is down regulated in aggressive prostate cancers and is prognostic for poor clinical outcome. Proc Natl Acad Sci U S A. 2012;109:14977–82.
17. Hu H, Zhang H, Ge W, Liu X, Loera S, Chu P, Chen H, Peng J, Zhou L, et al. Secreted protein acidic and rich in cysteines-like 1 suppresses aggressiveness and predicts better survival in colorectal cancers. Clin Cancer Res. 2012;18:5438–48.
18. Sullivan MM, Sage EH. Hevin/SC1, a matricellular glycoprotein and potential tumor suppressor of the SPARC/BM-40/osteonectin family. Int J Biochem Cell Biol. 2004;36:991–6.
19. Cao F, Wang K, Zhu R, Hu YW, Fang WZ, Ding HZ. Clinicopathological significance of reduced SPARCL1 expression in human breast cancer. Asian Pac J Cancer Prev. 2013;14:195–200.
20. Kondo Y, Iijima T, Noguchi M. Evaluation of immunohistochemical staining using whole-slide imaging for HER2 scoring of breast cancer in comparison with real glass slides. Pathol Int. 2012;62:592–9.
21. Gasparini G, Harris AL. Clinical importance of the determination of tumor angiogenesis in breast carcinoma: much more than a new prognostic tool. J Clin Oncol. 1995;13:765–82.
22. Gagliardi F, Narayanan A, Mortini P. SPARCL1 a novel player in cancer biology. Crit Rev Oncol Hematol. 2017;109:63–8.
23. Lau CP, Poon RT, Cheung ST, Yu WC, Fan ST. SPARC and Hevin expression correlate with tumour angiogenesis in hepatocellular carcinoma. J Pathol. 2006;210:459–68.
24. Li T, Liu X, Yang A, Fu W, Yin F, Zeng X. Associations of tumor suppressor SPARCL1 with cancer progression and prognosis. Oncol Lett. 2017;14:2603–10.
25. Shen C, Chen H, Yin Y, Chen J, Han L, Zhang B, Chen Z, Chen J. Endoscopic versus open resection for small gastric gastrointestinal stromal tumors: safety and outcomes. Medicine (Baltimore). 2015;94:e376.
26. Hara R, Kikuchi H, Setoguchi T, Miyazaki S, Yamamoto M, Hiramatsu Y, Kamiya K, Ohta M, Baba S, et al. Microarray analysis reveals distinct gene set profiles for gastric and intestinal gastrointestinal stromal tumors. Anticancer Res. 2015;35:3289–98.
27. Li P, Qian J, Yu G, Chen Y, Liu K, Li J, Wang J. Down-regulated SPARCL1 is associated with clinical significance in human gastric cancer. J Surg Oncol. 2012;105:31–7.
28. Yu Y, Chen Y, Ma J, Yu X, Yu G, Li Z. SPARCL1 is a novel predictor of tumor recurrence and survival in hilar cholangiocarcinoma. Tumour Biol. 2016;37:4159–67.
29. Hanahan D, Weinberg RA. Hallmarks of cancer: the next generation. Cell. 2011;144:646–74.
30. Bayraktar UD, Bayraktar S, Rocha-Lima CM. Molecular basis and management of gastrointestinal stromal tumors. World J Gastroenterol. 2010;16:2726–34.
31. DeMatteo RP, Lewis JJ, Leung D, Mudan SS, Woodruff JM, Brennan MF. Two hundred gastrointestinal stromal tumors: recurrence patterns and prognostic factors for survival. Ann Surg. 2000;231:51–8.
32. Isler SG, Ludwig CU, Chiquet-Ehrismann R, Schenk S. Evidence for transcriptional repression of SPARC-like 1, a gene downregulated in human lung tumors. J Oncol. 2004;25:1073–9.

19

HPV positive, wild type *TP53*, and p16 overexpression correlate with the absence of residual tumors after chemoradiotherapy in anal squamous cell carcinoma

Paulo C. Soares[1,2*], Eliana S. Abdelhay[3], Luiz Claudio S. Thuler[3], Bruno Moreira Soares[4], Samia Demachki[5], Gessica Valéria Rocha Ferro[5], Paulo P. Assumpção[5], Leticia Martins Lamarão[6], Luis Felipe Ribeiro Pinto[3] and Rommel Mario Rodríguez Burbano[1,4]

Abstract

Background: Anal residual tumors are consensually identified within six months of chemoradiotherapy and represent a persistent lesion that may have prognostic value for overall survival. The aim of this study was to evaluate the association of HPV and HIV status, p16 expression level and *TP53* mutations with the absence of residual tumors (local response) in Squamous Cell Carcinoma (SCC) of the anal canal after chemoradiotherapy.

Methods: We performed a study on 78 patients with SCC of the anal canal who submitted to chemoradiotherapy and were followed for a six-month period to identify the absence or presence of residual tumors. HPV DNA was identified by polymerase chain reaction and direct sequencing, HIV RNA was detected by TaqMan amplification, p16 expression was detected by western blotting, and the mutational analysis of *TP53* was performed by direct sequencing; additionally, samples carrying mutations underwent fluorescent in sit hybridization. The evaluation of the tumor response to treatment was conducted six months after the conclusion of chemoradiotherapy. The following classifications were used to evaluate the outcomes: a) no response (presence of residual tumor) and b) complete response (absence of residual tumor).

Results: The significant variables associated with the absence of residual tumors were HPV positive, p16 overexpressed, wild-type *TP53*, female gender, and stages I and II. Only the presence of HPV was independently correlated with the clinical response; this variable increased the chances of a response within six months by 31-fold.

Conclusions: The presence of HPV in tumor cells was correlated with the absence of a residual tumor. This correlation is valuable and can direct future therapeutic approaches in the anal canal.

Keywords: HPV, HIV, p16, *TP53*, Anal squamous cell carcinoma

Background

Squamous cell carcinoma (SCC) of the anal canal has an annual incidence in western countries of 1.0 to 2.5 per 100,000 people, with a female predominance of 2:1. It is strongly associated with human papillomavirus (HPV) and human immunodeficiency virus (HIV) infection and is also significant in immunosuppressed patients following solid organ transplantation [1].

Understanding prognostic biomarkers provides information on how biological factors mediate disease progression and response. The integration of this understanding may allow identification of treatments and facilitate a new therapeutic intervention for all patients with SSC. The use of predictive biomarkers of response may also facilitate the modulation of chemoradiotherapy components and the early detection of relapse, which would facilitate rescue surgery. In addition, there is the potential to

* Correspondence: psoares19@hotmail.com
[1]Hospital Ophir Loyola, Belém, Pará 66060-281, Brazil
[2]Universidade do Estado do Pará, Belém, Pará, Brazil
Full list of author information is available at the end of the article

investigate whether underlying genomic factors modulate the transformation of HPV-induced tumor [2].

Some studies have sought to identify predictive onco-biological factors of local response, disease-free time, and overall survival. Of particular note are the papers that emphasize the role of HPV high-risk genotypes, p16 protein expression and *TP53* gene disruption in oropharyngeal and anogenital SCC [3–11]. These studies demonstrate that patients with positive HPV tumors have a better response to standard therapy, as well as those who over-express p16 and do not have a *TP53* mutation.

There is still no consensus on the best time to define the lack of clinical response to the treatment of carcinomas. Some prospective studies evaluated the response within 4 weeks after completion of chemoradiation, performing biopsies for pathologic determination within 4 to 6 weeks, rather than longer periods for better evaluation of local tumor regression. An 80% regression after chemoradiation may predict colostomy-free survival and disease-free survival. Most randomized studies, however, assess the tumor response between 6 and 12 weeks after chemoradiation. Disparities in response rates in several studies may be partially explained by differences in how and when response to treatment was performed [1]. Results from more recent studies show that the proportion of people with a complete clinical response 6 months after initiation of treatment is more strongly associated with progression and mortality compared to any assessment in less time [12].

The current literature concerning local clinical response after treatment indicates that, when there is a suspicion of a residual tumor, digital rectal examination, anoscopy, biopsy, and less frequent imaging techniques, such as endorectal ultrasound, MRI or PET/CT, should always be performed. This is because the most common recurrence sites are near the primary tumour site (75%), compared to metastatic sites such as presacral, iliac (21%) and inguinal (4%) lymph nodes [13, 14].

Even though PET/CT is not a commonly used imaging exam (in the Brazilian public health system) to observe how anal tumors behave, it has been considered an alternative method to evaluate clinical response and disease relapse [15]. A full metabolic response consists of the absence of FDG (2-Deoxy-2-[18F] fluoro-D-glucose) detection in regions where tumors were detected in pre-treatment investigations, while a partial response is defined as an increase or persistence of FDG captations by tumor cells in the same sites. A partial response assessed by post-therapy PET/CT is significantly associated with disease-free survival (22% versus 95%). The elevated negative predictive value (ranging between 94 and 98%) of PET/CT is important and avoids unnecessary biopsies or surgeries in patients with irradiated tissue [13, 16].

To the best of our knowledge, this type of study has not been conducted in South America. Thus, the objective of this study was to identify the presence of various HPV genotypes, as well as HIV and *TP53* mutations, to quantify the p16 expression levels in patients with SCC of the anal canal and to analyze the associations of the variables with local clinical responses to chemoradiotherapy.

Methods

Clinical data retrieval

Clinical details were retrieved for 78 patients treated with radical chemoradiotherapy for stages I, II, IIIa and IIIb SCC of the anal canal between 2003 and 2014. The staging was based on the American Joint Committee on Cancer tumor–node–metastasis (TNM) staging system. The treatment used for all patients was the Nigro protocol [17], which consisted of 50.4 Gray of external radiation divided into 28 daily doses and concurrent treatment with 5-flourouracil and mitomycin.

Study design

- Seventy-eight patients diagnosed with SCC of the anal canal underwent chemoradiation.
- Three months after the end of treatment, all 78 patients made the first evaluation of local response with standard anoscopy, digital rectal examination, and clinical examination of the inguinal region. The objective was to identify if any patient was presenting a lesion progression.
- Six months after the end of treatment, all 78 patients underwent a new evaluation with computer tomography (CT) of the chest, magnetic resonance imaging (MRI) of the abdomen and pelvic, digital rectal examination, high-resolution anoscopy, and clinical examination of the inguinal region. Those who were suspected of a residual lesion underwent a new biopsy to confirm histopathological suspicion of the residual lesion.
- Patients who had residual lesions confirmed by biopsy were referred for surgical treatment.
- The results of the HPV, HIV, *TP53* and p16 analyses of all 78 patients were only known after 6 months of treatment (blind to those who evaluated the response and to those who did the molecular analyses).

Analysis of the clinical response

The evaluation of the tumor response to treatment was conducted six months after the conclusion of chemoradiotherapy for all patients and consisted of chest CT, abdomen and pelvic MRI, digital rectal exam, high-resolution anoscopy and clinical examination of the inguinal region. The following classifications were used to evaluate the outcomes: a) no response (presence of residual tumor) and b) complete response (absence of residual tumor). Only patients who showed a complete absence of an ulcerative or vegetative lesion were classified as responding. When a suspicious lesion was detected in the anorectal mucosa, biopsy, and histopathology were conducted. All patients followed-up every three and six months.

Pathology review

Haematoxylin and eosin stained slides of formalin-fixed paraffin-embedded (FFPE) samples were reviewed to confirm the presence of tumors in the blocks. The samples were microdissected by a pathologist and selected for the study.

DNA extraction

DNA extraction was performed using a QIAGEN (Venlo, Netherlands) QIAamp DNA FFPE Tissue kit.

HPV analysis by direct sequencing

Samples were submitted to polymerase chain reaction (PCR) using viral gene-specific primers, which amplified a 150 bp fragment of the *L1* gene corresponding to a conserved region of the virus genome. After PCR, virus identification was performed by direct sequencing of the PCR product using a capillary sequencer 3730XL DNA Analyzer (Thermo Fisher Scientific, USA).

HIV detection

Viral RNA was extracted using a QIAGEN (Venlo, Netherlands) QIAamp Viral RNA Mini Kit and transferred to COBAS TaqMan HIV-1 Test, v2.0 (Roche, Pleasanton, CA) for amplification and detection.

TP53 mutation analysis by nucleotide sequencing

The *TP53* gene has 11 exons. Exon 1 is non-coding in the human p53 protein and for this reason was not analyzed in this study. Exons 2–11 of the *TP53* gene were separately amplified by PCR using the specific primer sets described in Faria et al. [18] The direct sequencing analysis of the amplified products was performed using the automatic sequencer ABI Prism 3130 (Thermo Fisher Scientific, USA). The resulting sequences were directly edited on the Sequencing Analysis Software on a computer linked to a 3730XL DNA Analyzer (Thermo Fisher Scientific, USA).

Fluorescent in situ hybridization

Only tumor samples carrying mutations in the *TP53* gene were analyzed by fluorescent in situ hybridization (FISH). To determine the chromosome 17 and *TP53* copy numbers, the cells were hybridized using a dual-colour direct labelled probe (Abbott/Vysis, USA) specific for the chromosome 17 α-satellite (SpectrumGreen; p11.1-q11.1) and the *TP53* gene region (SpectrumOrange; 17p13.1). Nuclei were counterstained with DAPI/antifade. For each tumor, 200 interphase nuclei were analyzed and scored using the criteria from Hopman et al. [19]

Western blotting

The analysis was performed as previously described by Leal et al. [20] Reduced protein from each sample was electroblotted onto a polyvinylidene fluoride (PVDF) membrane (GE, USA). The PVDF membrane was blocked and incubated with the primary antibodies: anti-p16 (dilution 1:10; Thermo Fisher Scientific, USA) and anti-ACTB (dilution 1:250; Thermo Fisher Scientific, USA). After washing, a peroxidase-conjugated secondary antibody was added for 1 h at room temperature. Immunoreactive bands were visualized using the Western blotting Luminol reagent, and the images were acquired using an ImageQuant 350 digital image system (GE, USA). Beta-actin (ACTB) was used as a loading reference control.

Statistical analysis

This study was a descriptive observational study with a blind laboratory analysis for response to treatment. The mean and standard deviation were calculated for the age variable, and the absolute and relative frequency distributions were calculated for the categorical variables. The association between the independent variables and the presence of a clinical response after six months was analyzed by univariate analysis using Pearson's Chi-square tests or Fisher's exact tests for categorical variables; SPSS version 21.0 (IBM, USA) was used for statistical analysis. To estimate the independent factors associated with a clinical response at 6 months, all the variables with p-values < 0.20 in the univariate analysis were used in the Cox regression. Only variables with p-values < 0.05 were retained in the model.

Results

Study population

The age of the 78 patients with SCC of the anal canal ranged from 34 to 86 years (mean 63.4 ± 10.3), and 64 patients (82.1%) were female. Analysis of their clinical stage (TNM) showed that the majority of the patients were stage II (60.3%). For the variable T, we found that 30 patients were T2 (38.5%) and 30 were T3 (38.5%). Thus, more than 2/3 (77.0%) of the patients had tumors classified as T2 or T3. Sixty patients (76.9%) clinically evaluated by imaging did not have metastases in their lymph nodes (N0), whereas 18 (23.1%) were positive for lymph node metastases. Analysis of the degree of cellular differentiation showed a predominance of grade II (74.4%). HIV was detected in 18 of the investigated biopsies (23,07%). Nine (64.28%) males and 9 (14.06%) females were HIV positive.

HPV was detected in 59 of the analyzed biopsies (75.6%). HPV 16 was most common and was detected in 49 (62.8%) tumors, followed by HPV 18 in 10 (12.8%) tumors. Nineteen patients (24.4%) did not have detectable HPV infections, and no other type of HPV was found.

Overexpression of p16 was found in 57 patients (73.1%). Overexpression was defined as 50% higher expression of the protein in the tumor tissue than in the normal anal mucosal tissues used as the control. Overexpression was not detected in 19 patients (24.4%) because the amount of protein detected in the tumour was 49% or less compared to the control. Borderline overexpression was found in two patients (2.6%) because protein expression in the tumor was 47% and 50% more than the control.

Analysis of the clinical response at six months showed a complete response in 47 patients (60.3%), and a residual tumor detectable by clinical exam and confirmed by histopathological analysis was found in 31 (39.7%) patients.

Mutational status and *TP53* copy number and p16 protein expression analyses

TP53 was wild type in 57 patients (73.1%) and mutated in 21 (26.9%) patients. All cases with p16 overexpression had wild-type *TP53* (73.1%) and vice versa. All the patient characteristics studied are shown in Table 1.

Of the 78 patients analyzed, 21 had mutations in exons 5, 6, 7 or 8 of the *TP53* gene. All the mutations identified were homozygous and consisted of both non-functional (80.5%) and partially functional (19.05%) variants (Fig. 1). Because the homozygous state of the mutations may be due to a loss of one allele, cases with mutations in *TP53* were analyzed for copy number by FISH (Table 2).

Aneuploidies in chromosome 17, where the *TP53* gene is located, were analyzed to establish a relationship between the number of *TP53* alleles and the number of chromosome 17 copies. Table 2 shows that two chromosome 17 copies and a single allele of the *TP53* gene (2/1) were present between 49.5% and 15% of the cells in cases 50 (Fig. 2) and 60, respectively.

Several other changes were also observed in this analysis (Table 2), including the presence of only one chromosome 17 and one allele of the *TP53* gene (1/1) between 1.5% and 10,5% of the cells in cases 29 and 57, respectively. Additional changes, such as three chromosome 17 copies and two alleles of the *TP53* gene (3/2) and other combinations, were observed in small cellular clones.

Another phenomenon worth highlighting is that 90% of the mutations in the *TP53* gene occurred in tumors that were both HPV negative and did not overexpress the p16 protein, whereas the other 10% occurred in tumors testing positive for HPV and containing borderline overexpression of this protein.

Factors correlated to the clinical response

The variables with significant associations with the clinical response were HPV, p16, *TP53*, female gender, and stage I or II cancer. Therefore, HPV was highly associated with patients with a complete response to chemotherapy (absence of a residual tumor), with a p-value < 0.001. HPV positive tumors showed p16 overexpression 79.7% of the time (p-value = 0.003), had borderline overexpression 2.7% of the time and were under expressed 24.4% of the time. Figure 3 shows a representative western blot of p16. The *TP53* gene was wild type in 78.9% (p-value = 0.003) of the tumors positive for HPV (Tables 3 and 4).

After adjusting for variables with a p-value < 0.20 in the univariate analysis (Table 4), only the presence of HPV was independently correlated with the clinical response. This variable increased the chances of a response within six months by 31-fold.

Discussion

Tumors affecting the anal canal generally regress slowly after chemoradiotherapy [21]. Favorable clinical outcome at three months seems to be more important than the initial T and N stages, and the magnitude of tumor regression (over 80%) is a better predictor of both colostomy and disease-free survival [22]. In our study, we observed that the female gender ($p = 0.022$) and clinical stages I and II ($p = 0.008$) were predictive variables for a good local response and significantly increased the chances of responding to treatment compared to males and the more advanced stages III A and III B. In our analysis, tumor size and lymph node metastases were not identified as independent predictive variables.

The evaluation of complete response after six months of chemoradiotherapy and the correlation with the biomarkers analyzed in this study is a significant parameter, but it is not definitive. A 3-year locoregional control rate would be considered the most relevant evaluation because it provides information on recurrences (local and distant), which occur predominantly in the first year after treatment [23]. We did not follow-up for three years because most of the patients who participated in this study did not return to the hospital after the six-month visit.

HPV status is recognized as prognostic factor in head and neck carcinomas, where it is agreed that positive HPV patients react well to chemoradiotherapy. Interest in identifying the role of HPV in SCC of the anal canal has increased because patients with HPV positive tumors in the head and neck region, especially the oropharyngeal region, have better overall survival. Thus, the role of high risk HPV in the aetiology of SCC of the anal canal is well established [4, 5, 21, 24–29].

Table 1 Patient characteristics

Characteristics	N	%	*HPV Positive N (%)*	*HPV Negative N (%)*	*p*-value
Age					*0.361*
< 65 years old	44	56.4%			
≥ 65 years old	34	43.6%	*35 (59.3)*	*9 (47.4)*	
Gender			*24 (40.7)*	*10 (52.6)*	**0.004**
Female	64	82.1			
Male	14	17.9	*53 (89.8)*	*11 (57.9)*	
Degree of Cellular Differentiation			*6 (10.2)*	*8 (42.1)*	*0.351*
G I	6	7.7			
G II	58	74.4	*6 (10.2)*	*0 (0)*	
G III	11	14.1	*42 (71.2)*	*16 (84.2)*	
G IV	3	3.8	*8 (13.6)*	*3 (15.8)*	
Clinical Stage (UICC)			*3 (5.1)*	*0 (0)*	**0.031**
I	5	6.4			
II	47	60.3	*5 (8.5)*	*0 (0)*	
IIIA	16	20.5	*39 (66.1)*	*8 (42.1)*	
IIIB	10	12.8	*8 (13.6)*	*8 (42.1)*	
N Stage			*7 (11.9)*	*3 (15.8)*	*0.354*
Negative	60	76.9			
Positive	18	23.1	*47 (79.7)*	*13 (68.4)*	
T Stage			*12 (20.3)*	*6 (31.6)*	**0,012**
T1 (≤ 2 cm)	6	7.7			
T2 (> 2 and ≤5 cm)	30	38.5	*6 (10.2)*	*0 (0)*	
T3 (> 5 cm)	30	38.5	*27 (45.8)*	*3 (15.8)*	
T4 (tumour invading adjacent organ)	12	15.4	*20 (33.9)*	*10 (52.6)*	
HPV			*6 (10.2)*	*6 (31.6)*	*NA*
16	49	62.8			
18	10	12.8	*49 (62.8)*	*0 (0)*	
Negative	19	24.4	*10 (12.8)*	*0 (0)*	
HIV			*19 (24.4)*	*0 (0)*	*1.000*
Positive	19	24.4			
Negative	59	75.6	*14 (23.7)*	*5 (26.3)*	
P16			*45 (76.3)*	*14 (73.7)*	**< 0.001**
Positive	57	73.1			
Negative	19	24.4	*57 (96.6)*	*0 (0)*	
Borderline	2	2.6	*0 (0)*	*19 (100.0)*	
Clinical response at 6 months			*2 (3.4)*	*0 (0)*	**< 0.001**
Yes	47	60.3			
No	31	39.7	*47 (79.7)*	*0 (0)*	
TP53			*12 (20.3)*	*19 (100.0)*	**< 0.001**
Mutated	21	26.9			
Wild type	57	73.1	*2 (3.4)*	*19 (100.0)*	
Total	78	100.0	*57 (96.6)*	*0 (0)*	

NA = Not available
Statistically significant p-values are shown in bold

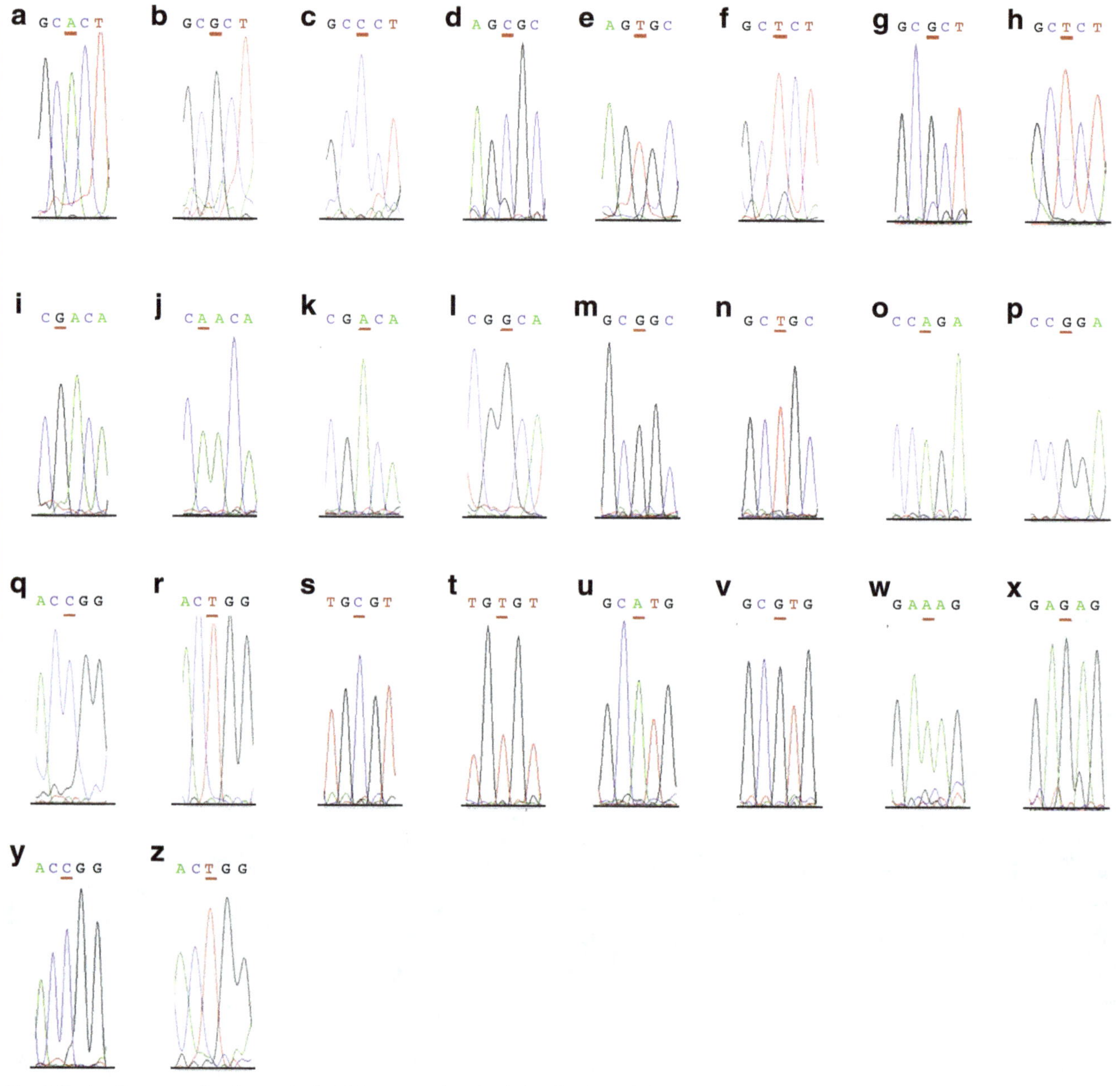

Fig. 1 Electropherograms for changes in the *TP53* gene codons (underlined). **a** R175; **b** R175H; **c** R175P; **d** R181; **e** R181C; **f** R181H; **g** R181; **h** R181L; **i** R213; **j** R213G; **k** G245; **l** G245D; **m** G245; **n** G245S; **o** R248; **p** R248Q; **q** R248; **r** 248 W; **s** R273; **t** R273C; **u** R273; **v** R273H; **w** C277; **x** C277F; **y** R282; **z** R282W

A complete clinical response, i.e. the absence of residual tumour after six months of the end of treatment with chemoradiation, is considered an excellent predictor of local control. In fact, several studies have shown that after this period, an 80% regression in T3 and T4 tumors is predictive of disease-free survival in two years: 66% versus 20% for responders and non-responders, respectively [22, 28].

In this study, the presence of HPV increased the chance of absence of residual tumors, within six months, by 31-fold. HPV was detected in 75.6% of the biopsies; of these, 79.7% ($p = 0.018$) showed complete local regression, and 20.3% had residual tumors after six months. However, all the patients with HPV negative biopsies (24.4%) had residual tumors, which is higher than expected when compared to data published in international studies [6, 7, 10, 11, 30]. All patients who had detectable residual lesions underwent a CT of the chest and MRI of their abdomen and pelvis to analyze the distant metastasis and regional lymph node chains.

In a retrospective study, Yhim et al. found similar results. They analyzed the prognostic significance of HPV

Table 2 Mutational status and copy number analysis for the *TP53* gene and quantification of the centromeres of chromosome 17 in anal canal tumours according to HPV infection status and p16 expression

HPV negative /p16 negative				FISH chromosome 17/ gene *TP53* (%)							
Case	Protein Change	Functional Consequence	Exon	*2/2*	*2/1*	*1/1*	*3/2*	*3/1*	*3/3*	*4/2*	*4/1*
6	R282W	Non-functional	8	60.5	28.0	10.0	1.5	–	–	–	–
7	R181L	Partially functional	5	52.5	43.0	4.5	–	–	–	–	–
11	R273H	Non-functional	8	69.0	23.0	4.5	3.5	–	–	–	–
16	G245S	Non-functional	7	67.5	28.5	2.0	2.0	–	–	–	–
19	R273H	Non-functional	8	70.0	24.5	4.0	1.5	–	–	–	–
23	R175P	Non-functional	5	72.0	20.0	6.0	2.0			–	–
31	R175H	Non-functional	5	67.0	23.0	7.0	3.0	–	–	–	–
34	G245D	Non-functional	7	64.5	20.5	10.0	3.0	2.0	–	–	–
49	R181C	Partially functional	5	48.0	44.0	8.0	–	–	–	–	–
50	R181H	Partially functional	5	44.5	49.5	6.0	–	–	–	–	–
59	R213Q	Non-functional	6	64.0	26.0	6.5	3.5	–	–	–	–
60	R248W	Non-functional	7	76.5	15.0	7.5	0.5	0.5	–	–	–
63	R175H	Non-functional	5	68.0	22.5	5.5	4.0	–	–	–	–
64	C277F	Non-functional	8	63.4	17.0	8.0	4.2	4.2	1.6	1.6	–
70	R273C	Non-functional	8	63.0	19.0	7.5	7.5	2.0	1.0	–	–
72	R248Q	Non-functional	7	65.0	17.5	9.5	4.0	1.5	1.5	1.0	–
75	R248Q	Non-functional	7	67.0	18.5	7.5	3.0	1.5	1.5	1.0	–
76	R213Q	Non-functional	6	65.0	25.5	5.5	4.0	–	–	–	–
77	R273C	Non-functional	8	62.7	24.3	2.7	5.5	2.7	1.6	0.5	–
HPV positive/p16 borderline				*2/2*	*2/1*	*1/1*	*3/2*	*3/1*	*3/3*	*4/2*	*4/1*
29	G245S	Non-functional	7	54.0	24.0	1.5	5.0	5.5	2.5	6.0	1.5
57	R181H	Partially functional	5	59.0	23.0	10.5	1.5	2.0	1.0	1.5	1.5

type 16 after an oncological follow-up of 51.7 months in patients with SCC of the anal canal treated with chemoradiation and found a disease progression-free period in 63.1% of the HPV positive patients compared to 15.6% of the HPV-negative patients and an overall survival of 84.6% versus 39.8%, respectively [6].

Other studies have also analyzed HPV and p16 expression as markers of the prognostic outcome in patients with SCC of the anal canal and corroborated the results found in this study. Koerber et al. analyzed the HPV and p16 statuses in 105 patients with SCC of the anal canal in a study cohort. The average follow-up was 48.6 months, and the analysis showed that the overall survival and progression-free times were three years longer in the HPV positive patients than in the HPV-negative patients. The authors also concluded that HPV detection and p16 expression together represented a prognostic marker in patients with SCC of the anal canal [8]. Mai et al. conducted a study that analyzed the prognostic relevance of HPV combined with p16 expression and observed that locoregional clinical control was significantly higher in stage T1/T2, female, HPV positive, and p16-overexpressing patients [9].

Meulendijks et al. performed a cohort study in 107 patients with SCC of the anal canal undergoing standard treatments. They demonstrated that the HPV and p16 statuses were strong predictors of locoregional clinical control and overall survival. The outcomes of patients with HPV negative/non-p16-overexpressing tumors were considerably worse than those of patients with HPV positive/p16-overexpressing tumors. Similar to our study, they found a high frequency of p53 mutations in the HPV negative/non-p16-overexpressing tumors (80%) and a sporadic frequency in the HPV positive/p16-overexpressing tumors (6%) [10]. However, unlike our results, they observed that 4 of the 16 HPV negative tumors had p16 overexpression (25%). Similarly, in a population of 135 patients, Serup-Hansen et al. found that 6 out of 15 HPV negative tumors (40%) showed overexpression of the p16 protein [30].

TP53 sequence analysis of the 78 tumor samples showed that 21 patients had tumors with homozygous mutations in this gene (Table 2). Therefore, the copy number analysis by FISH was performed on *TP53* mutations to verify whether the mechanism of the loss of heterozygosity (LOH) was involved in the carcinogenicity of

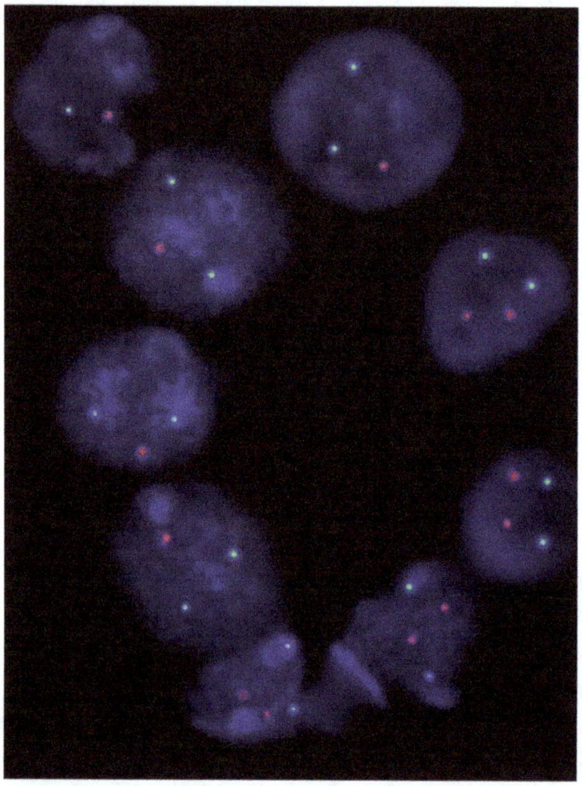

Fig. 2 Interphase nuclei from SCC of anal canal cells after FISH analysis. Green points correspond to centromeres of chromosome 17, and red points correspond to alleles of the *TP53* gene

the anus, i.e. to confirm whether the mutation is homozygous. This was visualized by the Sanger sequencing method, to determine if it originated from the two mutated alleles or because only one allele was sequenced since the other allele was lost by deletion and gave the false impression of homozygous [31, 32].

The FISH analysis (Table 2) revealed the presence of two chromosome 17 copies and a single allele of the *TP53* gene (2/1) in 15% to 49.5% of the analyzed tumor cells, indicating that LOH is a mechanism for the activation of this tumour suppressor gene. Another population of cells with homozygous mutations in the *TP53* gene that could be explained by a similar mechanism was the clone with only one chromosome 17 and one allele of the *TP53* gene (1/1) that was found in 1.5% to 10.5% of the cells in the analyzed samples.

Additionally, the typical diploid ratio of normal somatic human cells was also observed in 44.5% to 76.5% of the cells in the 21 analyzed cases. For these cellular clones, which represent most of the cells in the tumor, there are two other mechanisms to explain the homozygosity of the mutations. The first explanation is the occurrence of sporadic mutations in the two alleles of the tumor cells, and the second is gene conversion [33].

Other changes, such as the presence of three chromosome 17 copies and two *TP53* alleles (3/2) and other combinations, were observed in small clones of cells. These homozygous mutations can also be explained by the two mechanisms cited above.

Another significant phenomenon is that 100% of the HPV negative tumours had mutations in the *TP53* gene. This change in the genome of the anal mucosal cells could cause the formation of the tumor because the loss of p53 suppression might be directly related to carcinogenesis in some types of cancer [34].

TP53 mutations may explain the process of carcinogenesis in the anal canal in 3.4% of the HPV positive tumors. Additionally, the mechanism of carcinogenesis might be related to the dysregulation of *TP53* by the viral oncogene E6 in the 96.6% of the tumors that were HPV positive but did not have mutations in this gene [35].

The SCC model of the anal canal may also explain why the presence of the virus gives a better response to

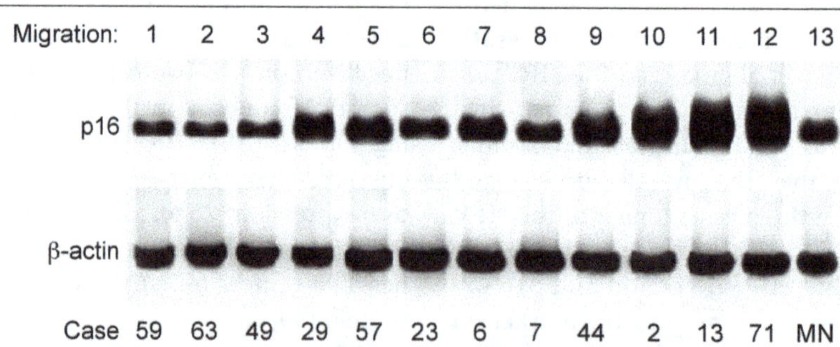

Fig. 3 Representative western blot of p16 (upper gel) and beta-actin (lower gel), which was used as an endogenous marker for normalization. Lanes are labelled at the top of the figure, and the case numbers for the patients analyzed are labelled at the bottom. Lanes 1–3 correspond to cases with mutations in *TP53* that are negative for the HPV virus and p16 overexpression. Lanes 4 and 5 correspond to HPV positive cases with mutated *TP53* and borderline p16 overexpression. Lanes 6, 7 and 8 correspond to cases with mutated *TP53* that are negative for HPV and do not overexpress p16 (p16 expression similar to the normal anal mucosa tissue). Lanes 9–12 corresponded to samples with wild-type *TP53* that are positive for HPV and exhibit p16 overexpression. Line 13 corresponds to a pool of p16 proteins extracted from five normal anal mucosal (NM) tissues

Table 3 Presence of a clinical response at 6 months by selected factors

Characteristics	Clinical response (%)	No clinical response (%)	*p*-value
Age			*0.488*
< 65 years old	28 (63.6)	16 (36.4)	
≥ 65 years old	19 (55.9)	15 (44.1)	
Gender			**< 0.001**
Female	46 (71.9)	18 (28.1)	
Male	1 (7.1)	13 (92.9)	
Degree of Cell Differentiation			*0.387*
G I / G II	40 (62.5)	24 (37.5)	
G III / G IV	7 (50.0)	7 (50.0)	
Clinical Stage (UICC)			**< 0.001**
I - II	31 (86.1)	5 (13.9)	
III A - III B	16 (38.1)	26 (61.9)	
T stage			**< 0.001**
T 1 (≤2 cm)	1 (16.7)	5 (83.3)	
T 2 (> 2 and ≤5 cm)	4 (13.3)	26 (86.7)	
T 3 (> 5 cm)	15 (50.0)	15 (50.0)	
T 4 (tumour invading adjacent organ)	11 (91.7)	1 (8.3)	
N stage			**0.035**
Negative	40 (66.7)	20 (33.3)	
Positive	7 (38.9)	11 (61.1)	
HPV			**< 0.001**
Positive	47 (79.7)	12 (20.3)	
Negative	0 (0.0)	19 (100.0)	
HIV			*0.063*
Positive	8 (42.1)	11 (57.9)	
Negative	39 (66.1)	20 (33.9)	
P16			**< 0.001**
Positive	45 (78.9)	12 (21.1)	
Negative/borderline	2 (9.5)	19 (90.5)	
TP53			**< 0.001**
Mutant	2 (9.5)	19 (90.5)	
Wild type	45 (78.9)	12 (21.1)	

Statistically significant *p*-values are shown in bold

Table 4 Univariate and multiple analyses of factors associated with the clinical response at 6 months

Characteristics	OR	95% CI	*p*	aOR	95% CI	*p*
HPV positive	31.1	1.8–531.1	**0.018**	31.1	1.8–531.1	**0.018**
Female gender	10.1	1.4–73.0	**0.022**			
P16 positive	8.3	2.0–34.2	**0.003**			
Age < 65 years	1.1	0.6–2.0	0.662			
Degree of cell differentiation I and II	1.3	0.6–2.5	0.586			
Clinical stage I and II	2.5	1.3–5.0	**0.008**			
T 2/3	1.2	0.5–3.1	0.675			
TP53 mutated	0.1	0.03–0.5	**0.003**			

OR = Odds ratio; aOR = Adjusted odds ratio
Statistically significant *p*-values are shown in bold

therapy across the spectrum of HPV associated tumors (oropharynx, cervix, vulva, penis) [2]. The presence of *TP53* mutations is associated with worse outcomes after chemoradiotherapy and is inversely correlated with the presence of p16 / HPV [7]. Mutations of *TP53* and HPV involvement are, for the most part, mutually exclusive in SCC of the anal canal [10] and in head and neck cancer [36]. HPV positive tumors develop through the production of the E6 oncoprotein and chemoradiotherapy can disrupt this process causing significant DNA damage. In the absence of E6 (i.e., HPV negative cases), the *TP53* mutation is irreversible and the DNA-damage-response (DDR) mechanisms are no longer orchestrated by the p53 protein, which can cause increasingly aberrant cells after treatment [2, 37].

The difference between these two mechanisms to inactivate the activity of the p53 protein may explain why HPV negative patients generally do not respond to treatment within 6 months. Our hypothesis proposes that the mutations in *TP53* found in the tumor cells of HPV negative patients produce abnormal proteins that confer chemoresistance to the administered treatment. Conversely, the majority of HPV positive tumors (79.7%) responded well to chemotherapy, which is explained under our hypothesis by their production of wild-type p53; even though p53 was degraded by the viral E6 oncoprotein, other proteins were concurrently generated to maintain a basal level of the protein that likely prevented the onset of chemoresistance.

Patients with SCC anal canal tumors with mutations of *TP53* gene are associated with short-term disease-free survival and decreased local responses [3, 38–42]. These observations are consistent with our results, where a significant majority of the mutant *TP53* tumors did not show a local response, although we did not analyze disease-free survival.

Individuals infected with HIV are at increased risk of infection with both low-risk and high-risk HPV types. Chronic immunosuppression provides an environment for persistent HPV infection which carries a higher risk of malignant transformation [43]. In this study, HIV infection was not associated with the presence of HPV and/or clinical response in SCC, reinforcing the hypothesis that HPV infection is only one of the mechanisms of anal canal carcinogenesis.

The explanation for the favorable clinical outcome of chemoradiotherapy in HPV16 positive patients is evident in tumors harboring strong infiltration of immune cells. These tumors present tumor-infiltrating lymphocytes (TILs) with a strong expression of CD8 and the immunological markers Programmed Cell Death Protein-1 (PD-1) and its ligand (PD-L1) [44, 45] Patients with SSC of the anal canal with high levels of infiltration of TILs present a relapse-free rate higher than those with low levels of infiltration of TILs [46]. For this reason it is important that the immune recognition in SSC of the anal canal is measured systemically.

Conclusions

Only the presence of HPV increased the chance of absence of residual tumors, within six months, by 31-fold. This correlation is valuable and can direct future therapeutic approaches in SCC of the anal canal.

Abbreviations

ACTB: Beta-actin; CMT: Combined Modality Therapy; CT: Computer Tomography; FDG: 2-Deoxy-2-[18F] fluoro-D-glucose; FFPE: Formalin-Fixed Paraffin-Embedded; FISH: Fluorescent In Situ Hybridization; HIV: Human Immunodeficiency Virus; HOL: Hospital Ophir Loyola; HPV: Human Papillomavirus; MRI: Magnetic Resonance Imaging; NM: Normal Anal Mucosal; PCR: Polymerase Chain Reaction; PET/CT: Positron Emission Tomography–Computed Tomography; PVDF: Polyvinylidene Fluoride; SCC: Squamous Cell Carcinoma; TNM: Cancer Tumour–Node–Metastasis

Acknowledgements

The authors thank all patients who participated in the study. We thank all laboratory personnel working at the Laboratório de Biologia Molecular do Hospital Ophir Loyola and the support of PROPESP / UFPA.

Funding

Funding for this study was provided as grants and fellowships from the Hospital Ophir Loyola (to PCS and RRB) and the Conselho Nacional de Desenvolvimento Científico e Tecnológico (to RRB # 305220/2013–6). The institutions and granters had no role in the study design, data collection and analysis, decision to publish, or preparation of the manuscript.

Authors' contributions

PCS, LCST, PPA and LFRP conceived and designed the study. PCS, BMS, SD, GVRF, LFRP and LML conducted the study and participated in the laboratory analysis. PCS, BMS, SD, GVRF, LCST, ESFW, and RRB analyzed the data. PCS, BMS, LCST, LFRP, ESFW and RRB wrote the paper. All authors read and approved the final manuscript.

Competing interests

The authors declare that they have no competing interests.

Author details

[1]Hospital Ophir Loyola, Belém, Pará 66060-281, Brazil. [2]Universidade do Estado do Pará, Belém, Pará, Brazil. [3]Instituto Nacional de Câncer, Rio de Janeiro, Brazil. [4]Laboratório de Citogenética Humana, Instituto de Ciências Biológicas, Belém, Pará, Brazil. [5]Núcleo de Pesquisas em Oncologia, Universidade Federal do Pará, Belém, Pará, Brazil. [6]Fundação de Hematologia e Hemoterapia do Pará, Belém, Pará, Brazil.

References

1. Glynne-Jones R, Renehan A. Current treatment of anal squamous cell carcinoma. Hematol Oncol Clin North Am. 2012;26:1315–50.
2. Jones CM, Goh V, Sebag-Montefiore D, Gilbert DC. Biomarkers in anal cancer: from biological understanding to stratified treatment. Br J Cancer. 2017;116:156–62.
3. Lampejo T, Kavanagh D, Clark J, Goldin R, Osborn M, Ziprin P, Cleator S. Prognostic biomarkers in squamous cell carcinoma of the anus: a systematic review. Br J Cancer. 2010;103:1858–69.
4. Ang KK, Harris J, Wheeler R, Weber R, Rosenthal DI, Nguyen-Tân PF, Westra WH, Chung CH, Jordan RC, Lu C, Kim H, Axelrod R, Silverman CC, Redmond KP, Gillison ML. Human papillomavirus and survival of patients with oropharyngeal cancer. N Engl J Med. 2010;363:24–35.
5. Rischin D, Young RJ, Fisher R, Fox SB, Le QT, Peters LJ, Solomon B, Choi J, O'Sullivan B, Kenny LM, McArthur GA. Prognostic significance of p16INK4A and human papillomavirus in patients with oropharyngeal cancer treated on TROG 02.02 phase III trial. J Clin Oncol. 2010;28:4142–8.
6. Yhim HY, Lee NR, Song EK, Kwak JY, Lee ST, Kim JH, Kim JS, Park HS, Chung IJ, Shim HJ, Hwang JE, Kim HR, Nam TK, Park MR, Shim H, Park HS, Kim HS, Yim CY. The prognostic significance of tumor human papillomavirus status for patients with anal squamous cell carcinoma treated with combined chemoradiotherapy. Int J Cancer. 2011;129:1752–60.
7. Gilbert DC, Williams A, Allan K, Stokoe J, Jackson T, Linsdall S, Bailey CM, Summers J. p16INK4A, p53, EGFR expression and KRAS mutation status in squamous cell cancers of the anus: correlation with outcomes following chemo-radiotherapy. Radiother Oncol. 2013;109:146–51.
8. Koerber SA, Schoneweg C, Slynko A, Krug D, Haefner MF, Herfarth K, Debus J, Sterzing F, von Knebel Doeberitz M, Prigge ES, Reuschenbach M. Influence of human papillomavirus and p16(INK4a) on treatment outcome of patients with anal cancer. Radiother Oncol. 2014;113:331–6.
9. Mai S, Welzel G, Ottstadt M, Lohr F, Severa S, Prigge ES, Wentzensen N, Trunk MJ, Wenz F, von Knebel-Doeberitz M, Reuschenbach M. Prognostic relevance of HPV infection and p16 overexpression in squamous cell anal cancer. Int J Radiat Oncol Biol Phys. 2015;93:819–27.
10. Meulendijks D, Tomasoa NB, Dewit L, Smits PH, Bakker R, van Velthuysen ML, Rosenberg EH, Beijnen JH, Schellens JH, Cats A. HPV-negative squamous cell carcinoma of the anal canal is unresponsive to standard treatment and frequently carries disruptive mutations in TP53. Br J Cancer. 2015;112:1358–66.
11. Rödel F, Wieland U, Fraunholz I, Kitz J, Rave-Fränk M, Wolff HA, Weiss C, Wirtz R, Balermpas P, Fokas E, Rödel C. Human papillomavirus DNA load and p16INK4a expression predict for local control in patients with anal squamous cell carcinoma treated with chemoradiotherapy. Int J Cancer. 2015;136:278–88.
12. Glynne-Jones R, Sebag-Montefiore D, Meadows HM, Cunningham D, Begum R, Adab F, Benstead K, Harte RJ, Stewart J, Beare S, Hackshaw A, Kadalayil L. ACT II study group. Best time to assess complete clinical response after chemoradiotherapy in squamous cell carcinoma of theanus (ACT II): a post-hoc analysis of randomised controlled phase 3 trial. Lancet Oncol. 2017;18:347–56.
13. Vercellino L, Montravers F, de Parades V, Huchet V, Kerrou K, Bauer P, Touboul E, Talbot JN. Impact of FDG PET/CT in the staging and the follow-up of anal carcinoma. Int J Color Dis. 2011;26:201–10.
14. Benson AB 3rd, Arnoletti JP, Bekaii-Saab T, Chan E, Chen YJ, Choti MA, Cooper HS, Dilawari RA, Engstrom PF, Enzinger PC, Fakih MG, Fleshman JW Jr, Fuchs CS, Grem JL, Leong LA, Lin E, May KS, Mulcahy MF, Murphy K, Rohren E, Ryan DP, Saltz L, Sharma S, Shibata D, Skibber JM, Small W Jr, Sofocleous CT, Venook AP, Willett C, Freedman-Cass DA. National Comprehensive Cancer Network.. Anal carcinoma, version 2.2012: featured updates to the NCCN guidelines. J Natl Compr Cancer Netw. 2012;10:449–54.
15. Schwarz JK, Siegel BA, Dehdashti F, Myerson RJ, Fleshman JW, Grigsby PW. Tumor response and survival predicted by post-therapy FDG-PET/CT in anal cancer. Int J Radiat Oncol Biol Phys. 2008;71:180–6.
16. Saboo SS, Zukotynski K, Shinagare AB, Krajewski KM, Ramaiya N. Anal carcinoma: FDG PET/CT in staging, response evaluation, and follow-up. Abdom Imaging. 2013;38:728–35.
17. Nigro ND, Vaitkevicius VK, Considine B. Combined therapy for cancer of the anal canal: a preliminary report. Dis Colon rectum. 1974;17:354–6.
18. Faria MH, Neves Filho EH, Alves MK, Burbano RM, de Moraes Filho MO, Rabenhorst SH. TP53 mutations in astrocytic gliomas: an association with histological grade, TP53 codon 72 polymorphism and p53 expression. APMIS Acta Pathol Microbiol Immunol Scand. 2012;120:882–9.
19. Hopman AH, Ramaekers FC, Raap AK, Beck JL, Devilee P, van der Ploeg M, Vooijs GP. In situ hybridization as a tool to study numerical chromosome aberrations in solid bladder tumors. Histochemistry. 1988;89:307–16.
20. Leal MF, Calcagno DQ, Demachki S, Assumpção PP, Chammas R, Burbano

RR, Smith Mde A. Clinical implication of 14-3-3 epsilon expression in gastric cancer. World J Gastroenterol. 2012;18:1531–7.
21. Salati SA, Al KA. Anal cancer - a review. Int J Health Sci. 2012;6:206–30.
22. Goh V, Gollub FK, Liaw J, Wellsted D, Przybytniak I, Padhani AR, Glynne-Jones R. Magnetic resonance imaging assessment of squamous cell carcinoma of the anal canal before and after chemoradiation: can mri predict for eventual clinical outcome? Int J Radiat Oncol Biol Phys. 2010;78:715–21.
23. RD J, Glynne-Jones R, Meadows HM, Cunningham D, Myint AS, Saunders MP, Maughan T, McDonald A, Essapen S, Leslie M, Falk S, Wilson C, Gollins S, Begum R, Ledermann J, Kadalayil L, Sebag-Montefiore D. Mitomycin or cisplatin chemoradiation with or without maintenance chemotherapy for treatment of squamous-cell carcinoma of the anus (ACT II): a randomised, phase 3, open-label, 2 × 2 factorial trial. Lancet Oncol. 2013;14:516–24.
24. Cardesa A, Nadal A. Carcinoma of the head and neck in the HPV era. Acta Derm Venerol Alp Pannonica Adriat. 2011;20:161–73.
25. Coutlée F, de Pokomandy A, Franco EL. Epidemiology, natural history and risk factors for anal intraepithelial neoplasia. Sex Health. 2012;9:547–55.
26. Szmulowicz UM, Wu JS. Squamous cell carcinoma of the anal canal: a review of the aetiology, presentation, staging, prognosis and methods available for treatment. Sex Health. 2012;9:593–609.
27. G E, Foo M, Harrow S, McGregor G, Hay J. Outcomes of salvage surgery for epidermoid carcinoma of the anus following failed combined modality treatment. Am J Surg. 2011;201:628–33.
28. Chapet O, Gerard JP, Riche B, Alessio A, Mornex F, Romestaing P. Prognostic value of tumor regression evaluated after first course of radiotherapy for anal canal cancer. Int J Radiat Oncol Biol Phys. 2005;63:1316–24.
29. Poggio JL. Premalignant lesions of the anal canal and squamous cell carcinoma of the anal canal. Clin Colon Rect Surg. 2011;24:177–92.
30. Serup-Hansen E, Linnemann D, Skovrider-Ruminski W, Høgdall E, Geertsen PF, Havsteen H. Human papillomavirus genotyping and p16 expression as prognostic factors for patients with American joint committee on cancer stages I to III carcinoma of the anal canal. J Clin Oncol. 2014;32(17):1812.
31. Charlton J, Pavasovic V, Pritchard-Jones K. Biomarkers to detect Wilms tumors in pediatric patients: where are we now? Future Oncol. 2015;11:2221–34.
32. Sidow A, Spies N. Concepts in solid tumor evolution. Trends Genet. 2015;31:208–14.
33. Chen JM, Cooper DN, Chuzhanova N, Férec C, Patrinos GP. Gene conversion: mechanisms, evolution and human disease. Nat Rev Genet. 2007;8:762–75.
34. Haupt S, Raghu D, Haupt Y. Mutant p53 drives cancer by subverting multiple tumor suppression pathways. Front Oncol. 2016;6:12.
35. Boulenouar S, Weyn C, Van Noppen M, Moussa Ali M, Favre M, Delvenne PO, Bex F, Noël A, Englert Y, Fontaine V. Effects of HPV-16 E5, E6 and E7 proteins on survival, adhesion, migration and invasion of trophoblastic cells. Carcinogenesis. 2010;31:473–80.
36. WH W, Taube JM, Poeta ML, Begum S, Sidransky D, Koch WM. Inverse relationship between human papillomavirus-16 infection and disruptive p53 gene mutations in squamous cell carcinoma of the head and neck. Clin Cancer Res. 2008;14:366–9.
37. Williams AB, Schumacher B. p53 in the DNA-Damage-Repair Process. Cold Spring Harb Perspect Med. 2016;6
38. Allal AS, Waelchli L, Prognostic BMA. Value of apoptosis-regulating protein expression in anal squamous cell carcinoma. Clin Cancer Res. 2003;9:6489–96.
39. Bonin SR, Pajak TF, Russell AH, Coia LR, Paris KJ, Flam MS, Sauter ER. Overexpression Of p53 protein and outcome of patients treated with chemoradiation for carcinoma of the anal canal: a report of randomized trial RTOG 87-04. Radiation therapy oncology group. Cancer. 1999;85:1226–33.
40. Indinnimeo M, Cicchini C, Stazi A, Giarnieri E, French D, Limiti MR, Ghini C, Vecchione A. Human Papillomavirus infection and p53 nuclear overexpression in anal canal carcinoma. J Exp Clin Cancer Res. 1999;18:47–52.
41. Tanum G, Holm R. Anal carcinoma: a clinical approach to p53 and RB gene proteins. Oncologia. 1996;53:369–73.
42. Wong CS, Tsao MS, Sharma V, Chapman WB, Pintilie M, Cummings BJ. Prognostic Role of p53 protein expression in epidermoid carcinoma of the anal canal. Int J Radiat Oncol Biol Phys. 1999;45:309–14.
43. Burd EM, Dean CL. Human Papillomavirus. Microbiol Spectr. 2016;4:4.
44. Balermpas P, Martin D, Wieland U, Rave-Fränk M, Strebhardt K, Rödel C, Fokas E, Rödel F. Human papilloma virus load and PD-1/PD-L1, CD8+ and FOXP3 in anal cancer patients treated with chemoradiotherapy: rationale for immunotherapy. Oncoimmunology. 2017;6:e1288331.
45. Martin D, Rödel F, Winkelmann R, Balermpas P, Rödel C, Fokas E. Peripheral leukocytosis is inversely correlated with Intratumoral CD8+ T-cell infiltration and associated with worse outcome after Chemoradiotherapy in anal cancer. Front Immunol. 2017;8:1225.
46. Gilbert DC, Serup-Hansen E, Linnemann D, Høgdall E, Bailey C, Summers J, Havsteen H, Thomas GJ. Tumour-infiltrating lymphocyte scores effectively stratify outcomes over and above p16 post chemo-radiotherapy in anal cancer. Br J Cancer. 2016;114:134–7.

Mitotic and apoptotic activity in colorectal neoplasia

Darina Kohoutova[1*], Jaroslav Pejchal[2] and Jan Bures[1]

Abstract

Background: Colorectal cancer (CRC) is third most commonly diagnosed cancer worldwide. The aim of the prospective study was to evaluate mitosis and apoptosis of epithelial cells at each stage of colorectal neoplasia.

Methods: A total of 61 persons were enrolled into the study: 18 patients with non-advanced colorectal adenoma (non-a-A), 13 patients with advanced colorectal adenoma (a-A), 13 patients with CRC and 17 controls: individuals with normal findings on colonoscopy. Biopsy samples were taken from pathology (patients) and healthy mucosa (patients and healthy controls). Samples were formalin-fixed paraffin-embedded and stained with haematoxylin-eosin. Mitotic and apoptotic activity were evaluated in lower and upper part of the crypts and in the superficial compartment. Apoptotic activity was also assessed using detection of activated caspase-3.

Results: In controls, mitotic activity was present in lower part of crypts, accompanied with low apoptotic activity. Mitotic and apoptotic activity decreased (to almost zero) in upper part of crypts. In superficial compartment, increase in apoptotic activity was observed. Transformation of healthy mucosa into non-a-A was associated with significant increase of mitotic activity in lower and upper part of the crypts and with significant increase of apoptotic activity in all three compartments; $p < 0.05$. Transformation of non-a-A into a-A did not lead to any further significant increase in apoptotic activity, but was related to significant increase in mitotic activity in upper part of crypts and superficial compartment. A significant decrease in apoptotic activity was detected in all three comparments of CRC samples compared to a-A; $p < 0.05$. No differences in mitotic and apoptotic activity between biopsies in healthy controls and biopsy samples from healthy mucosa in patients with colorectal neoplasia were observed. Detection of activated caspase-3 confirmed the above findings in apoptotic activity.

Conclusions: Significant dysregulation of mitosis and apoptosis during the progression of colorectal neoplasia, corresponding with histology, was confirmed. In patients with sporadic colorectal neoplasia, healthy mucosa does not display different mitotic and apoptotic activity compared to mucosa in healthy controls and therefore adequate endoscopic/surgical removal of colorectal neoplasia is sufficient.

Keywords: Mitosis, Apoptosis, Colorectal adenoma, Colorectal carcinoma

Background

Colorectal cancer (CRC) is the third most commonly diagnosed cancer with incidence of 1.36 million and mortality of 694,000 cases worldwide [1]. The etiopathogenesis of CRC is multifactorial, nevertheless, dysregulation of mitosis and apoptosis contribute to the pathogenesis of CRC significantly. Abnormalities in apoptosis are also responsible for poor response or resistance of CRC cells to chemotherapeutic agents and radiotherapy [2, 3].

The colorectal mucosa is formed into the crypts of Lieberkühn, which increase in number between the birth and adulthood [4]. In each colonic crypt there are four to six stem cells at the bottom producing the enormous number of colonocytes, which move from the lower to the upper part of crypts and reach the colonic lumen. At the lumen, they are eliminated by apoptosis [5–7]. The intestinal epithelium is fully replaced within 3–5 days [8] and the total proliferation rate is 3–10 billion

* Correspondence: darina.kohoutova@fnhk.cz
[1]Charles University, Faculty of Medicine in Hradec Kralove, University Hospital Hradec Kralove, 2nd Department of Internal Medicine - Gastroenterology, Sokolska 581, 500 05 Hradec Kralove, Czech Republic
Full list of author information is available at the end of the article

colonocytes per day [5, 9]. Therefore, cell production, differentiation and apoptosis have to be regulated precisely [8].

Colorectal carcinomas arise in 70–80% sporadically [10], usually through the "non-advanced adenoma - advanced adenoma - carcinoma" sequence. Advanced colorectal adenoma is defined as a neoplasia larger than 10 mm and/or containing villous component and/or containing high grade dysplasia [11].

The aim of our prospective study was to evaluate the degree of mitotic and apoptotic activity at each stage of colorectal neoplasia.

Methods

Patients

A total of 18 patients with non-advanced colorectal adenoma (13 men, 5 women, aged 41–84, mean 66 ± 12; 8/18 right sided neoplasia), 13 patients with advanced colorectal adenoma (10 men, 3 women, aged 58–79, mean 67 ± 7; 4/13 right sided neoplasia) and 13 patients with colorectal carcinoma (5 men, 8 women, aged 50–87, mean 66 ± 10; CRC: 4/13 right sided neoplasia) were included into the prospective study. Inclusion criteria for those with colorectal neoplasia were: sporadic neoplasia, absence of previous colorectal surgery, negative history of inflammatory bowel disease, absence of any type of colitis (including inflammatory bowel disease, pseudomembranous colitis, ischaemic colitis), absence of serrated lesion, absence of hyperplastic polyps proximal to the rectosigmoid colon, absence of diverticulitis and postradiation proctopathy. Two patients with well differentiated carcinoma and 11 patients with moderately differentiated carcinoma were included. A total of 7 patients with dedifferentiated carcinoma were excluded from the original group of 20 patients with CRC as mitotic and apoptotic activity could not be evaluated due to presence of excessive necrotic tissue. A total of 17 controls, individuals with normal findings on colonoscopy, with no previous history of colorectal neoplasia or inflammatory bowel disease (6 men, 11 women, aged 25–75, mean 55 ± 14), were enrolled into the study.

Collection of samples

Biopsy samples were taken during diagnostic and/or therapeutic colonoscopy. Paired biopsies were obtained in patients with colorectal neoplasia: one sample was taken from the pathology and the second sample was taken from a healthy mucosa, 10 cm distally from the side of neoplasia. In healthy individuals, one biopsy sample was obtained, usually in the rectum, after the exclusion of a colorectal neoplasia in the colon and the rectum.

All biopsy samples were formalin-fixed (10% formalin), embedded into paraffin (Paramix, Holice, the Czech Republic), and tissue sections 5 µm thick were cut (Microtome model SM2000 R, Leica, Heidelberg, Germany). Sections were stained with haematoxylin-eosin (Merck, Kenilworth, NJ, USA) and evaluated using a BX-51 microscope (Olympus Czech Group, Prague, Czech Republic). The grade of mitosis, conveyed as a mitotic index [mitotic index (%) = number of mitotic figures × 100 / number of all evaluated cells] and grade of apoptosis, conveyed as an apoptotic index [apoptotic index (%) = number of apoptotic cells × 100 / number of all evaluated cells] were assessed in three different compartments: in the superficial compartment (which is in the direct contact with the lumen of the large intestine), in the upper part of intestinal crypts and in the lower part of intestinal crypts. Single apoptotic fragments of similar size, when compared to the adjacent non-apoptotic cells, or a cluster of at least three small apoptotic bodies were considered to be apoptotic cells. A minimal amount of 750 cells were evaluated in each compartment in each biopsy sample.

Apoptotic activity was also assessed immunohistochemically by detection of activated (cleft) caspase-3, which is a key element regulating the apoptotic process. For that, a rabbit monoclonal antibody (1:200; Cell Signaling Technology, Danvers, MA, USA) and standard peroxidase technique in 5 µm thick tissue sections were used [12]. After the detection of activated caspase-3, samples were counterstained with haematoxylin (Fig. 1). Clusters of ≥3 apoptotic bodies would have been positive in haematoxylin-eosin staining, but might not have shown activated caspase-3 positivity, as apoptotic bodies

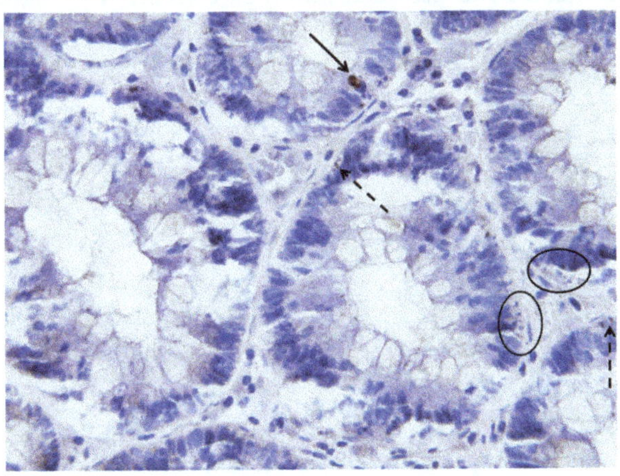

Fig. 1 Immunohistochemical detection of activated caspase-3 counterstained with haematoxylin. Original magnification: × 500. Apoptotic cell with sufficient cytoplasmatic material and strong activated caspase-3 positivity (arrow); small apoptotic body with with weak activated caspase-3 positivity (dashed arrow); apoptotic bodies without cytoplasmatic material that would have been positive in samples stained with haematoxylin-eosin, but are not dysplaying any positivity in activated caspase-3 immuno-stained samples (circled)

were seen if the cytoplasmatic tissue was maintained. If the apoptotic body contained nuclear material only, positivity was not observed.

The original effort was to evaluate apoptosis similarly to the samples stained with haematoxylin-eosin. Nevertheless, high false positivity in marginal areas was observed (Fig. 2), probably due to trauma when biopsy sample was taken. Mild intensity of trauma does not seem to induce necrotic cell death, however, it seems to be sufficient enough to result in a rapid activation of apoptotic signaling pathways. Subsequently, some samples (especially of small size) could not be assessed at all. In the remaining samples, apoptotic activity could not have been evaluated in the superficial compartment and at the outfall of the crypts. At least 1500 cells per compartment in each biopsy sample were analysed. Therefore, after an exclusion of false positive areas, apoptotic activity was evaluated in the upper and lower part of crypts. Firm conclusion were drawn from the upper cryptal compartment as sufficient numbers for statistics were obtained from this compartment only.

Preliminary data without controls in each group of patients with colorectal neoplasia and without any data on mitosis have been published previously [13].

Statistical analysis

Obtained data were tested statistically by means of descriptive statistics and Mann-Whitney rank sum test using Statistica software, version 13, 2013, Tulsa, OK, USA.

Ethical issues

All patients included in the study were given the necessary information and provided informed consent via a signed form. The project was approved by the Joint Ethical Committee (Charles University, Faculty of Medicine in Hradec Kralove, University Hospital Hradec Kralove); approval number: 201107 S54. For all obtained data, all personal identification information was removed in compliance with the Czech laws for protection of confidentiality.

Results

In healthy controls, mitotic activity was observed in the lower part of crypts, where it was accompanied by low apoptotic activity. Both activities decreased (to almost zero) in the upper part of crypts (Fig. 3), whereas apoptotic activity increased again in the superficial compartment (Figs. 5, 6 and 7).

Transformation of healthy mucosa into a non-advanced adenoma (non-a-A) was associated with a significant increase of apoptotic activity in all three compartments (Figs. 5, 6 and 7); $p < 0.05$. The most significant increase was present in the upper part of crypts, where it was associated with a significant increase in mitotic activity (Fig. 6); $p < 0.05$.

Transformation of a non-a-A into an advanced adenoma (a-A) did not affect apoptotic activity (Figs. 5, 6 and 7) significantly, nevertheless, differences were found in mitotic activity: when compared to non-a-A group, significantly higher mitotic activity in the upper part of crypts and in the superficial compartment of a-A group was confirmed (Figs. 6, 7 and 4); $p < 0.05$.

Finally, there was a statistically significant decrease in apoptotic activity in all three compartments of carcinoma samples (CRC) compared to a-A group (Figs. 5, 6 and 7); $p < 0.05$.

Further statistical analysis was conducted in order to compare mitosis and apoptosis of neoplastic epithelial cells between the right (caecum, ascending colon, transverse colon) and the left colon (descending colon,

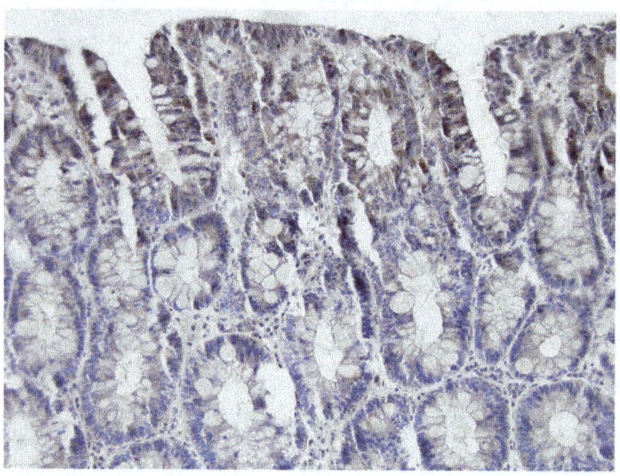

Fig. 2 Falsely positive immunohistochemical detection of activated caspase-3 in the superficial compartment and at the outfall of crypts. The sample was counterstained with haematoxylin. Original magnification: × 200

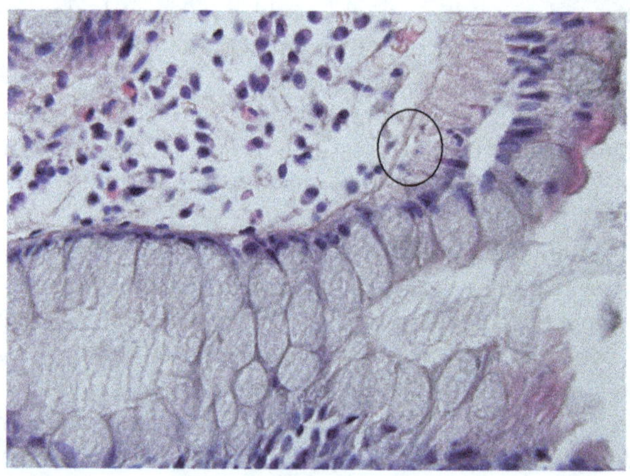

Fig. 3 Control sample showing the upper part of the crypt with details of the cryptal orificium. No mitotic and apoptotic activity is observed in the upper part of the crypts. A cluster of apoptotic bodies is present in the superficial compartment (circled). Haematoxylin-eosin, original magification: × 600

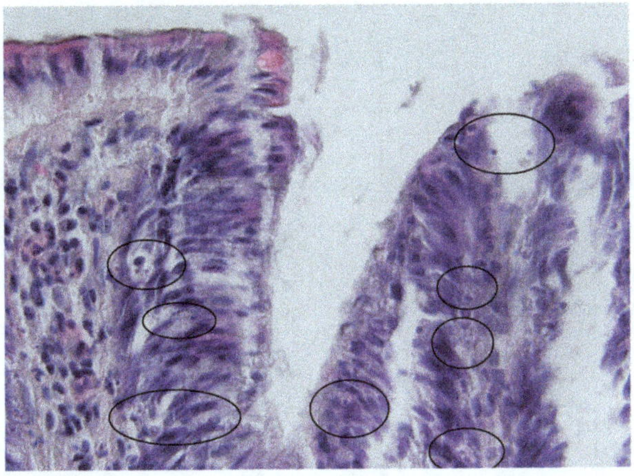

Fig. 4 Advanced adenoma: apoptotic activity in the upper part of crypts (apoptotic bodies: circled). Haematoxylin-eosin, original magnification: × 600

sigmoid colon and rectum): no differences were found in each pathology; p > 0.05, Figs. 8 and 9.

Mitotic and apoptotic activity in biopsies from the normal tissue taken in patients with colorectal neoplasia in the right and left colon was assesed: there were no differences, p > 0.05.

No differences in mitotic and apoptotic activity between controls from healthy individuals and control samples in each group of patients with colorectal neoplasia in each compartment were found; p > 0.05, Figs. 10 and 11.

A total of eight CRC patients had the neoplasia localised in the rectosigmoid junction or in the rectum and the biopsy from the healthy mucosa was taken in the rectum. Mitotic and apoptotic activity from these samples were compared with mitotic and apoptotic activity of eight randomly chosen controls, whose biopsies were taken in the rectum: no differences were found out; p > 0.05.

No differences in mitotic and apoptotic activity between females and males were observed; p > 0.05.

Immunohistochemical detection of activated caspase-3 showed significant increase in apoptotic activity in the upper part of the crypts during the transformation of healthy mucosa into a non-a-A and an a-A; p < 0.05. This was followed by a significant decrease of activated caspase-3 positivity in the same compartment in CRC samples when compared to a non-a-A and an a-A; p < 0.05 (Table 1).

Discussion

Dysregulation of epithelial proliferation and apoptosis is typical for a neoplastic process. Recently, therapeutic strategies involving induction of apoptosis have become an effective part of therapy of an established carcinoma [14–18], but it is not yet a tool to prevent development of carcinoma from precancerous lesions.

The "programmed cell death" was first proposed by Lockshin and Williams in 1965 [19]. The term "apoptosis" was first introduced by Kerr et al. in 1972, who suggested, that this process involves a controlled cell deletion, which plays a complementary, but opposite role to mitosis [20].

In healthy mucosa, mitotic activity was observed in the lower part of crypts only, where it was accompanied by a certain level of apoptotic activity. Apoptotic activity

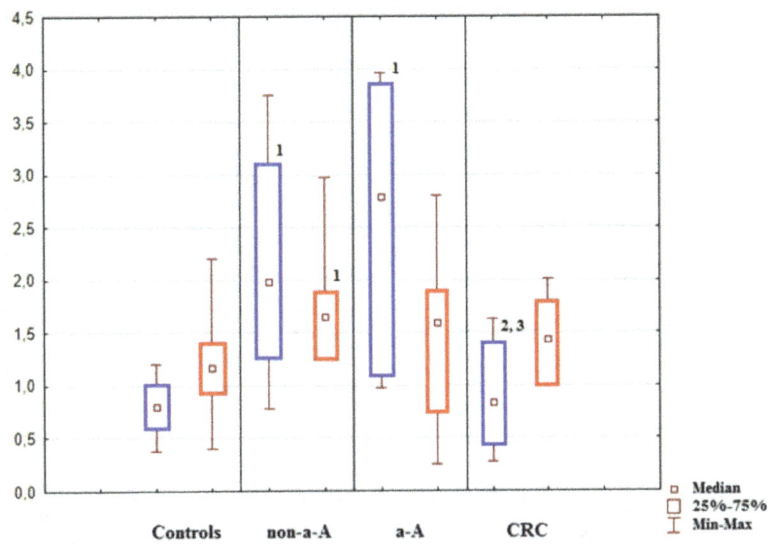

Fig. 5 Lower part of crypts: apoptosis (in blue) conveyed as an apoptotic index (%) and mitosis (in red) conveyed as a mitotic index (%). 1: statistically significant difference when compared to control: $p < 0.05$. 2: statistically significant difference when compared to non-advanced adenoma (non-a-A): $p < 0.05$. 3: statistically significant difference when compared to advanced adenoma (a-A): $p < 0.05$

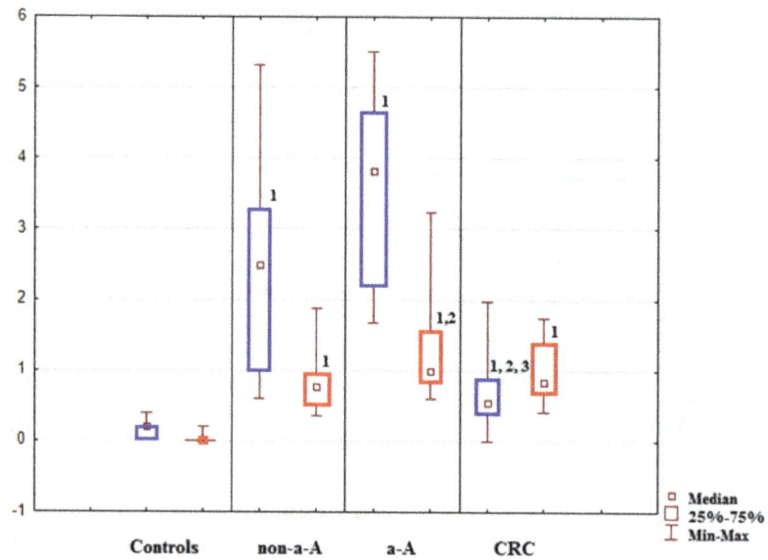

Fig. 6 Upper part of crypts: apoptosis (in blue) conveyed as an apoptotic index (%) and mitosis (in red) conveyed as a mitotic index (%). 1: statistically significant difference when compared to control: $p < 0.05$. 2: statistically significant difference when compared to non-advanced adenoma (non-a-A): $p < 0.05$. 3: statistically significant difference when compared to advanced adenoma (a-A): $p < 0.05$

in this part of crypts might be a mechanism contributing to the maintenance of genetic information providing stability of mutiplying stem cells and progenitors [21, 22]. The upper part of a crypt is a compartment where the cells undergo differentiation [23] and mitotic and apoptotic activity decrease to almost zero in healthy controls. Apoptotic activity increases in the superficial compartment again, where the cells are eliminated physiologically. Our study confirmed these findings in all control samples taken from both healthy individuals and patients with colorectal neoplasia.

In this study, mitosis and apoptosis increased significantly almost in all evaluated compartmens of non-advanced and advanced adenomas. Resembling trends in both neoplasias suggest that both these processes are triggered by genetic alterations. On the contrary, mitotic activity remained unaffected at the luminal surface of non-advanced adenomas indicating

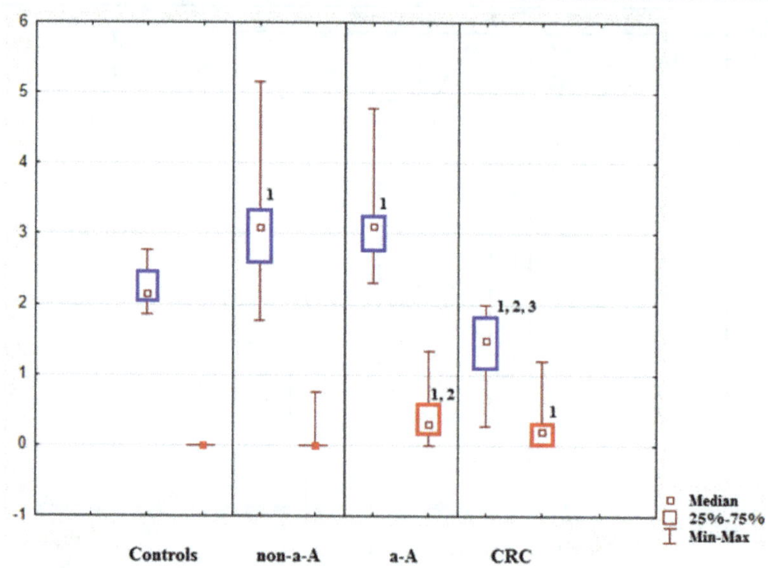

Fig. 7 Superficial compartment: apoptosis (in blue) conveyed as an apoptotic index (%) and mitosis (in red) conveyed as a mitotic index (%). 1: statistically significant difference when compared to control: $p < 0.05$. 2: statistically significant difference when compared to non-advanced adenoma (non-a-A): $p < 0.05$. 3: statistically significant difference when compared to advanced adenoma (a-A): $p < 0.05$

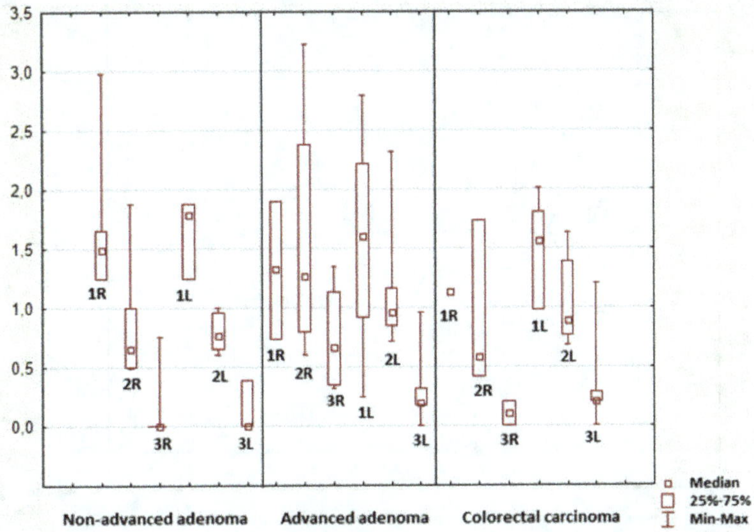

Fig. 8 Mitotic index in the lower part of the crypts (1), upper part of the crypts (2) and superficial compartment (3) in the right and left (R, L) colon

maintenance of terminal differentiation in this compartment despite altered morphology, which is in agreement with the literature [24]. This was not observed in advanced adenomas. The transformation of a non-advanced adenoma into an advanced form was associated with increased mitotic activity in the upper cryptal and superficial compartment, which implies further distortion of mucosal spatial differentiation. The final step of adenoma – carcinoma sequence was related to decrease in apoptosis in all compartments, whereas increased mitotic activity remained unchanged. Amplified production of "incompetent" cells, which are neither eliminated sufficiently, contribute to further progression of growth and development of invasive colorectal carcinoma. In our study, activation of caspase-3 correlated with morphological findings in the upper part of crypts, i.e. the compartment with the most profound dysregulation of mitotic and apoptotic activity in all selected colonic neoplasms.

Apoptosis is regulated by two major mechanisms: Bcl-2 family, which consists of pro- and antiapoptotic

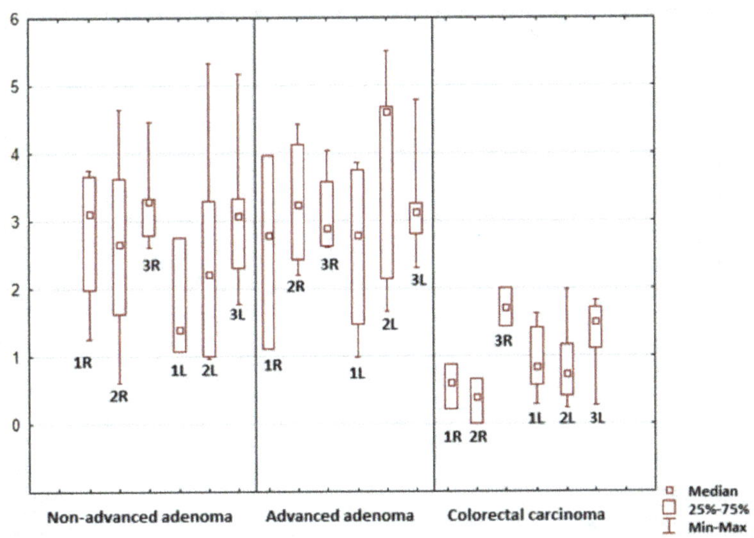

Fig. 9 Apoptotic index in the lower part of the crypts (1), upper part of the crypts (2) and superficial compartment (3) in the right and left (R, L) colon

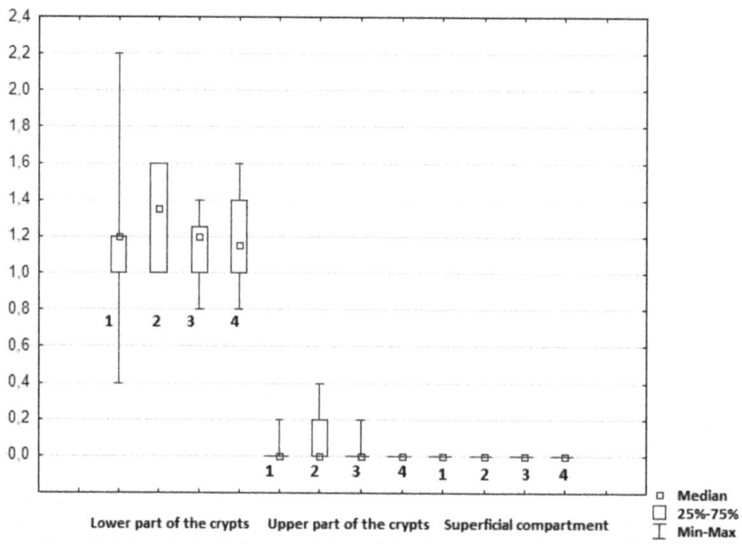

Fig. 10 Mitotic index in controls from healthy individuals (1) and control samples in each group of patients with colorectal neoplasia (2: non-advanced adenoma; 3: advanced adenoma; 4: colorectal carcinoma)

members and Inhibitor of apoptosis (IAP) family [25]. Survivin is the smallest member of the IAP family of proteins and is involved in inhibition of apoptosis, regulation of cell cycle and resistence to chemotherapy. Survivin is highly expressed during embryonal period, absent in majority of differentiated tissues, but upregulated in different human cancers [26]. Soreide et al. documented that survivin is an independent predictor for metachronous colorectal carcinoma development in patients with a sporadic colorectal adenoma [27]. Hernandez et al. looked at expression of survivin in colorectal adenomas and carcinomas and confirmed not only overexpression of survivin in these tissue samples, but interestingly, increase in expression of survivin during the normal mucosa-adenoma-carcinoma sequence [28]. Konturek et al. reported that a 14-day therapy with celecoxib, inhibitor of cyclooxygenase-2, lead to a significant decrease of survivin in tumour tissue and normal rectal mucosa of patients with rectal adenocarcinoma [29]. Survivin

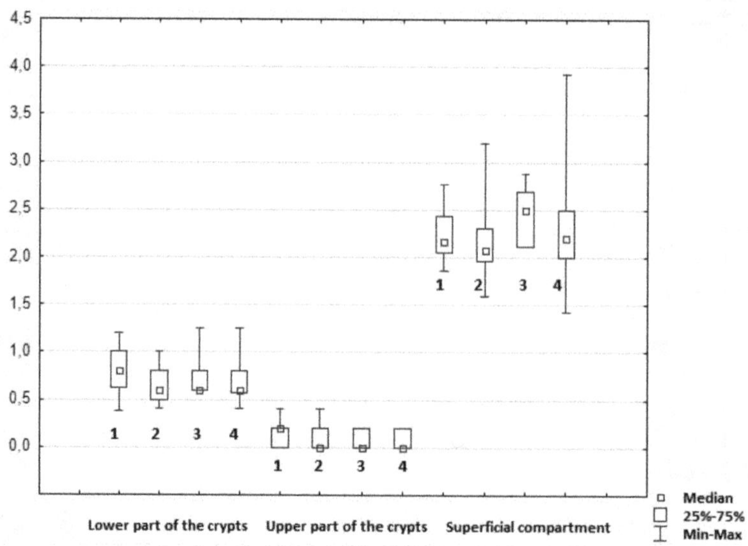

Fig. 11 Apoptotic index in controls from healthy individuals (1) and control samples in each group of patients with colorectal neoplasia (2: non-advanced adenoma; 3: advanced adenoma; 4: colorectal carcinoma)

Table 1 Immunohistochemical detection of activated caspase-3 positive cells in the upper part of crypts

	Apoptotic index of activated caspase-3 positive cells in the upper part of crypts (%)
Controls	Median 0.00, IQR 0 (13)
Non-advanced-adenoma	Median 1.37, IQR 1.42–1.18 (8) [1]
Advanced adenoma	Median 1.84, IQR 2.03–1.72 (10) [1, 2]
Colorectal carcinoma	Median 0.86, IQR 1.05–0.77 (9) [1, 2, 3]

Results are conveyed as median and interquartile range (IQR) of apoptotic indices. Number of compartments evaluated in particular group are in brackets
1: statistically significant difference when compared to control: $p< 0.05$
2: statistically significant difference when compared to non-advanced adenoma (non-a-A): $p< 0.05$
3: statistically significant difference when compared to advanced adenoma (a-A): $p< 0.05$

therefore seems to be an ideal tumour marker and potential therapeutic target [30, 31].

Mutations in the WNT/beta-catenin pathway are typical for sporadic colorectal cancer and apoptosis in CRC cells with these mutations is induced by histone deacetylase inhibitors [32]. Butyrate, a short-chain fatty acid which is produced from dietary fiber by intestinal microbiota, is the most well-known inhibitor of histone deacetylase [33, 34]. Butyrate is the preferred source of energy for healthy colonocytes [35] nevertheless, due to its different concentration in each compartment, the effect of butyrate is diverse: low concentrations of butyrate, which are typical for the base of colonic crypts, are quickly metabolized and stimulate cell proliferation. Higher concentrations of butyrate, which are present near the intestinal lumen, exceed the metabolic capacity of colonocytes. This results in accumulation of butyrate in the nucleus where it acts as a histone deacetylase inhibotor and induces apoptosis [36]. Our study, when contemplating the degree of mitosis and apoptosis in the lower part of crypts and in the superficial compartment, fulfills these theoretical prerequisites derived from the effect of butyrate.

Due to Warburg effect, the cells of colorectal neoplasia prefer glucose as the energy source. Butyrate therefore accumulates in the nuclei of cancerous colonocytes and induces apoptosis via the inhibition of histone deacetylase [36]. Our study showed that apoptosis increased significantly in all compartments in non-advanced and advanced adenomas, which is in agreement with a study conducted by Strater et al. [7]. Nevertheless, significant decrease in apoptosis was observed during the transformation of advanced colorectal adenomas into carcinomas. This finding is in agreement with a study performed by Kikuchi et al. [37], but the assumptions derived from Warburg effect are not fulfilled. This could be explained by the fact, that adenoma cells are known to be very sensitive to the effects of butyrate on apoptosis and proliferation suppression, more when compared to carcinoma cells (32). Further, there are other components regulating apoptosis, such as antiapoptotic survivin. Pathways induced by mitogens secreted from apoptotic cells, such as AKT, JAK/STAT and ERK, play a key role in the complex process of apoptosis, too [28, 32, 38, 39].

No differences in mitotic and apoptotic activity were found between right sided and left sided neoplasias, between normal tissue obtained in patients with right sided and left sided neoplasias, and between males and females. Still, we are very carefull to draw any firm conclusions - despite a very high number of cells (> 750) were evaluated in each compartment - as the numbers of participants in each subgroup (especially those with a right sided advanced adenoma and CRC (4/13) and women in the group with advanced adenoma (3/13)) were small.

Another limitation worth noting is that most of the samples taken from healthy patients were from the rectum and we are aware that rectal samples do not have to be fully representative of the entire colorectum. Yet, based on our study, the observation of no difference in mitotic and apoptotic activity between controls from healthy individuals and control samples in each group of patients with colorectal neoplasia is of a very high clinical significance: adequate endoscopic/surgical removal of colorectal neoplasia is warranted, but should be sufficient in case that we deal with a sporadic colorectal neoplasia in a patient without inflammatory bowel disease.

Conclusions

Significant dysregulation of mitosis and apoptosis during the progression of colorectal neoplasia, corresponding with histology, was confirmed. In patients with sporadic colorectal neoplasia, healthy mucosa does not display different mitotic and apoptotic activity compared to mucosa in healthy controls and therefore adequate endoscopic/surgical removal of colorectal neoplasia is sufficient.

Abbreviations

a-A: Advanced colorectal adenoma; CRC: Colorectal carcinoma; non-a-A: Non-advanced colorectal adenoma

Acknowledgements

The study was supported by the Project PROGRES from Charles University (Q40 – 15). Funding was used for consumables needed for collection of samples (biopsy forceps, tubes with formalin) and further for haematoxylin-eosin and activated caspase-3.

Authors' contributions

DK: conception and design of the study; analysis and interpretation of the data; drafting of the article. JP: conception and design of the study; analysis and interpretation of the data; drafting of the article; critical revision of the article for important intellectual content. JB: conception and design of the study; final approval of the article. All authors read and approved the final manuscript.

Competing interests

The authors declare that they have no competing interests.

Author details

[1]Charles University, Faculty of Medicine in Hradec Kralove, University Hospital Hradec Kralove, 2nd Department of Internal Medicine - Gastroenterology, Sokolska 581, 500 05 Hradec Kralove, Czech Republic. [2]University of Defence, Faculty of Military Health Sciences, Hradec Kralove, Czech Republic.

References

1. Ferlay J, Soerjomataram I, Dikshit R, et al. Cancer incidence and mortality worldwide: sources, methods and major patterns in GLOBOCAN 2012. Int J Cancer. 2015;136(5):E359–86.
2. Arora H, Qureshi R, Rizvi MA, et al. Study of apoptosis-related interactions in colorectal cancer. Tumour Biol. 2016;37(11):14415–25.
3. Abraha AM, Ketema EB. Apoptotic pathways as a therapeutic target for colorectal cancer treatment. World J Gastrointest Oncol. 2016;8(8):583–91.
4. Maskens AP, Dujardin-Loits RM. Kinetics of tissue proliferation in colorectal mucosa during post-natal growth. Cell Tissue Kinet. 1981;14(5):467–77.
5. Raskov H, Pommergaard HC, Burcharth J, et al. Colorectal carcinogenesis-update and perspectives. World J Gastroenterol. 2014;20(48):18151–64.
6. Zhao R, Michor F. Patterns of proliferative activity in the colonic crypt determine crypt stability and rates of somatic evolution. PLoS Comput Biol. 2013;9:e1003082.
7. Sträter J, Koretz K, Günthert AR, et al. In situ detection of enterocytic apoptosis in normal colonic mucosa and in familial adenomatous polyposis. Gut. 1995;37(6):819–25.
8. van der Wath RC, Gardiner BS, Burgess AW, et al. Cell organisation in the colonic crypt: a theoretical comparison of the pedigree and niche concepts. PLoS One. 2013;8(9):e73204.
9. Potten CS, Kellett M, Roberts SA, et al. Measurement of in vivo proliferation in human colorectal mucosa using bromodeoxyuridine. Gut. 1992;33(1):71–8.
10. Karoui M, Tresallet C, Brouquet A, et al. Colorectal carcinogenesis. 1. Hereditary predisposition and colorectal cancer. J Chir (Paris). 2007;144(1): 13–8.
11. Kohoutova D, Smajs D, Moravkova P, et al. Escherichia coli strains of phylogenetic group B2 and D and bacteriocin production are associated with advanced colorectal neoplasia. BMC Infect Dis. 2014;14:733.
12. Pejchal J, Pejchal J, Novotný J, et al. Activation of p38 MAPK and expression of TGF-β1 in rat colon enterocytes after whole body γ-irradiation. Int J Radiat Biol. 2012;88(4):348–58.
13. Kohoutova D, Pejchal J, Cyrany J et al. Apoptosis in the development of colorectal neoplasia. Gastroenterol and Hepatol. 2016;70(4):313–318. [Article in Czech].
14. Hassan M, Watari H, AbuAlmaaty A, et al. Apoptosis and molecular targeting therapy in cancer. Biomed Res Int. 2014;2014:150845.
15. Leiszter K, Galamb O, Sipos F, et al. Sporadic colorectal cancer development shows rejuvenescence regarding epithelial proliferation and apoptosis. PLoS One. 2013;8(10):e74140.
16. Plati J, Bucur O, Khosravi-Far R. Apoptotic cell signaling in cancer progression and therapy. Integr Biol (Camb). 2011;3(4):279–96.
17. Koehler BC, Jäger D, Schulze-Bergkamen H. Targeting cell death signaling in colorectal cancer: current strategies and future perspectives. World J Gastroenterol. 2014;20(8):1923–34.
18. Wang H, Sun X, Li M. Apoptosis-induction is a novel therapeutic strategy for gastrointestinal and liver cancers. Curr Gene Ther. 2015;15(2):193–200.
19. Lockshin RA, Williams CM. Programmed cell death - II. Endocrine potentiation of the breakdown of the intersegmental muscles of silkmoths. J Ins Physiol. 1964;10:643–9.
20. Kerr JF, Wyllie AH, Currie AR. Apoptosis: a basic biological phenomenon with wide-ranging implications in tissue kinetics. Br J Cancer. 1972;26(4): 239–57.
21. Harfouche G, Martin MT. Response of normal stem cells to ionizing radiation: a balance between homeostasis and genomic stability. Mutat Res. 2010;704:167–74.
22. Umar S. Intestinal stem cells. Curr Gastroenterol Rep. 2010;12:340–8.
23. Dhawan P, Ahmad R, Srivastava AS, et al. Cancer stem cells and colorectal cancer: an overview. Curr Top Med Chem. 2011;11(13):1592–8.
24. Roostaee A, Benoit YD, Boudjadi S, et al. Epigenetics in intestinal epithelial cell renewal. J Cell Physiol. 2016;231(11):2361–7.
25. Singh N. Apoptosis in health and disease and modulation of apoptosis for therapy: an overview. Indian J Clin Biochem. 2007;22(2):6–16.
26. Garg H, Suri P, Gupta JC, et al. Survivin: a unique target for tumor therapy. Cancer Cell Int. 2016;16:49.
27. Søreide K, Gudlaugsson E, Skaland I, et al. Metachronous cancer development in patients with sporadic colorectal adenomas-multivariate risk model with independent and combined value of hTERT and survivin. Int J Color Dis. 2008;23(4):389–400.
28. Hernandez JM, Farma JM, Coppola D, et al. Expression of the antiapoptotic protein survivin in colon cancer. Clin Colorectal Cancer. 2011;10(3):188–93.
29. Konturek PC, Rembiasz K, Burnat G, et al. Effects of cyclooxygenase-2 inhibition on serum and tumor gastrins and expression of apoptosis-related proteins in colorectal cancer. Dig Dis Sci. 2006;51(4):779–87.
30. Cai Y, Ma W, Huang X, et al. Effect of survivin on tumor growth of colorectal cancer in vivo. Int J Clin Exp Pathol. 2015;8(10):13267–72.
31. Pennati M, Folini M, Zaffaroni N. Targeting survivin in cancer therapy: fulfilled promises and open questions. Carcinogenesis. 2007;28(6):1133–9.
32. Bordonaro M, Drago E, Atamna W, et al. Comprehensive suppression of all apoptosis-induced proliferation pathways as a proposed approach to colorectal cancer prevention and therapy. PLoS One. 2014;9(12):e115068.
33. Davie JR. Inhibition of histone deacetylase activity by butyrate. J Nutr. 2003; 133(7 Suppl):2485S–93S.
34. Candido EP, Reeves R, Davie JR. Sodium butyrate inhibits histone deacetylation in cultured cells. Cell. 1978;14(1):105–13.
35. Csordas A. Butyrate, aspirin and colorectal cancer. Eur J Cancer Prev. 1996; 5(4):221–31.
36. Bultman SJ. Molecular pathways: gene-environment interactions regulating dietary fiber induction of proliferation and apoptosis via butyrate for cancer prevention. Clin Cancer Res. 2014;20(4):799–803.
37. Kikuchi Y, Dinjens WN, Bosman FT. Proliferation and apoptosis in proliferative lesions of the colon and rectum. Virchows Arch. 1997;431:111–7.
38. Hong MY, Turner ND, Murphy ME, et al. In vivo regulation of colonic cell proliferation, differentiation, apoptosis, and P27Kip1 by dietary fish oil and butyrate in rats. Cancer Prev Res (Phila). 2015;8(11):1076–83.
39. Drago E, Bordonaro M, Lee S, et al. Propolis augments apoptosis induced by butyrate via targeting cell survival pathways. PLoS One. 2013;8(9):e73151.

21

Comparison of AIMS65, Glasgow–Blatchford and Rockall scoring approaches in predicting the risk of in-hospital death among emergency hospitalized patients with upper gastrointestinal bleeding

Lei Gu[1†], Fei Xu[2,3†] and Jie Yuan[1*]

Abstract

Background: This study aims to compare the performance of AIMS65, Glasgow–Blatchford (GBS) and Rockall scores (RS) in predicting the death risk among emergency-hospitalized patients with upper gastrointestinal bleeding (UGIB) in regional China.

Methods: A retrospective study was implemented between January 2014 and December 2015. Eligible participants were those who were hospitalized with UGIB. The outcome variable was in-hospital death, while explanatory variables were AIMS65, GBS and RS scores. Odds ratios (OR) and 95% confidence interval (CI) were estimated to assess the association of AIMS65, GBS and RS with death risk using multivariate logistic regression models. The areas under the receiver operating characteristics curve (AUC) of three scoring systems were computed to compare their predictive power.

Results: Among 799 UGIB participants, 674 were non-variceal bleeding (NVUGIB) and 125 variceal bleeding (VUGIB) patients. AIMS65 (OR = 14.72, 95% CI = 6.48, 33.43) and RS (OR = 1.60, 95% CI = 1.20, 2.13) were positively associated with the risk of in-hospital death. Moreover, AIMS65 (AUC = 0.91, 95% CI = 0.84, 0.98) performed the best in predicting in-hospital death, followed by RS (AUC = 0.79, 95% CI = 0.72, 0.86) and GBS (AUC = 0.71, 95% CI = 0.59, 0.83) among overall UGIB participants. AIMS65 was also the best indicator to predict in-hospital death among either NVUGIB participants (AUC = 0.89, 95% CI = 0.80, 0.98) or VUGIB participants (AUC = 0.94, 95% CI = 0.89, 1.00).

Conclusions: AIMS65, GBS and RS scoring approaches were all acceptable for predicting in-hospital death among UGIB patients irrespective of the subtype of UGIB in China. The AIMS65 might be the most powerful predictor.

Keywords: Upper gastrointestinal bleeding, Rockall score, Glasgow-Blatchford score, AIMS65 score, In-hospital death, China

* Correspondence: jim0790@sina.com
†Lei Gu and Fei Xu contributed equally to this work.
[1]Department of Gastroenterology, Nanjing First Hospital, Nanjing Medical University, 68, Changle Road, Nanjing 210006, China
Full list of author information is available at the end of the article

Background

Upper gastrointestinal bleeding (UGIB) refers to the acute bleeding caused by upper gastrointestinal tract lesions beyond the ligament of Treitz, including non-variceal upper gastrointestinal bleeding (NVUGIB) and variceal upper gastrointestinal bleeding (VUGIB) [1]. Over the past decades, the treatment and management of UGIB have been substantially improved, however the death rate among UGIB patients did not decline notably. The death rate was approximately 10% within overall UGIB patients and even as high as 35% among those with acute and chronic co-morbidities in Western countries [2–4]. In China, UGIB-specific death rate was estimated to be 4–14%, showing a heavy disease burden caused by UGIB [5].

The scenarios of prognosis are different for UGIB patients. Some patients with minor bleeding might get completely recovered without clinical treatment, while others with severe clinical symptoms might lose lives if they could not receive appropriate and effective clinical treatment timely. Therefore, it is of particular importance for clinical practitioners to effectively identify those UGIB patients who are at high risk of experiencing subsequent adverse outcomes. Recently, some scoring approaches have been developed to predict the subsequent outcomes for patients with UGIB, including Rockall score (RS), Glasgow Blatchford Score (GBS), Baylor Bleeding score, Cedars-Sinai Medical Center predictive index, Almela score and AIMS65 score. Among the above mentioned scoring approaches, RS and GBS are the most often-used [6–10]. However, they were not applied as widely as expected in clinical practice due to the complicated score calculation. Fortunately, the AIMS65 scoring system has recently been developed and validated to predict in-hospital death by Harvard Medical School in 2011 [11], which was more easily-calculated relative to either GBS or RS.

Considering that there are approximately 1 million UGIB patients visiting hospital each year and high mortality among these UGIB patients in China [5], it is of great significance to identify those UGIB patients who are at high risk of death (or other severe adverse outcomes) and provide them appropriate clinical treatment in time. Therefore, an effective and easily-used scoring approach is urgently needed for identifying those UGIB patients at high risk of death in China. Using hospital-based retrospective data, we aimed to evaluate the performance of AIMS65, GBS and RS scoring approaches in predicting the risk of death for hospitalized UGIB patients in China.

Methods

Participants

This was a retrospective hospital-based observational study. Participants were UGIB patients who visited the Department of Gastroenterology of Nanjing First Hospital with related signs and symptoms (i.e., melena, hematemesis, coffee ground vomiting, and/or abdominal pain) and were hospitalized for clinical treatment between January 2014 and December 2015. Those patients were excluded from the study if they (1) did not receive endoscopy examination as they had severe clinical symptoms and needed emergent clinical treatment to save their lives ($n = 7$), and/or (2) had missing data regarding calculation of GBS, RS and AIMS65. Finally, 799 of 814 UGIB patients were successfully included in this study. Prior to data collection, written informed consent was obtained from each alive participant or from his/her next of kin for the died. This study was approved by the Academic and Ethical Committee of Nanjing First Hospital.

Data collection

For each participant, the following information were collected: age, gender, symptoms and signs on admission (including hematemesis, coffee ground vomiting, melena, syncope, mental status, blood pressure and pulse), co-morbidities (e.g., ischemic heart disease, diabetes mellitus, congestive cardiac failure, liver disease), profiles from laboratory tests (e.g., albumin level, urea, international normalized ratio, creatinine, hemoglobin), endoscopy examination records and subsequent clinical outcome events (in-hospital death or being alive).

Study variables

Outcome variables

The primary outcome variable was in-hospital death ("Yes" or "No"), defined as any death occurred during the period of hospitalization due to UGIB attack.

Explanatory variables

Explanatory variables were GBS, RS and AIMS65 scores, which were used as continuous and categorical measures, separately, in our analysis. There were 8, 5 and 5 risk factors involved to compute the score of GBS, RS and AIMS65, respectively. Table 1 presented all the specific risk factors and scoring algorithms included in each scoring system.

Statistical analysis

First, we conducted descriptive analysis using t-test (continuous variables) or Chi-square test (categorical variables). Then, using logistic regression models, we examined the relationship between outcome events and scores, separately. Two models were introduced: model 1 was a univariate analysis with each score as the single predictor; model 2 was a multivariate regression model with adjustment for participants' age and/or gender and/or other potential clinical confounders (including albumin, urea, international normalized ratio, hemoglobin, blood pressure, pulse, comorbidity, mental status [12, 13], blood

Table 1 Factors and scoring algorithms included in GBS, RS and AIMS65

	Admission clinical factor	Parameter	Score
GBS	BUN (mmol/L)	6.5–7.9	2
		8.0–9.9	3
		10.0–24.9	4
		≥ 25.0	6
	Hemoglobin level (g/dL)	Male: ≥ 12 to < 13	1
		Female: ≥ 10 to < 12	1
		Male: ≥ 10 to < 12	3
		Male: < 10, female: < 10	6
	SBP (mm Hg)	≥ 100 to < 109	1
		≥ 90 to < 100	2
		< 90	3
	Other marker	HR ≥ 100 bpm	1
		Melena	1
		Syncope	2
		Hepatic disease or cardiac failure	2
RS	Age (yr)	< 60	0
		60–79	1
		≥ 80	2
	Shock	HR > 100 bpm	1
		SBP < 100 mmHg	2
	Comorbidity	IHD, CHF, any major comorbidity renal failure, liver failure	2
		metastatic malignancy	3
	Endoscopic finding	Mallory-Weiss tear or no lesion	0
		Peptic ulcer disease, erosive esophagitis	1
		Malignancy	2
	Stigmata of recent hemorrhage	Clean-based ulcer, flat pigmented spot	0
		Blood in upper gastrointestinal tract, clot, visible vessel, bleeding	2
AIMS65	Albumin (g/dL)	< 3.0	1
	INR	> 1.5	1
	Mental status	Altered	1
	SBP (mm Hg)	≤ 90	1
	Age (yr)	≥ 65	1

GBS glasgow-blatchford score, *BUN* blood urea nitrogen level, *SBP* systolic blood pressure, *HR* heart rate, *RS* rockall risk score, *IHD* ischemic heart disease, *CHF* congestive heart failure, *INR* international normalized ratio, AIMS65 AIMS65 score

platelet count, prothrombin time or bleeding causes based on endoscopy exam) with consideration of specific variables included in each scoring system. Next, we used receiver operator characteristic curve (ROC) analysis, a widely used approach, to compare the predictive power of each scoring system on the risk of experiencing outcome events [14, 15]. ROC curve is a graphic representation of the relation between sensitivity and specificity for a diagnostic test. The areas under the receiver operating characteristics curve (AUC) were calculated with sensitivity as y-axis against 1-specifity as x-axis. With AUC, ROC curve can estimates and compares the predictive power of different tests or measures, which can assist with the choice of one test over the others. Generally, a perfect test will have an AUC of 1.0 and an AUC = 0.5 means the test performs no better than chance. Sensitivity and specificity of each scoring system were calculated at all possible cut-off points. The optimal cut-off value was identified based on the maximum sum of sensitivity and specificity for each scoring system. Data were double-entered and cleaned with EpiData 3.0 (The Epidata Association, Odense, Denmark) and analyzed using SPSS 21.0 (IBM Corp, Armonk, NY, USA).

Results

Selected participants' characteristics

Among the total 814 patients with UGIB, 799 participants were eligibly included in this study, with a mean (SD) age of 57.46 (18.04) years and 612 (76.60%) of men. Table 2 displayed the selected characteristics for 799 participants in this study. There were only 15 patients (1.8%) excluded from our analysis due to incomplete information. No death case was observed among those 15 excluded patients. The 15 patients excluded from our analysis (mean ± SD: 73.93 ± 14.84, $p < 0.05$) were significantly older than those 799 participants included in this study. However there was no statistical difference in gender proportion between the 15 excluded (60% of men) and 799 included patients (76.60% of men, $p = 0.13$).

Of those 799 UGIB patients, 125 (15.60%) were with variceal bleeding and 674 (84.40%) with nonvariceal bleeding. With respect to the causes of bleeding for these 799 patients, 484 (60.58%) participants were with peptic ulcer bleeding, 65 (8.14%) with cancer bleeding, 40 (5.01%) with Mallory-Weiss syndrome, 9 (1.13%) with erosive esophagitis and 201 (25.16%) with other diseases (e.g., gastro-oesophageal varices, acute gastric mucosal lesions, Dieulafoy's lesion, or diverticular bleeding).

Associations of RS, GBS and AIMS65 scores with the risk of in-hospital death

The death rate was 3.1% (25/799) among UGIB patients in this study. Table 3 presented the associations of RS, GBS and AIMS65 scores with the risk of in-hospital death among overall 799 participants. After adjustment for potential confounders, AIMS65 (OR = 14.72, 95% CI = 6.48, 33.43) and RS (OR = 1.60, 95% CI = 1.20, 2.13) scores were examined

Table 2 Selected demographic and clinical characteristics of participants ($N = 799$)

Characteristics	n (%)
Men (%)	612 (77.22)
Age, yr. (mean ± SD)	57.46 ± 18.04
Clinical symptoms	
Melena	671 (84.0)
Coffee ground vomiting	90 (11.3)
Mental status or syncope	77 (9.6)
Signs and Laboratory Examinations (mean ± SD)	
Systolic blood pressure, mm Hg	118.37 ± 17.87
Pulse, bpm	85.17 ± 13.53
Hemoglobin, g/dL	9.48 ± 2.89
Urea, mmol/L	9.84 ± 5.50
Albumin, g/dL	3.37 ± 0.57
INR	1.10 ± 0.49
Comorbidities	
Ischemic heart disease	120 (15.0)
Diabetes mellitus	98 (12.3)
Congestive cardiac failure	25(3.1)
Liver disease	130 (16.3)
Liver failure	123 (15.4)
Chronic renal impairment	11 (1.4)
Endoscopic finding	
Mallory-Weiss tear	40 (5.0)
Peptic ulcer disease	484 (60.6)
Malignancy	65 (8.1)
Erosive esophagitis	9 (1.1)
Other diagnoses	201 (25.2)
Stigmata of recent hemorrhage	
Clean-based ulcer	462 (57.7)
Flat pigmented spot	279 (34.9)
Blood in upper gastrointestinal tract,	30 (3.8)
Clot	3(0.4)
Visible vessel	6(0.8)
Bleeding	19 (2.4)

to be positively associated with the risk of death among the overall participants, while marginally significant link (OR = 1.09, 955CI = 0.93, 1.27) was observed between GBS score and death risk.

Table 4 showed the associations of RS, GBS and AIMS65 scores with in-hospital death by type of UGIB. Among participants with NVUGIB, the scenarios of the associations of RS, GBS and AIMS65 scores with in-hospital death were similar to those within overall participants. However, for patients with VUGIB, only AIMS65 was examined to be positively associated with the likelihood of death.

Predictive power of RS, GBS and AIMS65 scoring approaches on the risk of experiencing in-hospital death based on ROC analysis

Figure 1 displayed the AUCs of RS, GBS and AIMS65 scoring systems to predict in-hospital death among overall participants. AIMS65 (AUC = 0.91, 95% CI = 0.84, 0.98) performed the best in predicting in-hospital death, followed by RS (AUC = 0.79, 95% CI = 0.72, 0.86) and GBS (AUC = 0.71, 95% CI = 0.59, 0.83).

Figures 2 and 3 showed the AUCs of RS, GBS and AIMS65 scoring systems to predict in-hospital death among NVUGIB and VUGIB participants, separately. Among the NVUGIB participants, AIMS65 (AUC = 0.89, 95% CI = 0.80, 0.98) performed the best to predict in-hospital death, then RS (AUC = 0.81, 95% CI = 0.73, 0.88) and GBS (AUC = 0.65, 95% CI = 0.50, 0.80), while AIMS65 (AUC = 0.94, 95% CI = 0.89, 1.00) was also the best predictor of in-hospital death, and then GBS (AUC = 0.78, 95% CI = 0.54, 0.93) and RS (AUC = 0.67, 95% CI = 0.50, 0.84) among VUGIB participants.

Optimal cutoff values of RS, GBS and AIMS65 scoring approaches for predicting in-hospital death

In this study, we estimated the optimal cutoff values of RS, GBS and AIMS65 scoring system, separately, for predicting in-hospital death among overall participants based on our ROC analysis (Table 5). The optimal cutoffs were identified to be 3, 12 and 2 for RS, GBS and AIMS65, respectively, and the largest sum of sensitivity (true positive rate) and specificity (true negative rate) produced for each scoring approach was 146% (RS), 140% (GBS) and 172% (AIMS65), separately, based on the corresponding estimated optimal cutoffs in this study.

Discussion

In this retrospective study, significantly positive associations were identified between either RS or AIMS65 score and the risk of in-hospital death but marginally statistical link was observed for GBS scores among UGIB patients in Nanjing, China. Furthermore, based on AUCs, AIMS65 was the best approach, against the other two scoring systems, to predict in-hospital death (AIMS65 > RS > GBS for overall participants) among overall participants. Finding from this study suggested that these three scoring systems might be acceptable to predict in-hospital death for emergency hospitalized UGIB patients in China, which also added further evidence to existing literature.

The majority (91.7%) of the 799 UGIB patients were those with peptic ulcer bleeding, gastro-oesophageal varices, cancer bleeding, Mallory-Weiss syndrome or acute gastric mucosal lesions in our study. This was

Table 3 The associations of RS, GBS and AIMS65 scores with the risk of in-hospital death among 799 UGIB participants in Nanjing, China

Scoring system	Death	*n* (%)	Score values (Mean ± SD)	Unadjusted odds ratio (95% CI)	Adjusted odds ratio (95% CI)
RS	No	774 (96.9)	2.86 ± 1.78	1	1
	Yes	25 (3.1)	4.88 ± 1.90	1.72 (1.38, 2.13)	1.60 (1.20, 2.13)[a]
GBS	No	774 (96.9)	8.31 ± 3.64	1	1
	Yes	25 (3.1)	11.24 ± 4.02	1.31 (1.14, 1.50)	1.09 (0.93, 1.27)[b]
AIMS65	No	774 (96.9)	0.69 ± 0.99	1	1
	Yes	25 (3.1)	2.00 ± 1.00	8.24(4.67, 14.54)	14.72 (6.48, 33.43)[c]

[a]RS: Adjusted for gender, Hb, Albumin, BUN, INR, Mental status/ Syncope, PT and PLT
[b]GBS: Adjusted for age, gender, Albumin, INR, PT, PLT and endoscopic findings
[c]AIMS65: Adjusted for gender, Hb, BUN, heart rate, co-morbidity, PT, PLT and endoscopic findings

consistent not only with that reported from Western societies [9] but also with findings from a survey among Chinese UGIB patients [16].

The death rate (3.10%) observed among UGIB patients in this study was lower relative to those documented in previous literatures from both China and UK [17, 18]. This might be explained, in part, by that application of proton pump inhibitors (PPIs) prior to endoscopy, which could reduce the risk of re-bleeding and death [1]. In addition, different from some previous studies, the outcome events (in-hospital death) assessed in this study were limited to those observed in the period of hospitalization, therefore the potential death cases after discharge were not investigated, which might have the number of death cases underestimated.

Some recent studies found that AIMS65 had similar power to RS or GBS in predicting death for UGIB patients [5, 19]. However, our study showed that AIMS65 was better than either GBS or RS in predicting in-hospital death. In addition to the interesting findings for overall participants, our study demonstrated that each of AIMS65, GBS and RS also could be used to assess the risk of in-hospital death in either NVUGIB or VUGIB patients. This was in line with the reports from previous retrospective studies [20, 21].

Only five variables are included to compute the AIMS65 score and the calculation of AIMS65 score is really simpler relative to GBS or RS. In our study, AIMS65 performed the best among these three scoring systems to predict in-hospital death for UGIB patients. Therefore, in terms of easy-use and predictive power, AIMS65 might be the most optimal instrument for predicting in-hospital death among UGIB patients in China.

A cut-off value is critically important for each scoring system in predicting clinical outcome events. Unfortunately, cutoffs were almost different for each of these three scoring systems in previous studies [6, 19]. It is really difficult to explain such inconsistency of cutoff values among different studies. However, this might be partly due to some differences in those studies: participants and ethnicity, bleeding cause based on endoscopy

Table 4 The associations of RS, GBS and AIMS65 scores with the risk of in-hospital death among participants by type of UGIB in Nanjing, China

Sub-group of participants	Scoring system	Mortality	*n* (%)	Score values (Mean ± SD)	Unadjusted odds ratio (95% CI)	Adjusted odds ratio (95% CI)
NVUGIB (*n* = 674)	RS	No	658(97.6)	2.27 ± 1.41	1	1
		Yes	16 (2.4)	3.94 ± 1.44	1.83 (1.38, 2.42)	1.79 (1.24, 2.58)[a]
	GBS	No	658(97.6)	7.82 ± 3.56	1	1
		Yes	16 (2.4)	10.06 ± 3.85	1.22 (1.04, 1.43)	0.99 (0.82, 1.18)[b]
	AIMS65	No	658(97.6)	0.58 ± 0.72	1	1
		Yes	16 (2.4)	2.31 ± 1.14	7.29(3.81, 13.94)	8.72 (3.54, 21.48)[c]
VUGIB (*n* = 125)	RS	No	116 (92.8)	2.86 ± 1.78	1	1
		Yes	9 (7.2)	4.88 ± 1.90	1.64 (0.88, 3.08)	1.95(0.79, 4.80)[a]
	GBS	No	116 (92.8)	8.31 ± 3.64	1	1
		Yes	9 (7.2)	11.24 ± 4.02	1.48 (1.07, 2.05)	1.26 (0.88, 1.82)[b]
	AIMS65	No	116 (92.8)	0.69 ± 0.99	1	1
		Yes	9 (7.2)	2.00 ± 1.00	28.88(3.76, 222.02)	244.11 (4.18, 14,266.12)[c]

[a]RS: Adjusted for gender, Hb, Albumin, BUN, INR, Mental status/Syncope, PT and PLT
[b]GBS: Adjusted for age, gender, Albumin, INR, PT, PLT and endoscopic findings
[c]AIMS65: Adjusted for gender, Hb, BUN, heart rate, co-morbidity, PT, PLT and endoscopic findings

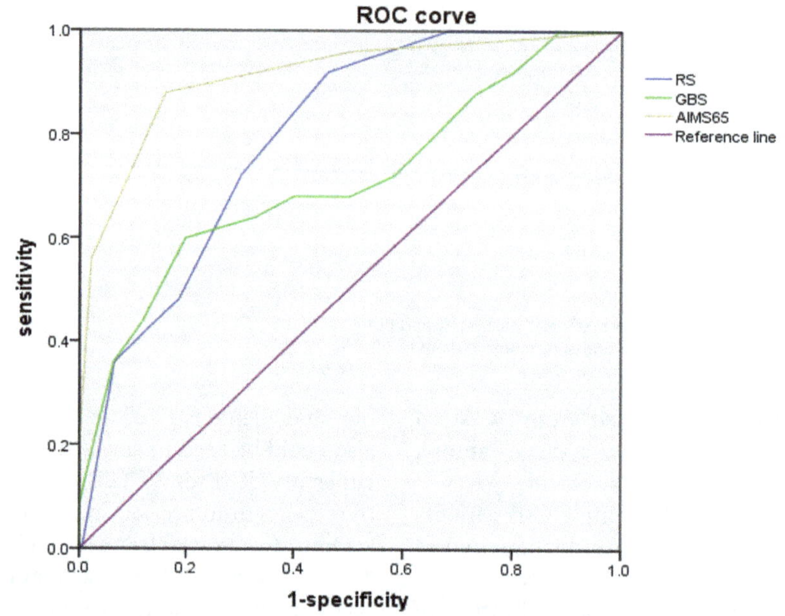

Fig. 1 The receiver operating characteristic curves for the predictive value of AIMS65, RS and GBS for in-hospital death (Overall)

exam, use of PPIs, time of endoscopy exam and adherence to guidelines regarding endoscopic therapy [19]. For example, a study from Spain found that the optimal cutoff value for predicting death among UGIB patients was 1 for AIMS65, 12 for GBS and 6 for RS [19]. An Australian study reported that the preferable cutoff was 3 for AIMS65, 15 for GBS and 7 for RS to predict death among UGIB patients [6]. And, our study suggested that the optimal cutoff value among Chinese UGIB patients was 2 for AIMS65, 12 for GBS and 3 for RS to predict in-hospital death. Therefore, the optimal cutoff of each scoring system should be specified for different population to maximize the power of identifying UGIB patients at high risk of death.

To the best of our knowledge, this is the first study conducted in China to compare the performance of GBS, RS and AIMS65 to predict the risk of in-hospital death among Chinese UGIB patients. The sample size

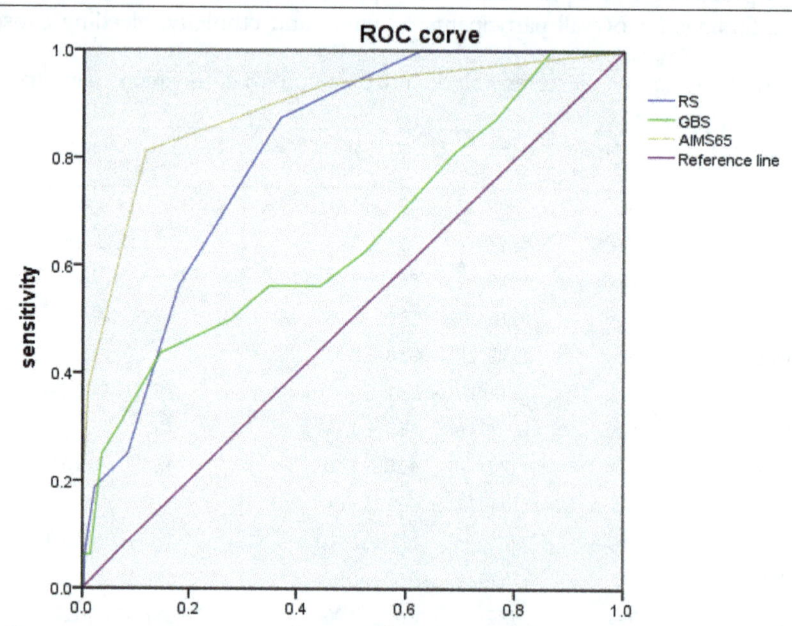

Fig. 2 The receiver operating characteristic curves for the predictive value of AIMS65, RS and GBS for in-hospital death (NVUGIB)

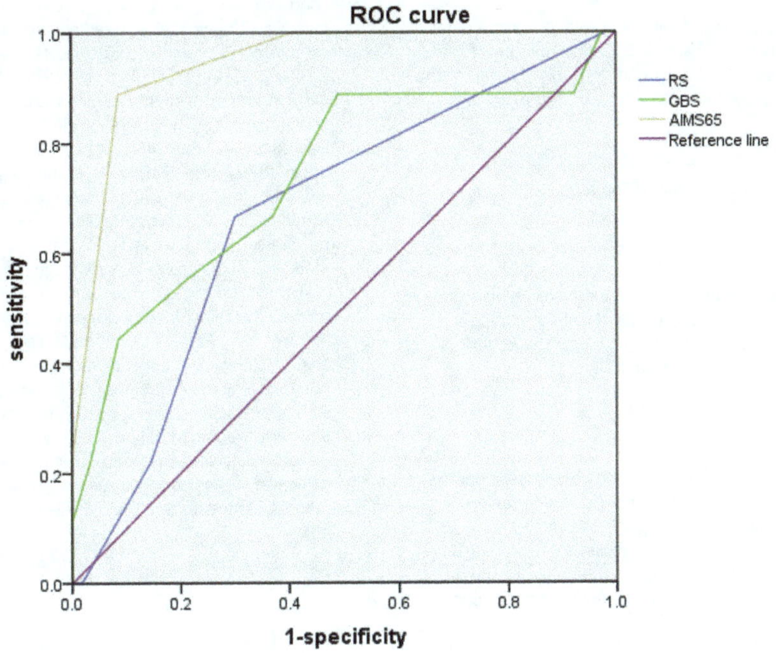

Fig. 3 The receiver operating characteristic curves for the predictive value of AIMS65, RS and GBS for in-hospital death (VUGIB)

was relatively large with sufficient number of VUGIB patients included, which allowed us to examine the predictive power of each scoring system within NVUGIB or VUGIB patients. Reasonable and appropriate statistical methods were used to investigate the association of scores generated by each instrument with the risk of death, to make comparison of predictive performance among the three scoring system, and to estimate the optimal cutoff for each scoring approach within this study.

Some limitations also need to be mentioned. First, this was a retrospective study, which implied potential information bias due to the study design, so the findings should be prudently interpreted. Second, 15 patients were excluded from our analysis due to incomplete data, which might cause potential bias in interpretation of the generalization of the present study findings. Third, only those UGIB patients died in hospital were included in this study and patients died after discharge were missed out. However, this might underpowered the effects of our analysis. In future, perspective studies are needed to further examine the performance of those scoring systems for predicting clinical outcome events among large scale representative sample population with UGIB in China.

Table 5 The estimated optimal cutoff values for AIMS65, GBS, and RS scoring system in this study

Scores	Cutoff value	Sensitivity	Specificity	Youden index
AIMS65	1	0.96	0.49	0.45
	2	0.88	0.84	0.72
	3	0.56	0.98	0.54
GBS	11	0.64	0.67	0.31
	12	0.60	0.80	0.40
	13	0.44	0.88	0.32
RS	2	1.0	0.32	0.32
	3	0.92	0.54	0.46
	4	0.72	0.70	0.42

Conclusions

AIMS65, GBS and RS were all acceptable for predicting in-hospital death among either overall UGIB, NVUGIB or VUGIB patients in China. Among the three scoring systems, AIMS65 might be the best to predict in-hospital death for hospitalized UGIB patients.

Abbreviations

AUC: Areas under the receiver operating characteristics curve; CI: Confidence interval; GBS: Glasgow–Blatchford; NVUGIB: Non-variceal upper gastrointestinal bleeding; OR: Odds ratios; ROC: Receiver operator characteristic curve; RS: Rockall scores; UGIB: Upper gastrointestinal bleeding; VUGIB: Variceal upper gastrointestinal bleeding

Acknowledgements

Our special thanks go to those staff who assisted us in data collection.

Funding

The work was supported by Nanjing Municipal Science and Technology Development Foundation (2007ZD011).

Authors' contributions
Conception and design: FX and JY; Analysis and interpretation of the data: LG, FX and JY; Drafting of the article: LG, FX and JY; Critical revision of the article for important intellectual content: LG, FX and JY; Final approval of the article: LG, FX and JY. All authors have read and approved the manuscript.

Competing interests
The authors declare that they have no competing interests.

Author details
[1]Department of Gastroenterology, Nanjing First Hospital, Nanjing Medical University, 68, Changle Road, Nanjing 210006, China. [2]Nanjing Municipal Center for Disease Control and Prevention, Nanjing, China. [3]The School of Public Health, Nanjing Medical University, Nanjing, China.

References

1. Chinese Association of Emergency Physicians. Expert consensus about the emergency diagnosis and treatment of acute upper gastrointestinal hemorrhage. Chin J Crit Care Med. 2015;35:865–73. (In Chinese).
2. Rockall TA, Logan RF, Devlin HB, Northfield TC. Incidence of and mortality from acute upper gastrointestinal haemorrhage in the United Kingdom. Steering committee and members of the National Audit of acute upper gastrointestinal Haemorrhage. BMJ. 1995;311:222–6.
3. Christensen S, Riis A, Norgaard M, Sorensen HT, Thomsen RW. Short-term mortality after perforated or bleeding peptic ulcer among elderly patients: a population-based cohort study. BMC Geriatr. 2007;7:8.
4. Zimmerman J, Siguencia J, Tsvang E, Beeri R, Arnon R. Predictors of mortality in patients admitted to hospital for acute upper gastrointestinal hemorrhage. Scand J Gastroenterol. 1995;30:327–31.
5. Zhong M, Chen WJ, Lu XY, Qian J, Zhu CQ. Comparison of three scoring systems in predicting clinical outcomes in patients with acute upper gastrointestinal bleeding: a prospective observational study. J Dig Dis. 2016;17:820–8.
6. Chen IC, Hung MS, Chiu TF, Chen JC, Hsiao CT. Risk scoring systems to predict need for clinical intervention for patients with nonvariceal upper gastrointestinal tract bleeding. Am J Emerg Med. 2007;25:774–9.
7. Masaoka T, Suzuki H, Hori S, Aikawa N, Hibi T. Blatchford scoring system is a useful scoring system for detecting patients with upper gastrointestinal bleeding who do not need endoscopic intervention. Journal of Gastroenterology & Hepatolog. 2007;22:1404–8.
8. Bryant RV, Kuo P, Williamson K, Yam C, Schoeman MN, Holloway RH, Nguyen NQ. Performance of the Glasgow-Blatchford score in predicting clinical outcomes and intervention in hospitalized patients with upper GI bleeding. Gastrointest Endosc. 2013;78:576–83.
9. Barkun AN, Bardou M, Kuipers EJ, Sung J, Hunt RH, Martel M, Sinclair P. International consensus recommendations on the Management of Patients with Nonvariceal Upper Gastrointestinal Bleeding. Ann Intern Med. 2010;152:101–13.
10. Li ZS. Guidelines for the diagnosis and treatment of acute non-variceal upper gastrointestinal bleeding. Chin J Dig. 2015;35:793–8. (In Chinese).
11. Saltzman JR, Tabak YP, Hyett BH, Sun X, Travis AC, Johannes RS. A simple risk score accurately predicts in-hospital mortality, length of stay, and cost in acute upper GI bleeding. Gastrointest Endosc. 2011;74:1215–24.
12. Thanapirom K, Ridtitid W, Rerknimitr R, Thungsuk R, Noophun P, Wongjitrat C, Luangjaru S, Vedkijkul P, Lertkupinit C, Poonsab S. Prospective comparison of three risk scoring systems in non-variceal and variceal upper gastrointestinal bleeding. Journal of Gastroenterology & Hepatology. 2016;31:761–7.
13. Hyett BH, Abougergi MS, Charpentier JP, Kumar NL, Brozovic S, Claggett BL, Travis AC, Saltzman JR. The AIMS65 score compared with the Glasgow-Blatchford score in predicting outcomes in upper GI bleeding. Gastrointest Endosc. 2013;77:551–7.
14. Hanley JA, Mcneil BJ. The meaning and use of the area under a receiver operating characteristic (ROC) curve. Radiology. 1982;143:29–36.
15. Greiner M, Pfeiffer D, Smith RD. Principles and practical application of the receiver-operating characteristic analysis for diagnostic tests. Preventive Veterinary Medicine. 2000;45:23–41.
16. Sung JJ, Tsoi KK, Ma TK, Yung MY, Lau JY, Chiu PW. Causes of mortality in patients with peptic ulcer bleeding: a prospective cohort study of 10,428 cases. Am J Gastroenterol. 2010;105:84–9.
17. Xu Q, Hu NZ, Cui XL. Etiology and clinical characteristic of upper gastrointestinal haemorrhage: analysis of 1520 cases. Chinese journal of general practice. 2010;8:1079–80. (In Chinese)
18. Hearnshaw SA, Logan RF, Lowe D, Travis SP, Murphy MF, Palmer KR. Acute upper gastrointestinal bleeding in the UK: patient characteristics, diagnoses and outcomes in the 2007 UK audit. Gut. 2011;60:1327–35.
19. Martínez-Cara JG, Jiménez-Rosales R, Úbeda-Muñoz M, de Hierro ML, de Teresa J, Redondo-Cerezo E. Comparison of AIMS65, Glasgow–Blatchford score, and Rockall score in a European series of patients with upper gastrointestinal bleeding: performance when predicting in-hospital and delayed mortality. United European Gastroenterol J. 2016;4:371–9.
20. Park SW, Song YW, Tak DH, Ahn BM, Kang SH, Moon HS, Sung JK, Jeong HY. The AIMS65 score is a useful predictor of mortality in patients with nonvariceal upper gastrointestinal bleeding: urgent endoscopy in patients with high AIMS65 scores. Clinical Endoscopy. 2015;48:522–7.
21. Budimir I, Gradišer M, Nikolić M, Baršić N, Ljubičić N, Kralj D, Budimir I Jr. Glasgow Blatchford, pre-endoscopic Rockall and AIMS65 scores show no difference in predicting rebleeding rate and mortality in variceal bleeding. Scand J Gastroenterol. 2016;51:1375–9.

Is perceived intolerance to milk and wheat associated with the corresponding IgG and IgA food antibodies? A cross sectional study in subjects with morbid obesity and gastrointestinal symptoms

Anne Stine Kvehaugen[1*], Dag Tveiten[2] and Per G. Farup[3,4]

Abstract

Background: Serum IgG and IgA food antibodies have been used for dietary advice to subjects with gastrointestinal symptoms and perceived food intolerance, but the role of these antibodies in mediating intolerance is controversial. The present study investigated associations between perceived gastrointestinal intolerance to milk-or wheat and the corresponding s-IgG and s-IgA food antibodies in subjects with morbid obesity.

Methods: Subjects with morbid obesity (BMI ≥ 40 kg/m^2 or ≥35 kg/m^2 with obesity-related complications) were included. Irritable Bowel Syndrome (IBS) was diagnosed based on the Rome III criteria. Severity of specific gastrointestinal symptoms were measured with the Gastrointestinal Symptom Rating Scale (GSRS)-IBS. S-IgG against cow's milk, cheese, wheat and gluten, and s-IgA against casein and gliadin were measured.

Results: Ninety-seven subjects (80 females) with mean age 45 (SD 8.4) years were included, 70 had gastrointestinal complaints, 25 had IBS, and 22 and 20 reported milk- and wheat- intolerance respectively. There were no significant differences in serum concentrations or proportions of subjects above defined cut-off values for the antibodies between subjects with and without gastrointestinal complaints. In the group with gastrointestinal complaints, no significant differences were found between subjects with and without perceived food intolerance. Except for a significant correlation between IgG against cheese and GSRS-diarrhea (*Rho*: -0.25, $P = 0.04$), no significant correlations were found between the antibodies and type or degree of gastrointestinal symptoms, including IBS.

Conclusions: The study showed no associations between perceived milk or wheat intolerance and the corresponding s-IgG and s-IgA food antibodies in subjects with morbid obesity.

Keywords: Antibodies, Immunoglobulin G, Immunoglobulin a, Milk, Wheat, Gastrointestinal, Hypersensitivity, Obesity

Background

Food-induced gastrointestinal (GI) symptoms are frequently reported in the population and associated with functional gastrointestinal disorders, in particular irritable bowel syndrome (IBS) [1]. Milk and dairy products, as well as wheat and/or gluten containing foods are among the foods often considered as triggers [2, 3]. Controversy still remains regarding the role of IgG food antibodies in mediating food intolerance. The measurement of serum concentrations of these antibodies has been and is still used by some laboratories as a guidance for dietary interventions [4]. Expert societies and guidelines on food allergy state that the evidence for the use of these tests is lacking; it has been proposed that the presence of IgG food antibodies merely reflects exposure to the corresponding foods and indicates immunological tolerance [4–7]. This view has been challenged by showing that IgG-guided elimination diets improved symptoms in

* Correspondence: akvehaugen@yahoo.no
[1]Department of Surgery, Innlandet Hospital Trust, Kyrre Greppsgate 11, 2819 Gjøvik, Norway
Full list of author information is available at the end of the article

different patient groups, including subjects with IBS and IBS with migraine [8–11]. However, there is a lack of studies investigating associations between perceived intolerance against particular foods and the corresponding s-IgG or s-IgA food antibodies in adults with GI symptoms. The present study addressed this issue in subjects with morbid obesity, a patient group with reportedly high prevalence of gastrointestinal symptoms, including IBS [12–14]. Interestingly, IBS and obesity also have several pathophysiological features in common, including increased gut permeability [15, 16], which could potentially result in increased translocation of food antibodies.

Aim of the present study was to explore the association between perceived intolerance to milk/dairy products and wheat and the serum concentrations (including cut-off values) of IgG and IgA against the corresponding food antigens in subjects with morbid obesity reporting GI complaints. Secondary aims were to investigate associations between 1) perceived intolerance to the foods in question; and 2) the IgGs and IgAs directed against these foods, with the following parameters; dietary intake of the offending foods, IBS, severity of specific GI symptoms and gut permeability.

Methods

Patients and study design

This cross-sectional study was performed at the unit for morbid obesity at Innlandet Hospital Trust, Gjøvik, Norway. Consecutive subjects referred for morbid obesity (BMI ≥ 40 kg/m^2 or BMI ≥ 35 kg/m^2 with obesity related complications (e.g. diabetes, hypertension, sleep apnoea, musculoskeletal problems) were included in a comprehensive study from December 2012 to September 2014. The patients were evaluated for bariatric surgery or non-surgical treatment of obesity, but had not started the weight reducing intervention at the time of study inclusion. A medical history was taken, a physical examination was performed, and a blood sample was collected for further analyses. The patients filled in paper-based questionnaires, including a case-report form and a food frequency questionnaire (FFQ). Subjects with major organic GI disorders (including celiac disease) or former major GI surgery, subjects who did not complete the FFQ or lacked blood samples for the biobank were excluded.

Case-report form

included questions on a large range of variables (e.g.demographics, previous or present co-morbidities (diabetes mellitus, polycystic ovary syndrome, hypertension, cardiovascular disease, gallstones, hypo–/ hyperthyroidism, fibromyalgia, osteoporosis, chronic bronchitis, hay-fever, asthma, psychological problems, GI diseases), different health scores, perception of overall state of health, GI symptoms (yes/no) and food-induced GI symptoms). IBS was diagnosed with a validated Norwegian translation of the Rome III criteria [17]; and the degree of specific GI complaints with the Gastrointestinal Symptom Rating Scale – IBS (GSRS-IBS) [18]. The GSRS-IBS questionnaire contained 13 questions with responses ranging from 1 to 7 (no discomfort at all to very severe discomfort). The questions were clustered into the following dimensions; GSRS-diarrhea, –constipation, –bloating, –pain and –satiety, and a mean value for the items in each dimension were calculated. Questions regarding food-induced GI symptoms were recorded with our own questionnaire, with focus on milk/dairy products and wheat. This questionnaire included questions regarding whether or not the patients related their GI symptoms to the intake of these foods, as well as visual analogue scales (range 0–100) asking *"how certain are you that; Milk/dairy products are the offending foods? Wheat is the offending food?"*

For convenience, further mention of intolerance to milk and dairy in the text will be mentioned as intolerance to milk only.

FFQ

The FFQ, designed to study the usual diet, has been prepared and validated by the University of Oslo [19, 20]. Daily intake of food, nutrients and energy was calculated by Department of Nutrition at the University of Oslo by their in-house calculation program (KBS, version 7.3, food database AE-14). The food composition database in the calculation program is based on the official Norwegian food composition table from 2016 [21] and is supplemented with additional food items.

Laboratory analyses

Analyses of food antibodies were performed by Lab1, Sandvika in accordance with the manufacturer's instructions. Serum zonulin, a marker of tight junction gut permeability (reference value < 48 ng/ml), and IgA against casein and gliadin were analyzed with Enzyme Linked Immunosorbent Assays (Zonulin ELISA Kit, Immundiagnostik AG, Bensheim, Germany, and; IgA gliadin/casein Screening ELISA test from Immunolab GmbH, Kassel, Germany). IgG antibodies against a panel of 44 common foods were measured with an enzyme immunoassay from R-Biopharm AG, Darmstadt, Germany (RIDASCREEN® Spec. IgG Foodscreen). From this panel of antibodies, only those related to the food intolerances in question were selected for statistical analyses. Four IgG food antibodies were considered relevant: IgG against cow's milk, cheese, wheat and gluten. The following cut-off values for the food antibodies, as recommended by the manufacturers, were defined as test positive: For IgG a value ≥ 7.5 μg/ml was considered mildly elevated and a value ≥ 20 μg/ml was considered strongly elevated. The corresponding cut-off values for IgA were ≥ 8.0 U/ml (mildly elevated) and ≥ 12 U/ml (strongly elevated). Values below the lowest detection limit for the IgG food antibodies (2.5 μg/ml) were assigned the value 2.4 μg/ml.

Statistical analyses

Data analyses were performed with IBM SPSS Statistics for Windows, Version 23 (IBM Corp., Armonk, N.Y., USA). For continuous data, comparisons between two groups were analyzed with the independent sample t-test if data were normally distributed or the non-parametric Mann Whitney U-test if data were skewed. Categorical data were analyzed with χ^2 statistics. Correlations between variables were tested with Spearman's correlation. Associations between perceived food intolerance and the corresponding food antibodies were adjusted for co-variates by use of logistic regression models (milk- or wheat intolerance as the dependent variable). A P-value < 0.05 was considered statistically significant.

Sample size and power calculations

No power-calculation was performed as we were not aware of previously published studies with a similar study population and design.

Results

In all, 97 out of 159 subjects were eligible for the present study (female/male: 80/17; mean age: 45 (SD 8.4) years). Of these, 70 had GI complaints. There were no significant differences between the groups with and without GI complaints regarding demographics, co-morbidity, blood tests, dietary intake or food antibodies (data not shown). All the presented analyses were based on the group with GI complaints. Twenty-two (31.4%) and 20 (28.6%) subjects related their symptoms to the intake of milk and wheat respectively; 11 (15.7%) had a perceived intolerance to both milk and wheat.

Table 1 shows the patient characteristics, biochemical and dietary data in subjects with and without perceived intolerance to milk or wheat. The presence of co-morbidities was not significantly different between those with and without perceived intolerance to either milk or wheat (data not displayed; all P-values > 0.05). The exception was IBS (Table 1) and hypothyroidism. The latter was significantly more common among subjects with than without perceived intolerance to wheat (5/18 (27.8%) vs. 2/48 (4.2%), $P = 0.014$). Alcohol consumption and smoking did not differ between those with and without milk or wheat intolerance (data not displayed; P-values > 0.05 for both).

Tables 2 and 3 show the serum concentrations of the relevant food antibodies in subjects with and without perceived intolerance to milk and wheat respectively, with comparisons between the groups, and the number and proportion of subjects with food intolerance in the groups with positive and negative tests for the given cut-off values. Comparisons between the groups in question did not reveal any significant differences (Table 2 and Table 3). The results remained non-significant after adjusting for the intake of the offending foods (data not shown, all P-values > 0.05). For wheat intolerance versus no intolerance, additional adjustments for differences in s-Zonulin ≥48 ng/ml (as shown in Table 1) and hypothyroidism did also not alter the non-significant relationship between the antibodies and the reported intolerance (P-values > 0.05).

Table 4 shows the correlations between the antibodies investigated and the variables addressed in Table 1. Additionally, because hypothyroidism was significantly more common among subjects with than without perceived intolerance to wheat, correlations between the antibodies and hypothyroidism were examined as post-hoc analyses. Results are included in Table 4.

Discussion

There is a lack of studies investigating the association between patient reported food intolerances and the corresponding IgG or IgA food antibodies in adults with GI symptoms. The novelty of the present study is that IgG and IgA antibodies directed against milk and wheat were compared between subjects who all reported GI complaints, but who did or did not perceive themselves as intolerant to these foods. Dietary intake of the offending foods was also estimated, as dietary restrictions have been suggested to affect serum concentrations of the antibodies in some studies [22–24]. Milk/dairy consumption was lower and close to the level of statistical significance in those with than without perceived milk intolerance. No differences in the intake of wheat containing foods were seen between those with and without perceived wheat intolerance. The measured food antibodies did however not discriminate between those with and without perceived food intolerances, either in unadjusted analyses, or adjusted for the intake of the offending foods. We think that our inclusion of symptomatic subjects only, represents the subjects likely to seek medical/nutritional advice and undergo antibody testing. On the other hand, initial analyses did not reveal any differences between those with and without GI complaints either, regardless of perceived intolerance to milk or wheat.

We are aware of only a few previous studies with a similar design as the present study. One is a study from our group which demonstrated poor correspondence between perceived intolerance against gluten and milk/cheese in patients with IBS and common tests for food intolerance, including IgG and IgA against gliadin and gluten, and IgA against lactalbumin, lactoglobulin and casein [3]. Another is a study by Anthoni et al., which opposed to the present study detected slightly higher titers of IgG against milk protein in subjects with than

Table 1 Patient characteristics, biochemical and dietary data in subjects with and without perceived milk-or wheat intolerance

	Perceived milk intolerance		*P*-value	Perceived wheat intolerance		*P*-value
	Yes ($n = 22$)	No ($n = 48$)		Yes ($n = 20$)	No ($n = 50$)	
Age, years	43.0 (7.39)	45.5 (8.91)	0.256 [d]	46.3 (8.05)	44.1 (8.65)	0.312[d]
Gender (Female), n (%)	19 (86.4)	38 (79.2)	0.742 [a]	18 (90.0)	39 (78.0)	0.322[a]
BMI, kg/m^2	42.3 (2.70)	41.4 (3.39)	0.233 [d]	42.0 (2.72)	41.5 (3.40)	0.631[d]
IBS (Rome III), n (%)	12/21 (57.1)	13/47 (27.7)	0.020 [b] *	10/18 (55.6)	15/50 (30.0)	0.054[b]
GSRS-IBS (range: 1–7)						
GSRS-Pain	2.50 (1.00–5.00)	1.50 (1.00–4.00)	0.014 [c] *	2.25 (1.00–5.00)	2.00 (1.00–4.00)	0.158[c]
GSRS-Bloating	2.33 (1.00–5.33)	2.50 (1.00–5.67)	0.493 [c]	2.67 (1.00–5.33)	2.33 (1.00–5.67)	0.337[c]
GSRS-Diarrhea	1.75 (1.00–4.75)	1.50 (1.00–4.75)	0.065 [c]	2.12 (1.00–4.75)	1.50 (1.00–4.75)	0.075[c]
GSRS-Constipation	1.00 (1.00–4.50)	1.00 (1.00–4.00)	0.916 [c]	1.00 (1.00–4.50)	1.50 (1.00–4.00)	0.746[c]
GSRS-Satiety	1.00 (1.00–4.00)	1.50 (1.00–4.50)	0.669 [c]	1.25 (1.00–4.50)	1.50 (1.00–4.00)	0.493[c]
S-Zonulin ≥48 ng/ml, n (%)	16 (72.7)	29 (60.4)	0.318 [b]	9 (45.0%)	36 (72.0)	0.033[b]*
Dietary intake, g/day						
Milk, cream and cheese	238 (7.00–1173)	469 (23.4–1801)	0.053 [c]	NA	NA	NA
Bread, cereals and cakes	NA	NA	NA	274 (26.4–734)	280 (138–707)	0.654[c]
How certain are you that milk/wheat is the offending food? (VAS-scale: 0–100; a high value indicates high degree of certainty)	77.5 (13.0–100)	NA	NA	67.0 (17.7–95.8)	NA	NA

Data are given as mean (SD), median (min-max) or n (%)
IBS Irritable Bowel Syndrome, *GSRS-IBS* Gastrointestinal Symptom Rating Scale-IBS, *NA* Not applicable, *VAS-scale* Visual Analogue Scale
*Statistically significant: $P < 0.05$
[a]Fisher's Exact Test
[b]Pearson Chi-Square
[c]Mann-Whitney U test
[d]Independent sample t-test

without self-reported milk-induced GI symptoms [22]. However, likewise to the present study, no significant positive associations were found between the IgG antibodies and either IBS or specific GI symptoms [22].

Other studies on the relationship between IBS and IgG food antibody levels have brought mixed results, but correlations between the antibodies and type or severity of symptoms were rarely demonstrated, or even inverse correlations were found [23, 25, 26]. This is in contrast to intervention studies showing that exclusion diets guided by elevated IgG serum concentrations improved symptoms in patients with IBS [8–11]. However, these studies were associated with various limitations, such as the lack of blinding and/or the lack of a control group, incomplete details about how the diets were designed, or intervention and control diets being too different. Importantly, none of the studies compared the effect of excluding the same foods in those with high versus low serum concentrations of the corresponding food antibodies. We speculate that the divergent findings, with

Table 2 Associations between the s-IgG and s-IgA milk antibodies and perceived milk intolerance

	Perceived milk intolerance		*P*-value †	Cut-off ‡	Perceived milk intolerance (22/70 (31.4))		*P*-value ‡
	Yes ($n = 22$)	No ($n = 48$)			Test positive	Test negative	
IgG total (μg/ml) ($n = 69$)	9.77 (2.19)	10.6 (2.08)	0.143				
IgG cow's milk (μg/ml)	15.1 (2.40–112)	10.9 (2.40–117)	0.713	≥ 7.5 ≥ 20	14/43 (32.6) 9/23 (39.1)	8/27 (29.6) 13/47 (27.7)	0.797[b] 0.332[b]
IgG cheese (μg/ml)	5.99 (2.40–72.0)	3.84 (2.40–88.9)	0.755	≥ 7.5 ≥ 20	8/23 (34.8) 3/14 (21.4)	14/47 (29.8) 19/56 (33.9)	0.672[b] 0.524[a]
IgA casein (U/ml)	5.05 (2.70–65.0)	5.15 (2.10–33.1)	0.556	≥ 8.0 ≥ 12	7/25 (28.0) 4/12 (33.3)	15/45 (33.3) 18/58 (31.0)	0.645[b] 1.000[a]

†Data are given as mean (SD) or median (min-max) and independent sample t-test or Mann-Whitney-U-test is performed
‡Positive test results as defined by cut-off values recommended by the manufacturer
‡Data are given as proportion (percent) and X^2-statistics is performed
[a]Fisher's Exact Test
[b]Pearson Chi-Square

Table 3 Associations between the s-IgG and s-IgA wheat antibodies and perceived wheat intolerance

	Perceived wheat intolerance		*P*-value †	Cut-off ‡	Perceived wheat intolerance (20/70 (28.6))		*P*-value ‡
	Yes (n = 20)	No (n = 50)			Test positive	Test negative	
IgG total (μg/ml) (*n* = 69)	10.3 (2.03)	10.3 (2.19)	0.939				
IgG wheat (μg/ml)	8.30 (3.23–84.6)	8.93 (2.40–126)	0.933	≥ 7.5 ≥ 20	12/41 (29.3) 5/13 (38.5)	8/29 (27.6) 15/57 (26.3)	0.878[b] 0.498[a]
IgG gluten (μg/ml)	11.6 (5.77–82.4)	11.4 (2.40–139)	0.459	≥ 7.5 ≥ 20	17/52 (32.7) 6/19 (31.6)	3/18 (16.7) 14/51 (27.5)	0.195[b] 0.734[b]
IgA gliadin (U/ml) (*n* = 69)	5.40 (3.40–8.70)	4.70 (3.00–15.9)	0.337	≥ 8.0 ≥ 12	3/7 (42.9) 0/1 (0)	16/62 (25.8) 19/68 (27.9)	0.384[b] 1.000[a]

†Data are given as mean (SD) or median (min-max) and independent sample t-test or Mann-Whitney-U-test is performed
‡Positive test results as defined by cut-off values recommended by the manufacturer
‡Data are given as proportion (percent) and X^2-statistics is performed
[a]Fisher's Exact Test
[b]Pearson Chi-Square

the lack of correlations with symptoms in this and most other cross-sectional studies on the one hand, and intervention trials showing symptomatic improvements on the other hand, may be due to the many potential triggering components of the same food item. With respect to milk and wheat, several components, separate or in combination, may provoke symptoms (e.g. different proteins, peptides, lactose and fructans) [27–29]. Lactose and fructans both belongs to the Fermentable Oligo-Di-Monosaccharides And Polyols (FODMAPs), which

Table 4 Correlations between the food antibodies and the patient characteristics, biochemical and dietary data

	IgG cow's milk	IgG cheese	IgA casein	IgG wheat	IgG gluten	IgA gliadin
Age, years	Rho: 0.05, P = 0.67	Rho: 0.11, P = 0.35	Rho: −0.04, P = 0.73	Rho: 0.09, P = 0.44	Rho: 0.03, P = 0.82	Rho: −0.02, P = 0.90
Gender (0 = female, 1 = male)	Rho: 0.14, P = 0.24	Rho: 0.20, P = 0.09	Rho: 0.14, P = 0.26	Rho: 0.04, P = 0.72	Rho: 0.03, P = 0.79	Rho: 0.15, P = 0.22
BMI, kg/m^2	Rho: 0.08, P = 0.53	Rho: −0.02, P = 0.87	Rho: 0.17, P = 0.15	Rho: 0.03, P = 0.81	Rho: 0.09, P = 0.46	Rho: 0.12, P = 0.33
IBS (0 = no, 1 = yes)	Rho: 0.04, P = 0.74	Rho: −0.03, P = 0.82	Rho: 0.04, P = 0.74	Rho: −0.16, P = 0.20	Rho: − 0.04, P = 0.72	Rho: 0.06, P = 0.62
GSRS-Pain (range: 1–7)	Rho: −0.04, P = 0.73	Rho: − 0.09, P = 0.47	Rho: − 0.10, P = 0.41	Rho: − 0.07, P = 0.57	Rho: 0.10, P = 0.40	Rho: 0.07, P = 0.59
GSRS-Bloating (range: 1–7)	Rho: −0.11, P = 0.36	Rho: − 0.08, P = 0.53	Rho: − 0.04, P = 0.72	Rho: − 0.14, P = 0.25	Rho: − 0.02, P = 0.85	Rho: − 0.08, P = 0.52
GSRS- Diarrhea (range: 1–7)	Rho: − 0.18, P = 0.14	Rho: − 0.25, P = 0.04*	Rho: −0.19, P = 0.13	Rho: − 0.11, P = 0.35	Rho: 0.01, P = 0.91	Rho: 0.05, P = 0.66
GSRS-Constipation (range: 1–7)	Rho: 0.06, P = 0.61	Rho: 0.05, P = 0.70	Rho: 0.06, P = 0.60	Rho: −0.07, P = 0.55	Rho: −0.05, P = 0.70	Rho: 0.03, P = 0.80
GSRS-Satiety (range: 1–7)	Rho: <−0.01, P = 0.98	Rho: −0.05, P = 0.70	Rho: − 0.20, P = 0.10	Rho: 0.02, P = 0.87	Rho: 0.11, P = 0.36	Rho: −0.20, P = 0.09
S-Zonulin ≥48 ng/ml	Rho: − 0.02, P = 0.89	Rho: 0.05, P = 0.69	Rho: 0.03, P = 0.80	Rho: −0.10, P = 0.40	Rho: − 0.10, P = 0.41	Rho: 0.27, P = 0.02*
Hypothyroidism (0 = no, 1 = yes)	Rho: 0.06, P = 0.63	Rho: 0.09, P = 0.47	Rho: 0.14, P = 0.25	Rho: 0.26, P = 0.04*	Rho: 0.22, P = 0.07	Rho: 0.15, P = 0.23
Dietary intake, g/day						
Milk, cream and cheese	Rho: 0.01, P = 0.94	Rho: −0.02, P = 0.84	Rho: − 0.06, P = 0.61	NA	NA	NA
Bread, cereals and cakes	NA	NA	NA	Rho: −0.12, P = 0.30	Rho: −0.09, P = 0.44	Rho: 0.13, P = 0.27
How certain are you that milk/wheat is the offending food? (VAS-scale: 0–100; a high value indicates high degree of certainty) †	Rho: 0.30, P = 0.18	Rho: 0.19, P = 0.41	Rho: 0.09, P = 0.68	Rho: 0.05, P = 0.83	Rho: −0.14, P = 0.57	Rho: −0.30, P = 0.23

NA Not applicable, *IBS* Irritable Bowel Syndrome, *GSRS* Gastrointestinal Symptom Rating Scale-IBS, *VAS-scale* Visual Analogue Scale
†Included only those with perceived milk or wheat intolerance respectively
*Statistically significant: *P* < 0.05

collectively have been shown to play a role in IBS [30]. In open, uncontrolled trials, the placebo effect can also not be excluded. The lack of standardized methods in IgG testing is also a problem that may have affected differences between studies.

Increased gut permeability could potentially result in elevated levels of the food antibodies. Increased gut permeability, reflected by s-zonulin (a marker of tight junction permeability in the gut) [31], did not predict either serum concentrations of the food antibodies or perceived food intolerance in the present study. An exception was IgA against gliadin, which correlated positively with increased levels of s-zonulin. In spite of this, and in line with a previous study [32], there was an inverse association between tight-junctional gut permeability and perceived wheat intolerance, suggesting other underlying mechanisms for the reported intolerance.

Although not among our main study hypotheses, the present study showed that hypothyroidism was more common among subjects with than without perceived intolerance to wheat. Hypothyroidism also correlated significantly with IgG against wheat, and marginally with IgG against gluten. Numerous reports have described a link between celiac disease and thyroid disease [33, 34], but associations between non-celiac gluten–/wheat sensitivity and autoimmune diseases, such as autoimmune thyroiditis, remain elusive [32, 35–37]. Although not specific for the condition, anti-gliadin antibodies, in particular of the IgG sub-class, has been reported as a frequent serological marker in non-celiac gluten sensitivity in several studies [32, 36, 37]. Much controversy still remains regarding the clinical entity of "non-celiac wheat –/non-celiac gluten sensitivity" [38]. Nevertheless, the present results, in light of previous findings, may deserve closer attention in future studies.

Strengths and limitations

It was a strength that the study was performed pragmatically in a routine clinical setting in conformity with daily clinical practice, and that food intolerance was based on perceived GI intolerance. The antibody tests have commonly been used in this way. The design, therefore, increased the external validity. Food intolerance based on double-blind placebo-controlled food provocation, which is considered the gold standard in diagnosing adverse food reactions [39], could have given other results.

Another strength was the clearly formulated questions asking specifically about food-induced GI symptoms and not about other adverse food reactions, then followed by separate questions regarding the relation to milk or wheat. The degrees of certainty of the perceived associations between the food item and the GI complaints were also assessed.

Patients with celiac disease were excluded from the study. If systematic testing and exclusion of patients with IgE-mediated food allergy and lactose intolerance had also been performed, this could have yielded different results. Based on European data, the prevalence of IgE sensitization in adults were found to be approximately 2% [40] to 4.5% [41] for wheat and 0.8% for milk [41], suggesting a minor influence of these conditions to the present results. The prevalence of lactose malabsorption in Norway is also low, approximating 4% both in the general population and in patients with IBS [42]. Eliminating a potential confounding effect of FODMAPs would require the use of a FODMAP restricted elimination and provocation diet and was not performed. To use the tests for food antibodies only after thorough examinations is however not according to everyday use of the tests.

Another consideration is that the study was accomplished in subjects with morbid obesity referred for weight-reducing interventions. The literature suggests that overweight and obese subjects have a high frequency of GI co-morbidity, including IBS [12–14]. We therefore considered this study population as suitable for the present study question. If the patients had been recruited primarily due to GI complaints and with more severe symptoms, the results might have been different.

The many statistical tests performed increased the risk of a type 1 statistical error. Inaccuracies in the dietary reports, including the risk of re-call bias, can also not be excluded. Moreover, the dietary data did not contain exact information about the amount consumed of the different grains/flour types, such as wheat; only surrogate markers such as bread, cakes and cereals which often contain wheat. These aspects could perhaps explain the lack of a correlation between the intake of the offending foods and the corresponding food antibodies in this study. The significance of the amount consumed of particular foods in increasing the serum concentrations of the corresponding food antibodies seems however inconclusive [22–24, 43].

Conclusion

The study showed no associations between perceived milk and wheat intolerance and the corresponding IgG and IgA food antibodies and gave no support for the use of these antibodies for dietary advice to an unselected group of subjects with morbid obesity and GI complaints.

Abbreviations

ELISA: Enzyme Linked Immunosorbant Assay; FFQ: Food Frequency Questionnaire; FODMAPs: Fermentable Oligo-Di-Monosaccharides And Polyols; GI: Gastrointestinal; GSRS-IBS: Gastrointestinal Symptom Rating Scale – IBS; IBS: Irritable Bowel Syndrome; Ig: Immunoglobulin

Acknowledgements

We are grateful for the assistance of Martin Aasbrenn (physician) and Anja Byfuglien (study nurse), both at Innlandet Hospital Trust, Gjøvik, in patient inclusion and practical work.

Funding
The study has received funding from Innlandet Hospital Trust, Brumunddal, Norway, and Lab1 AS, Sandvika, Norway.

Authors' contributions
ASK participated in the planning and design of the study, performed statistical analyses, interpreted the data and drafted the manuscript. DT participated in the planning and design of the study, was responsible for the administration of the laboratory analyses, interpreted the data and revised the manuscript critically for important intellectual content. PGF designed the project, supervised the accomplishment, interpreted the data, revised the manuscript critically for important intellectual content and is the guarantor of the study. All authors read and approved the final manuscript.

Competing interests
A.S.K. and P.G.F. declare that they have no competing interests. D.T. is the Managing Director and shareholder in Lab1, which performed the analyses of the antibodies.

Author details
[1]Department of Surgery, Innlandet Hospital Trust, Kyrre Greppsgate 11, 2819 Gjøvik, Norway. [2]Lab1 AS, Sandvika, Norway. [3]Department of Research, Innlandet Hospital Trust, Brumunddal, Norway. [4]Unit for Applied Clinical Research, Department of Clinical and Molecular Medicine, Faculty of Medicine and Health Sciences, Norwegian University of Science and Technology, Trondheim, Norway.

References

1. Lomer MC. Review article: the aetiology, diagnosis, mechanisms and clinical evidence for food intolerance. Aliment Pharmacol Ther. 2015;41:262–75.
2. Bohn L, Storsrud S, Tornblom H, Bengtsson U, Simren M. Self-reported food-related gastrointestinal symptoms in IBS are common and associated with more severe symptoms and reduced quality of life. Am J Gastroenterol. 2013;108:634–41.
3. Monsbakken KW, Vandvik PO, Farup PG. Perceived food intolerance in subjects with irritable bowel syndrome– etiology, prevalence and consequences. Eur J Clin Nutr. 2006;60:667–72.
4. Gocki J, Bartuzi Z. Role of immunoglobulin G antibodies in diagnosis of food allergy. Postepy Dermatol Alergol. 2016;33:253–6.
5. Carr S, Chan E, Lavine E, Moote W. CSACI position statement on the testing of food-specific IgG. Allergy Asthma Clin Immunol. 2012;8:12.
6. Stapel SO, Asero R, Ballmer-Weber BK, Knol EF, Strobel S, Vieths S, Kleine-Tebbe J. Testing for IgG4 against foods is not recommended as a diagnostic tool: EAACI task force report. Allergy. 2008;63:793–6.
7. Boyce JA, Assa'ad A, Burks AW, Jones SM, Sampson HA, Wood RA, Plaut M, Cooper SF, Fenton MJ, Arshad SH, Bahna SL, Beck LA, Byrd-Bredbenner C, Camargo CA Jr, Eichenfield L, Furuta GT, Hanifin JM, Jones C, Kraft M, Levy BD, Lieberman P, Luccioli S, KM MC, Schneider LC, Simon RA, Simons FE, Teach SJ, Yawn BP, Schwaninger JM. Guidelines for the diagnosis and Management of Food Allergy in the United States: summary of the NIAID-sponsored expert panel report. J Allergy Clin Immunol. 2010;126:1105–18.
8. Atkinson W, Sheldon TA, Shaath N, Whorwell PJ. Food elimination based on IgG antibodies in irritable bowel syndrome: a randomised controlled trial. Gut. 2004;53:1459–64.
9. Aydinlar EI, Dikmen PY, Tiftikci A, Saruc M, Aksu M, Gunsoy HG, Tozun N. IgG-based elimination diet in migraine plus irritable bowel syndrome. Headache. 2013;53:514–25.
10. Zar S, Mincher L, Benson MJ, Kumar D. Food-specific IgG4 antibody-guided exclusion diet improves symptoms and rectal compliance in irritable bowel syndrome. Scand J Gastroenterol. 2005;40:800 7.
11. Guo H, Jiang T, Wang J, Chang Y, Guo H, Zhang W. The value of eliminating foods according to food-specific immunoglobulin G antibodies in irritable bowel syndrome with diarrhoea. J Int Med Res. 2012;40:204–10.
12. Aasbrenn M, Hogestol I, Eribe I, Kristinsson J, Lydersen S, Mala T, Farup PG. Prevalence and predictors of irritable bowel syndrome in patients with morbid obesity: a cross-sectional study. BMC Obes. 2017;4:22.
13. Pickett-Blakely O. Obesity and irritable bowel syndrome: a comprehensive review. Gastroenterol Hepatol (N Y). 2014;10:411–6.
14. Acosta A, Camilleri M. Gastrointestinal morbidity in obesity. Ann N Y Acad Sci. 2014;1311:42–56.
15. Camilleri M, Madsen K, Spiller R, Greenwood-Van MB, Verne GN. Intestinal barrier function in health and gastrointestinal disease. Neurogastroenterol Motil. 2012;24:503–12.
16. Moreno-Navarrete JM, Sabater M, Ortega F, Ricart W, Fernandez-Real JM. Circulating zonulin, a marker of intestinal permeability, is increased in association with obesity-associated insulin resistance. PLoS One. 2012;7: e37160.
17. Longstreth GF, Thompson WG, Chey WD, Houghton LA, Mearin F, Spiller RC. Functional bowel disorders. Gastroenterology. 2006;130:1480–91.
18. Wiklund IK, Fullerton S, Hawkey CJ, Jones RH, Longstreth GF, Mayer EA, Peacock RA, Wilson IK, Naesdal J. An irritable bowel syndrome-specific symptom questionnaire: development and validation. Scand J Gastroenterol. 2003;38:947–54.
19. Andersen LF, Solvoll K, Johansson LR, Salminen I, Aro A, Drevon CA. Evaluation of a food frequency questionnaire with weighed records, fatty acids, and alpha-tocopherol in adipose tissue and serum. Am J Epidemiol. 1999;150:75–87.
20. Carlsen MH, Lillegaard IT, Karlsen A, Blomhoff R, Drevon CA, Andersen LF. Evaluation of energy and dietary intake estimates from a food frequency questionnaire using independent energy expenditure measurement and weighed food records. Nutr J. 2010;9:37.
21. Matvaretabellen 2016. Mattilsynet, Helsedirektoratet og Universitetet i Oslo. http://www.matvaretabellen.no/. Accessed 25 September: 2017.
22. Anthoni S, Savilahti E, Rautelin H, Kolho KL. Milk protein IgG and IgA: the association with milk-induced gastrointestinal symptoms in adults. World J Gastroenterol. 2009;15:4915–8.
23. Ligaarden SC, Lydersen S, Farup PG. IgG and IgG4 antibodies in subjects with irritable bowel syndrome: a case control study in the general population. BMC Gastroenterol. 2012;12:166.
24. Pelto L, Impivaara O, Salminen S, Poussa T, Seppanen R, Lilius EM. Milk hypersensitivity in young adults. Eur J Clin Nutr. 1999;53:620–4.
25. Zuo XL, Li YQ, Li WJ, Guo YT, Lu XF, Li JM, Desmond PV. Alterations of food antigen-specific serum immunoglobulins G and E antibodies in patients with irritable bowel syndrome and functional dyspepsia. Clin Exp Allergy. 2007;37:823–30.
26. Zar S, Benson MJ, Kumar D. Food-specific serum IgG4 and IgE titers to common food antigens in irritable bowel syndrome. Am J Gastroenterol. 2005;100:1550–7.
27. De GR VU, Gibson PR. Sensitivity to wheat, gluten and FODMAPs in IBS: facts or fiction? Gut. 2016;65:169–78.
28. Turpeinen A, Kautiainen H, Tikkanen ML, Sibakov T, Tossavainen O, Myllyluoma E. Mild protein hydrolysation of lactose-free milk further reduces milk-related gastrointestinal symptoms. J Dairy Res. 2016;83:256–60.
29. Gibson PR, Muir JG, Newnham ED. Other dietary confounders: FODMAPS et al. Dig Dis. 2015;33:269–76.
30. Varju P, Farkas N, Hegyi P, Garami A, Szabo I, Illes A, Solymar M, Vincze A, Balasko M, Par G, Bajor J, Szucs A, Huszar O, Pecsi D, Czimmer J. Low fermentable oligosaccharides, disaccharides, monosaccharides and polyols (FODMAP) diet improves symptoms in adults suffering from irritable bowel syndrome (IBS) compared to standard IBS diet: a meta-analysis of clinical studies. PLoS One. 2017;12:e0182942.
31. Fasano A. Intestinal permeability and its regulation by zonulin: diagnostic and therapeutic implications. Clin Gastroenterol Hepatol. 2012;10:1096–100.
32. Sapone A, Lammers KM, Casolaro V, Cammarota M, Giuliano MT, De RM SR, Mazzarella G, Tolone C, Russo MI, Esposito P, Ferraraccio F, Carteni M, Riegler G, de ML FA. Divergence of gut permeability and mucosal immune gene expression in two gluten-associated conditions: celiac disease and gluten sensitivity. BMC Med. 2011;9:23.
33. Lerner A, Jeremias P, Matthias T. Gut-thyroid axis and celiac disease. Endocr Connect. 2017;6:R52–8.
34. Sun X, Lu L, Yang R, Li Y, Shan L, Wang Y. Increased incidence of thyroid disease in patients with celiac disease: a systematic review and meta-analysis. PLoS One. 2016;11:e0168708.
35. Carroccio A, D'Alcamo A, Cavataio F, Soresi M, Seidita A, Sciume C, Geraci G, Iacono G, Mansueto P. High proportions of people with nonceliac wheat sensitivity have autoimmune disease or antinuclear antibodies. Gastroenterology. 2015;149:596–603.

36. Volta U, Tovoli F, Cicola R, Parisi C, Fabbri A, Piscaglia M, Fiorini E, Caio G. Serological tests in gluten sensitivity (nonceliac gluten intolerance). J Clin Gastroenterol. 2012;46:680–5.
37. Volta U, Bardella MT, Calabro A, Troncone R, Corazza GR. An Italian prospective multicenter survey on patients suspected of having non-celiac gluten sensitivity. BMC Med. 2014;12:85.
38. Gibson PR, Skodje GI, Lundin KE. Non-coeliac gluten sensitivity. J Gastroenterol Hepatol. 2017;32(Suppl 1):86–9.
39. Turnbull JL, Adams HN, Gorard DA. Review article: the diagnosis and management of food allergy and food intolerances. Aliment Pharmacol Ther. 2015;41:3–25.
40. Zuidmeer L, Goldhahn K, Rona RJ, Gislason D, Madsen C, Summers C, Sodergren E, Dahlstrom J, Lindner T, Sigurdardottir ST, McBride D, Keil T. The prevalence of plant food allergies: a systematic review. J Allergy Clin Immunol. 2008;121:1210–8.
41. Burney PG, Potts J, Kummeling I, Mills EN, Clausen M, Dubakiene R, Barreales L, Fernandez-Perez C, Fernandez-Rivas M, Le TM KAC, Kowalski ML, Lidholm J, Ballmer-Weber BK, Braun-Fahlander C, Mustakov T, Kralimarkova T, Popov T, Sakellariou A, Papadopoulos NG, Versteeg SA, Zuidmeer L, et al. The prevalence and distribution of food sensitization in European adults. Allergy. 2014;69:365–71.
42. Farup PG, Monsbakken KW, Vandvik PO. Lactose malabsorption in a population with irritable bowel syndrome: prevalence and symptoms. A case-control study. Scand J Gastroenterol. 2004;39:645–9.
43. Zeng Q, Dong SY, Wu LX, Li H, Sun ZJ, Li JB, Jiang HX, Chen ZH, Wang QB, Chen WW. Variable food-specific IgG antibody levels in healthy and symptomatic Chinese adults. PLoS One. 2013;8:e53612.

23

Multivisceral IgG4-related disease presenting as recurrent massive gastrointestinal bleeding

Xuexue Deng, Ronghua Fang*, Jianshu Zhang and Rongqiong Li

Abstract

Background: IgG4-related disease (IgG4-RD) is a newly recognized autoimmune systemic disorder characterized by elevated levels of serum IgG4 and abundant infiltration of IgG4-positive plasmacytes in the affected organs. The liver, biliary system and pancreas are the most commonly affected organs. However, involvement of the digestive tract is very rare. To date, only a few cases of isolated gastric IgG4-RD have been reported.

Case presentation: We present a case of IgG4-RD of the liver, gallbladder, pancreas and duodenum, which was clinically misinterpreted and thereafter over-treated. A 52-year-old male presented with obstructive jaundice for 3 years, melena for 5 months and hematemesis for 10 days. Three years prior, the patient had undergone biopsies of pancreatic lesions, liver lesions, cholecystectomy and choledochojejunostomy. Histopathology showed chronic inflammatory changes. Endoscopy at admission revealed a duodenal ulcer with active bleeding. Despite medical management, the patient presented with repeated gastrointestinal bleeding. Upon evaluation, serum IgG4 levels were found to be elevated. Histopathology of the duodenal ulcer biopsy and repeated examination of the gallbladder and pancreatic and liver biopsies confirmed IgG4 positive plasma cell infiltration. A definitive diagnosis of IgG4-RD was made and steroid administration was initiated. At last follow up, 11 months to-the-day after initiating steroid treatment, the patient was asymptomatic.

Conclusions: Notably, IgG4-RD of multiple digestive organs is still very rare. As a systemic disease, it is characterized by the infiltration of IgG4-bearing plasma cells and raised IgG4 levels. Histopathology findings remain the diagnostic gold standard for this disorder.

Keywords: IgG4-related disease, Plasma cells, Liver, Gallbladder, Duodenal, Pancreatic, Gastrointestinal bleeding

Background

IgG4-related disease (IgG4-RD) is a relatively recently recognized chronic multi-organ autoimmune disease of unknown origin with a tendency to develop lesions at multiple sites throughout the body [1]. It is known to affect various organs including the bile duct, pancreas, gallbladder, liver, lungs and salivary glands. It is characterized by elevated IgG4 levels in the serum and the affected tissues, lymphoproliferative infiltration and sclerotic fibrosis [2, 3]. Other typical features are occlusive phlebitis and rising IgG4-plasma cells levels [4, 5]. Clinically, it mimics malignancy in some patients, especially those with liver and pancreatic lesions and is often thought to necessitate surgical resection, sometimes leading to over-treatment [6, 7]. To date, only a few isolated cases of digestive IgG4-RD have been reported.

Case presentation

A 52-year-old male from southwest China presented with obstructive jaundice for 3 years, melena for 5 months and hematemesis for 10 days. The patient had been diagnosed with type 2 diabetes mellitus for 4 years, which was treated with metformin. The patient was a

* Correspondence: fangronghua@126.com
Department of General Medicine, West China Hospital, Sichuan University, No. 37 Guoxuexiang, Wuhou District, Chengdu City, Sichuan Province, China

Table 1 Comparison of IgG4 parameters and routine blood and markers for liver function before and after treatment

Parameter	Admission day	Confirmed day	After treatment 8 days	Follow up 1 month	Follow up 3 months	Follow up 6 months	Follow up 9 months
IgG4 (g/L)	–	29.20	18.40	9.86	4.74	1.87	1.70
IgG (g/L)	–	24.5	19.4	–	–	8.80	–
CRP (mg/ L)	5.46	–	–	–	2.62	1.32	–
TBIL (μmol/L)	12.1	11.7	56.4	23.4	14.1	7.7	–
DBIL (umol/L)	6.5	5.4	44.5	16.4	6.1	3.1	–
ALT (IU/L)	41	13	315	134	44	29	–
AST (IU/L)	40	24	167	57	28	26	–
ALB (g/L)	30	36.4	34.8	37.1	35.2	42.1	–
PLT(*10^9/L)	80	95	88	106	81	110	140
HGB (g/L)	75	61	98	71	122	114	123

IgG4 Immunoglobulin G4 subtype, *IgG* Immunoglobulin G, *CRP* C-reactive protein, *TBIL* total bilirubin, *DBIL* direct bilirubin, *ALT* alanine aminotransferase, *AST* aspartate aminotransferase, *ALB* albumin, *PLT* platelet, *HGB* hemoglobin

chronic tobacco (10 cigarettes per day) and alcohol consumer over the previous 20 years but had quit smoking and drinking for the past 3 years. Three years prior to admission to our hospital, he developed obstructive jaundice, which was investigated with abdominal computed tomography (CT) and revealed multiple hypodense lesions in the liver and pancreatic head mass. He underwent cholecystectomy, choledochojejunostomy and biopsies from the liver and pancreatic lesions. Histopathology revealed chronic cholecystitis with lymphocytic, plasmacytic and eosinophilic infiltration of the gallbladder, liver and pancreatic parenchyma.

The physical examination was unremarkable (height – 165 cm, weight – 50 kg). Laboratory tests revealed hemoglobin levels of 75 g/L, a platelet count of 80×10^9/L, 30.0 g/L albumin levels, and serum potassium levels of 3.20 mmol/L (Table 1). The fecal occult blood was positive.

On the day of admission, the patient developed repeated painless hematemesis of about 2100 mL, which was associated with hypotension and tachycardia. He was resuscitated with intravenous, blood and norepinephrine infusions. Laboratory tests revealed hemoglobin levels of 47.5 g/L, platelet count levels of 38×10^9 L and

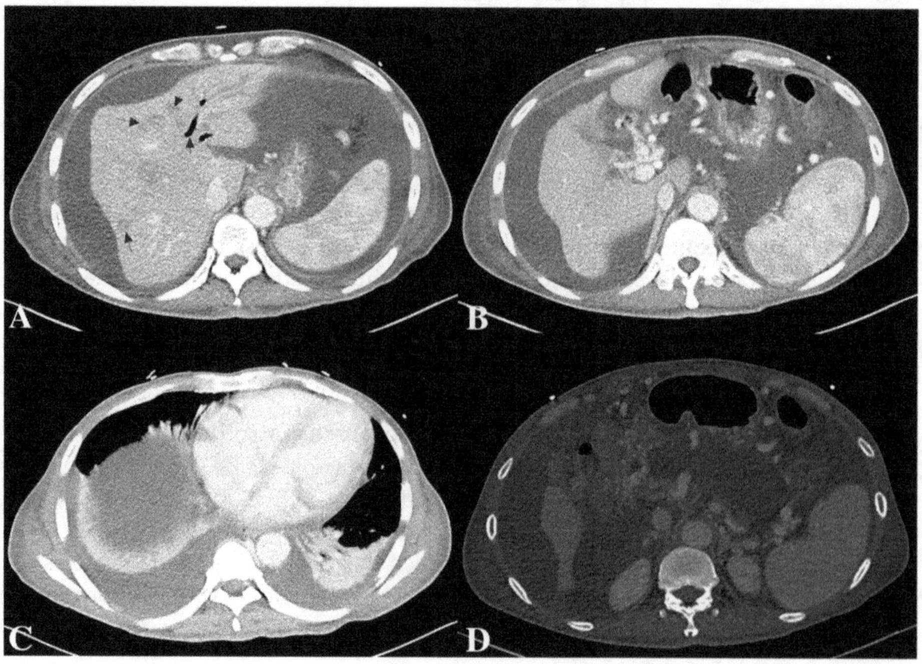

Fig. 1 Abdominal computed tomography. Images of the liver showed numerous hypodense nodules with mild contrast enhancement, ascites and intrahepatic bile duct dilatation (**a**). There were multiple enlarged lymph nodes in the hepatoduodenal ligament around the abdominal aorta (**b**). Mesenteric lymph nodes with bilateral pleural effusion (**c**). Multiple nodular dense shadows with dilatation of the main pancreatic duct in the tail region (**d**)

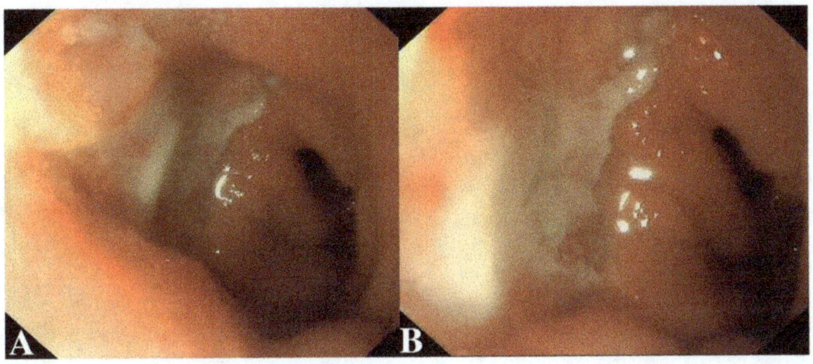

Fig. 2 Gastroscopy findings. An ulcer (1.5 cm × 1.2 cm) in the anterior wall of the duodenal bulb and a lot of white mosses in the fundus of stomach (**a**, **b**)

serum albumin 25.8 g /L. The day after admission, the patient again developed hematemesis of about 500 mL, for which he was treated with somatostatin, terlipressin and pantoprazole infusion. Sengstaken-Blakemore tube were placed to hemostasis by compression and tube feeding hemostatic medicine. After 4 days of medical intervention, the patient's gastrointestinal bleeding gradually stopped. Esophagogastroduodenoscopy revealed a duodenal ulcer (A1 stage) with active bleeding, gastric mucosal erosions and esophageal varices (mild). Contrast enhanced computed tomography of the abdomen with three-dimensional reconstruction exposed multiple nodular dense shadows with dilatation of the main pancreatic duct in the tail region (Fig. 1d). Images of the liver showed numerous hypodense nodules with mild contrast enhancement, ascites and intrahepatic bile duct dilatation (Fig. 1a). Additionally, there were multiple enlarged lymph nodes in the hepatoduodenal ligament around the abdominal aorta (Fig. 1b) and mesenteric lymph nodes with bilateral pleural effusion (Fig. 1c). In view of the liver disease with portal hypertension and esophagogastric varices, a transjugular intrahepatic

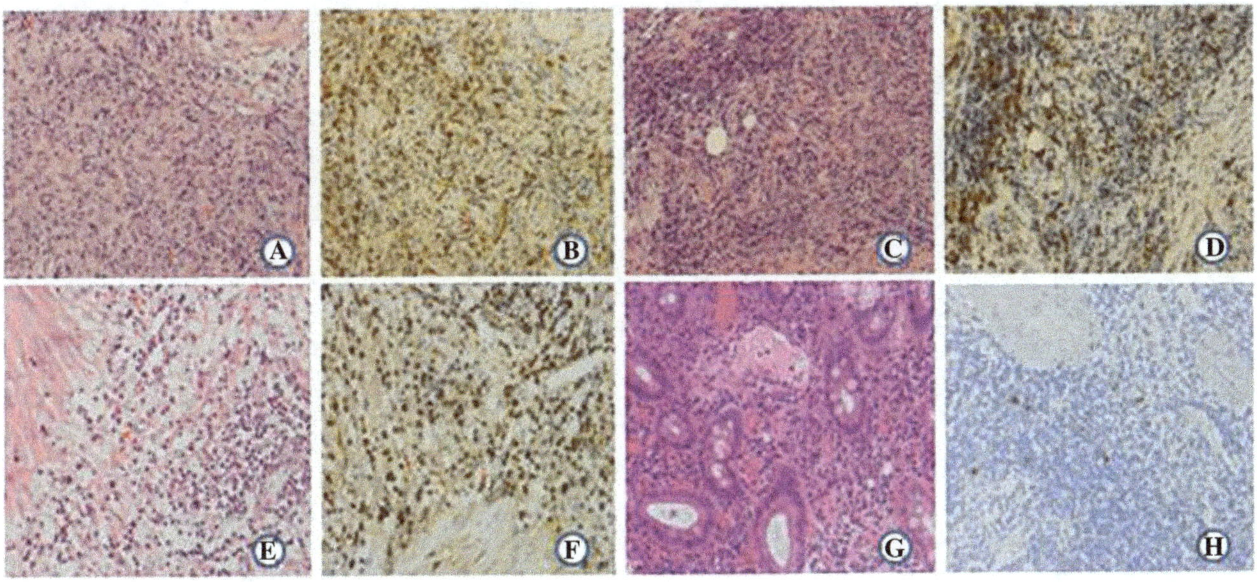

Fig. 3 Pathologic findings. **a** Diaminobenzidine staining of liver specimens revealed focal necrosis of the liver surrounded by fibrous tissue. The focal necrosis area revealed infiltration by lymphocytes, plasma cells and eosinophils. Peripheral hepatocytes were partially silt. **b** Immunoglobulin G (IgG) immunohistochemical staining showing increased numbers of IgG-positive plasma cells in the liver lesions (30–60/ high power field [HPF], × 400). **c** Diaminobenzidine staining of pancreas tissues revealed focal areas of glandular atrophy accompanied by lymphocyte, plasma cell and eosinophil infiltration and fibrous tissue hyperplasia. **d** IgG immunohistochemical staining showing increased numbers of IgG-positive plasma cells in the pancreas (30–80/HPF, × 400). **e** Diaminobenzidine staining of gallbladder tissue revealed chronic cholecystitis, focal lymphoid hyperplasia, formation of lymph follicles and infiltration of the gallbladder wall by the lymphocytes, plasma cells and eosinophils. **f** IgG immunohistochemical staining showing increased numbers of IgG-positive plasma cells in the gallbladder (30–80/HPF, × 400). **g** Hematin and yepin staining of duodenum tissue revealed lymphocytic, plasmacytic and neutrophilic infiltration of the inner layer of the duodenal mucosa with congestion and dilatation of the blood vessels. **h** IgG immunohistochemical staining showing increased numbers of IgG-positive plasma cells in the duodenum (> 100 /HPF, × 400)

Table 2 Summary of demographic, radiographic and clinical information from a review of 18 previously published cases of IgG4-Related gastrointestinal disorders

Study	Age, Gender	Clinical Symptoms	Laboratory	CNS Imaging (modality)	Biopsy Source	Organ Involvement	Treatment, Response
Fong et al., 2013 [11]	42, M	Obstructive jaundice, pruritus, pale stools, weight loss, tea-colored urine	Increased liver enzymes, IgG4 normal	Extrahepatic duct presented with a mural thickening (CT), stricture in the middle of bile duct with proximal biliary dilatation (ERCP)	Duodenal ampulla	Duodenal, liver	Marked
	79, M	Obstructive jaundice, weight loss	Not reported	Mild dilatation of the biliary tree (CT)	Not reported	Pancreas, biliary	Surgery
Rungsakulkij et al., 2017 [12]	56, M	Obstructive jaundice	Increased serum IgG4	Bile duct obstruction(CT); stricture of hepatic duct (ERCP)	Ampullary	Bile duct	Surgery
Cai et al., 2014 [13]	57, M	Jaundice, upper abdominal Discomfort	IgG4 serum normal	Mass observed in the hepatic duct (CT), hepatic duct and proximal bile duct dilatation (MRI)	Bile duct	Bile duct	Surgery
El Euch et al., 2017 [14]	70, M	Obstructive jaundice, anorexia, abdominal pain, \weight loss	Increased liver enzymes, and Serum IgG4	Diffuse pancreatic swelling and strictures of the main pancreatic duct (CT), thickened rim surrounding the pancreatic duct (MRI)	Not reported	Pancreatic	Marked
Miki et al., 2015 [15]	69, M	Jaundice, steatorrhea	Increased liver enzyme, and serum IgG4	Thickening of the bile duct wall, compressing the right portal vein (CT); bile duct lesions involving the left and right hepatic ducts (ERCP)	Bile duct	Bile duct	Surgery
Sivakumaran et al.., 2014 [16]	51, F	Jaundice, weight loss	Increased carbohydrate antigen 19–9	Intrahepatic duct dilatation and a hilar stricture (CT), a mass at the portal hepatitis (MRI)	Liver	liver	Surgery, Marked
Rodriguez et al., 2016 [17]	55, F	Abdominal pain, weight loss	IgG4 and other blood indices were normal	A mass in the pancreas(CT), hypermetabolic of the pancreas tail, bone marrow, and spleen, diffuse lymphadenopathy (PET)	Bone marrow	Pancreas	Marked
Kondo et al., 2016 [18]	78, M	Bilateral leg edema	Not reported	Sclerosing cholangitis (MRI)	Pleural	Pleura, bile duct, pericardium	Marked
Yang et al., 2015 [19]	60, M	Acid reflux	Increased serum IgG4	Multiple masses in the esophagus stomach, and liver (CT)	Esophagus, stomach	Esophagus, stomach and liver	Marked
Miyajima et al., 2017 [20]	50, M	Right upper pain, anorexia	Leucocytosis	Two liver masses (CT)	Liver	Liver	Surgery
Li et al., 2016 [21]	57, F	Pruritus	Increased liver enzymes and serum IgG4	Dilation of intrahepatic bile duct and lesions occupying the on head of pancreas, anastomotic stenosis (MRCP)	Biliary	Biliary	Surgery
Chen et al., 2016 [22]	58, M	Pruritus	Increased total bilirubin, direct	Stricture of the distal bile duct and dilatation of the	Not reported	Pancreas	Marked

Table 2 Summary of demographic, radiographic and clinical information from a review of 18 previously published cases of IgG4-Related gastrointestinal disorders *(Continued)*

Study	Age, Gender	Clinical Symptoms	Laboratory	CNS Imaging (modality)	Biopsy Source	Organ Involvement	Treatment, Response
			bilirubin, lipase, and serum IgG4	pancreatic duct (MRI); pancreatic duct with double duct sign (ERCP)			
Shimamura et al., 2015 [23]	74, M	Not reported	Increased serum IgG4	Low-density lesions, rim-like lesions in the bilateral kidneys (CT)	Gastric mass and Kidney	Stomach and kidney	Marked
Bulanov et al., 2016 [24]	62, F	Severe weakness and fatigue	Hemoglobin reduction, increased serum IgG4	Chronic ulcerative lesion, thickening of the stomach wall(CT)	Gastric mass and regional lymph nodes	Stomach, lymph nodes	Surgery
Takasumi et al., 2016 [25]	63, F	Not reported	thrombocytopenia, increased serum IgG4 and IgM	Enlargement of the submandibular glands, diffuse enlargement of the pancreas (CT)	Bone marrow, liver	Liver	Marked
Kim et al., 2016 [26]	61, M	Weakness, easy fatigability, weight loss	Increased liver enzymes and serum IgG4	Type IV hilar cholangiocarcinoma with periductal invasion into underlying hepatic parenchyma (MRI), multiple enlarged lymph nodes in left axillary (PET)		Intrahepatic bile duct	Marked
Matsunaga et al., 2014 [27]	72, M	Not reported	Increased hepatobiliary enzymes, serum IgG, and tumor markers	Enhancement in the pancreatic head, stenosis in the bile duct head and dilatation (CT), diffuse pancreatic ductal stenosis (MRI)	Duodenal papilla	Duodenum	Not reported
Van et al., 2017 [28]	26, M	Lymphadenopathy, splenomegaly	Increased IgG4, reduced T lymphocyte	Not reported	Pancreas	Pancreas	Not reported

CT computed tomography, *ERCP* endoscopic retrograde cholangiography, *MRI* magnetic resonance imaging, *PET* positron emission tomography

portosystemic shunt (TIPS) procedure was performed under local anesthesia and regional portal hypertension, splenic vein and portal vein obstruction were detected. Subsequently, the patient re-bleed both 14 days and 20 days after admission, about 600 mL and 400 mL, respectively. The patient was treated with somatostatin, pantoprazole infusion and blood transfusion. Gastroscopy identified an ulcer (1.5 cm × 1.2 cm) in the anterior wall of the duodenal bulb that was not actively bleeding (Fig. 2a, Fig. 2b). Pathological examination of the ulcer biopsy verified a moderate degree of chronic mucosal inflammation.

When investigating the recurrent bleeds, serum IgG4(0.035–1.500 g/L)and IgG(8~ 15.5 g/L)were found to be 29.200 g/L and 24.50 g/ L respectively and IgG4 disease was suspected (Table 1). The patient's prior surgical pathology specimens were retrieved for IgG4 immunohistochemical examination. Immunohistochemical staining revealed increased IgG-positive and IgG4-positive plasma cells in the liver lesions (IgG4 positive cells 30–60/ high power field (HPF); Fig. 3b), pancreas (IgG4 positive cells 30–80/HPF; Fig. 3d) and gallbladder (IgG4 positive cells 30–80/HPF; Fig. 3f). Staining of the duodenum ulcer biopsy also showed more than 100 IgG4-positive cells per HPF (Fig. 3h). Based on these findings, a definitive diagnosis of IgG4-RD was made.

The patient was administered 40 mg/d prednisone intravenously for 7 days without any side effects followed by oral prednisolone 40 mg/d for 1 week. Laboratory tests indicated a reduction in the serum IgG4 levels 8 days after initiating prednisone but the liver function continued to be impaired (Table 1). As the patient improved symptomatically, he was discharged on a regime of prednisolone and mycophenolate mofetil.

Since discharge until the time of writing, during the 11 monthly visits since starting steroid therapy, laboratory tests indicate significant improvements in the patient's serum IgG4 subtype, liver function and hemogram tests (Table 1).

Discussion and conclusions

IgG4-RD was first described in patients with sclerosing cholangitis, known as autoimmune pancreatitis (AIP) type I. Subsequently, IgG4-RD was found to affect other organs [6]. At present IgG4-RD is believed to be a systemic disease and diagnostic criteria for IgG4-RD [8, 9] include: (1) single or multiple organs with diffuse or localized swelling, masses, nodules and/or hypertrophic lesions; (2) elevated serum IgG4 levels (≥135 mg/dL); and (3) histopathologic features that include marked lymphocytic and plasma cell infiltration and fibrosis, with IgG4-positive plasma cell infiltration (IgG4/IgG positive cell ratio of 40% and IgG4-positive plasma cells exceeding 10/HPF). Diagnosis of IgG4-related is confirmed when all of the following are fulfilled: (1), (2) and (3). Diagnosis is likely if criteria (1) + (3) are fulfilled, possible if (1) + (2) are fulfilled and unlikely if only (1) presents.

Notably, the biliary tract and pancreas are the organs most frequently affected by IgG4-RD [10]. Few studies have reported isolated cases of IgG4-RD in other digestive organs, such as in the esophagus, stomach, liver or duodenum [7].

A recent review of IgG4-RD cases reporting on gastrointestinal lesions showed that most patients present with multiple organ disease involvement, including the stomach, duodenum, liver, bile duct, esophagus, jejunum, lymph nodes and pancreas (Table 2). Six patients presented with obstructive jaundice as the main clinical manifestation [11–16] and others presented with varied clinical symptoms [17–28]. Gastrointestinal bleeding was not reported in any of the studies. Our patient had recurrent gastrointestinal bleeding due to a duodenal ulcer. The ulcer failed to heal with standard treatment. Serum IgG4 was elevated in most of the cases reviewed, similar to our case, though was normal in three reports [11, 13, 17] and was not reported in two cases [11, 18]. The diagnosis of IgG4-RD was based on a combination of features that include clinical parameters, serology, immunohistochemistry, imaging and histopathology. In the present case, the diagnosis of IgG4-RD was initially missed in the histological analysis of the liver and pancreatic biopsy and gallbladder samples. When IgG4-RD was suspected based on the clinical and laboratory findings, IgG4 immunostaining was undertaken and the IgG4-RD diagnosis was confirmed. In our literature review, there were eight patients treated through surgery, 10 patients by corticosteroids, two were given corticosteroids after surgery, and in two patient studies, the treatment course was not reported (Table 2). Our patient responded partially to steroid therapy and required other immunosuppressive agents for a complete and successful response.

IgG4-RD can affect multiple gastrointestinal organs simultaneously or over different time periods. The clinical manifestations can mimic malignancy or other benign diseases such as portal hypertension, acid peptic disease. A high index of suspicion is required to make an accurate diagnosis and avoid unnecessary surgical interventions.

Abbreviations

ALT: Alanine aminotransferase; AST: Aspartate aminotransferase; ALB: albumin; CRP: C-reactive protein; CT: Computed tomography; DBIL: Direct bilirubin; ERCP: Endoscopic retrograde cholangiography;; HGB: Hemoglobin; IgG: Immunoglobulin G; IgG4: Immunoglobulin G4 subtype; IgG4-RD: IgG4-related disease; MRI: Magnetic resonance imaging; PET: positron emission tomography; PLT: Platelet; TBIL: Total bilirubin

Acknowledgements

We are grateful to Prof. Yin Gen of the Department of General Medicine, West China Hospital of Sichuan University for her contribution to the case.

Authors' contributions

DXX wrote the manuscript under the close supervision of FRH. FRH guaranteed the integrity of entire study. DXX prepared the literature search. DXX and FRH designed the study preliminarily and contributed to data acquisition and data analysis. ZJS and LRQ participated in the design and coordination of the study. All authors critically revised the manuscript and approved it.

Competing interests

The authors declare that they have no competing interests.

References

1. Decker L, Crawford AM. Orenzo GL, et al. IgG4-related Hypophysitis: case report and literature review. Cureus. 2016;8:e907.
2. Zhang W, Xue F, Liu MC, et al. 36 cases IgG4 related clinical analysis. [Chinese] Chinese. Journal of Nephrology. 2016;32:253–8.
3. Li YM, Wang H, Fang F, et al. IgG4 related clinical feature analysis. [Chinese] National Medical Journal of China. 2015;95:3281–4.
4. Stone JH, Zen Y, Deshpande V. IgG4-related disease. N Engl J Med. 2012; 366:539–51.
5. Woo CG, Yook JH, Kim AY, et al. IgG4-related disease presented as a muralmass in the stomach. J Pathol Transl Med. 2016;50:67–70.
6. Masaki Y, Shimizu H, Nakamura TS, et al. IgG4-related disease: diagnostic methods and therapeutic strategies in Japan. J Clin Exp Hematop. 2014;54: 95–101.
7. Koizumi S, Kamisawa T, Kuruma S, et al. Immunoglobulin G4-related gastrointestinal diseases, are they immunoglobulin G4-related diseases. WJG. 2013;19:5769–74.
8. Umehara H, Okazaki K, Masaki Y, et al. Comprehensive diagnostic criteria for IgG4-related disease (IgG4-RD), 2011. Modern Rheumatology. 2012;22:21–30.
9. Umemura T, Zen Y. IgG4-related Hepatopathy. In: Umehara H, Okazaki K, Stone J, Kawa S, Kawano M, editors. IgG4-Related Disease. Tokyo: Springer; 2014. p. 205–9.
10. Hubers LM, Maillette de Buy LJ, Wenniger ME, et al. IgG4-associated cholangitis: a comprehensive review. Clin Rev Allergy Immunol. 2015;48: 198–206.
11. Fong WW, Thumboo J, Azhar R, et al. IgG4-related disease in Singapore: a description of two cases and review of the literature. Int J Rheum Dis. 2013; 16:93–7.
12. Rungsakulkij N, Sornmayura P, Tannaphai P, et al. Isolated IgG4-related sclerosing cholangitis misdiagnosed as malignancy in an area with endemic cholangiocarcinoma: a case report. BMC Surg. 2017;17:17.
13. Cai J, Mou YP, Pan Y, et al. Immunoglobulin G4-associated cholangitis mimicking cholangiocarcinoma treated by laparoscopic choledochectomy with intracorporeal roux-en-Y hepaticojejunostomy. World J Surg Oncol. 2014; 12:363.
14. Euch ME, Hddad S, Mahfoudhi M, et al. A case of type 1 autoimmune pancreatitis (AIP), a form of IgG4-related disease (IgG4-RD). Am J Case Rep. 2017;18:822–5.
15. Miki A, Sakuma Y, Ohzawa H, et al. Immunoglobulin G4-related sclerosing cholangitis mimicking hilar cholangiocarcinoma diagnosed with following bile duct resection: report of a case. Int Surg. 2015;100:480–5.
16. Sivakumaran Y, Le Page PA, Becerril-Martinez G, et al. IgG4-related sclerosing cholangitis: the cholangiocarcinoma mimic. ANZ J Surg. 2014;84:486–7.
17. Rodriguez EA, Williams FK. A mass in the junction of the body and tail of the pancreas with negative IgG4 serology: IgG4-related disease with negative serology. Am J Case Rep. 2015;16:305–9.
18. Kondo T, Uehara T. Immunoglobulin G4-related disease with fibroinflammatory lesions in the pleura, bile ducts and pericardium. CMAJ. 2016;188:972.
19. Yang L, Jin P, Sheng JQ. Immunoglobulin G4-related disease (IgG4-RD) affecting the esophagus, stomach,and liver. Endoscopy. 2015;47:E96–7.
20. Miyajima S, Okano A, Ohana M. Immunoglobulin G4-related hepatic inflammatory pseudotumor invading the abdominal wall. Clin J Gastroenterol. 2017;10:57–62.
21. Li Y, Zhou L, Zhao X, et al. The importance of IgG4 screening in patients diagnosed with primary sclerosing cholangitis in the past: a case rediagnosed as IgG4-SC after 10 years. Medicine (Baltimore). 2016;95(50):e5628.
22. Chen CT, Chiang CL, Huang HH. IgG4-related double duct sign mimicking pancreatic head cancer. QJM. 2016;109:207–8.
23. Inoue K, Okubo T, Kato T, et al. IgG4-related stomach muscle lesion with a renal pseudotumor and multiple renal rim-like lesions: A rare manifestation of IgG4-related disease. Mod Rheumatol. 2018;28:188–92.
24. Bulanov D, Arabadzhieva E, Bonev S, et al. A rare case of IgG4-related disease: a gastric mass, associated with regional lymphadenopathy. BMC Surg. 2016;16:37.
25. Takasumi M, Miyata M, Kuroda M, et al. Overlap of IgG4-related disease and primary biliary cirrhosis complicated with autoimmune thrombocytopenia. Internal Med. 2016;55:1387–92.
26. Kim S, Bae H, Choi M, et al. Isolated mass-forming IgG4-related cholangitis as an initial clinical presentation of systemic IgG4-related disease. J Pathol Transl Med. 2016;50:300–5.
27. Matsunaga K, Hayashi R, Otsuka T, et al. A case of IgG4-related disease complicated by duodenal bulbitis with IgG4-positive plasma cell infiltration. Endoscopy. 2014;46:E408–10.
28. Van de Ven AAJM, Seidl M, Drendel V, et al. IgG4-related disease in autoimmune lymphoproliferative syndrome. Clin Immunol. 2017;180:97–9.

24

HLA-DQ2 and -DQ8 genotype frequency in Syrian celiac disease children: HLA-DQ relative risks evaluation

Hossam Murad[1*], Batoul Jazairi[1], Issam Khansaa[1], Doaa Olabi[2] and Lina Khouri[2]

Abstract

Background: Celiac disease (CD) is a common autoimmune disease in Syria which manifesting with inflammation of the small intestine and with various extra intestinal symptoms. The disease is associated with human HLA-DQ genes encoding HLA-DQ2 and DQ8 proteins.

Methods: In this study, 49 children patients of CD and 58 healthy control samples were genotyped for HLA-DQ genes using SSP-PCR technique. Relative risks for different genotypes were also evaluated.

Results: The DQB1*0201 allele was the most common in the patients (77.6%) followed by DQB1*0302 allele (10.2%). The highest HLA-DQB risk for CD development was found in patients carriers a DQ2.5/DQ8 genotype (1/10), followed by the patients carriers DQ2.5/DQ2.5 (1/12).

Conclusion: The significant differences in the frequency of HLA-DQ2 and HLA-DQ8 in Syrian patients in compared with controls and relative risks predicted demonstrated the importance role of these alleles in the development of CD in Syrian children patients.

Keywords: Celiac disease, HLA, Children, Syria

Background

Celiac disease is an immune-mediated disorder with a strong genetic predisposition and dietary gluten as an environmental trigger [1]. This disease causes inflammation in the small intestinal mucosa. The developing villus atrophy can impede the absorption of nutrients [2].

Several ways to diagnosis celiac disease using anti-tissue transglutaminase (anti-TG2) test, anti-endomysium (EMA) auto-antibodies and small bowel biopsy [3]. This disease is widespread in most Mediterranean countries [4], and it estimated that about more than 5 million patients will be affected in the next 10 years in the Mediterranean region [5]. The only effective therapy is gluten-free diet for life-long, which leads to complete remission of all clinical signs [6, 7]. Celia disease characterized by an interaction of a certain genes, gluten, and environmental influences [8]. The majority of patients with CD carrying the HLA class II genes: HLA-DQ2.5 (DQA1*05-DQB1*02) and HLA-DQ8 (DQA1*03-DQB1*0302) [9]. Strong association was observed between HLA-DQ2.5 and predisposition to CD, explained by its affinity to binding gluten proteins [10]. While, HLA-DQ2.2 contributes less to the risk of CD [11]. Moreover, the risk of CD is shown to be higher in individuals homozygous for the HLA-DQ2.5 or HLA-DQ2.5/DQ2.2 genotypes compared with those homozygous for HLA-DQ2.2 or heterozygous for HLA-DQ2.5 or DQ2.2 [12, 13].

HLA genotyping can be used as an efficient adjunct in the CD diagnostic as already confirmed by the New ESPGHAN guidelines for the diagnosis of CD [14, 15].

In Syria, previous reports indicated that Syrian population has high prevalence of the CD (1/62) in healthy blood donors [16, 17], but no published study about the link of HLA-DQ alleles and Syrian celiac patients; so, we aim to study the distribution of the CD genes: DQ2 and DQ8 in 49 children patients (age from 1 to 18 years old) in comparable with 58 control samples of the same ages.

* Correspondence: ascientific@aec.org.sy
[1]Molecular Biology and Biotechnology Department, Human Genetics Division, Atomic Energy Commission of Syria, P.O. Box 6091, Damascus, Syria
Full list of author information is available at the end of the article

Methods

Patients and controls

Forty nine CD patients (35 males and 14 females; mean age, 9.5 years; range (1–18) and fifty eight healthy controls (30 males and 28 females; mean age, 29 years; range, (18–40) with no history of CD, cancer or autoimmune diseases and were negative for CD serological screening, were selected from the blood transfusion center of Damascus University in Syria. All patients had positive tTGA and/or EMA antibodies and histology according to Rostami Marsh classification [3, 18].

This study was approved by the Ethics Committee of Atomic Energy Commission of Syria, and written informed consent was obtained from all participants. If participant was a minor, parental consent was taken.

HLA DQ2 and DQ8 genotyping

Peripheral blood was drawn on BD Vacutainer plus Blood Collection tubes K2 EDTA 18.0 mg (BD Biosciences, USA). Genomic DNA was extracted from peripheral blood cells using the salting-out method [19]. HLA-DQB1 genotype was performed by sequence-specific primer-polymerase chain reaction (SSP-PCR) method using published primers [20] and for HLA-DQA1 genotype [21].

Statistical analysis

Data were analyzed using SPSS software (version 22, SPSS Inc., Chicago, Illinois, USA). Odds ratios was applied to establish statistical significance with 95% confidence (P value ≤0.05). Relative risk of developing disease for specific genotypes were calculated as (% of allele in patients / % of allele in controls) x probability to be affected in general population [22].

Results

In this study, forty nine definite CD patients (25 males and 24 females) and 58 controls of Syrian origin were genotyped for HLA-DQ2 and DQ8 genes. The allele and genotype frequencies of DQ2 and DQ8 genes in CD were compared with the controls. The frequency of the DQB1*02:01 allele was very significantly increased in patients compared with the controls (77.6% vs. 58.6%; p value: 0.00). The frequency of the DQB1*03:02 allele was also elevated in patients versus controls, but uncorrected P value was borderline significant (10.2% vs. 8.6%; p value: 0.09), Table 1).

Genotype analysis of DQ2 and DQ8 genes shows that the 24 of 49 patients carrying DQ2.5 in homozygous genotype with high frequency 49%, whereas, this genotype was found in 6 controls (10.3%). The frequency of the DQ2.5/DQ2.2 or DQ2.5/DQ8 were increased in patients versus controls (10.2% vs. 3.4%), (10.2% vs. 1.7%) respectively. More genotype analysis demonstrated that

Table 1 HLA-DQ2 (DQB1*0201) and HLA-DQ8 (DQB1*0302) alleles frequency in patients and control

Allele	Patient (n = 49) (98 alleles)		Control (n = 58) (116 alleles)		P-value
	n	Fr (%)	n	Fr (%)	
DQB1*0201	76	77.6	34	29.3	< 0.01
DQB1*0302	10	10.2	5	4.3	0.09
DQ7	8	8.2	4	3.4	0.13
DQX	4	4.1	73	62.9	< 0.01

Fr frequency. *P*-values are results of Chi-square test; significance level is defined at ≤ 0.05

30.6% of patients carried another DQ genotypes, while 84.5% of controls had these genotypes (Table 2).

The highest HLA-DQB relative risk for CD development was found in patients carriers DQ2.5/DQ8 genotype (1/10), while, the patients carriers of DQ2.5/DQ2.5 or DQ2.5/DQ2.2 genotype had a relative risk about 1/12.5 and 1/20 respectively (Table 2).

Based on the Marsh Score, forty-two of 49 CD patients with biopsy result were classified into Marsh I, Marsh II and Marsh III as indicated in Table 3.

The frequency of the patients with mild form of CD (Marsh I) carrying DQ2 allele was 9.5%, whereas, the frequency was 23.8% for the patients with Marsh II having DQ2. While, 26 patients from 42 (52.4%) were classified into Marsh III, 22 out of them carrying DQ2 allele, all this results indicated the involvement of DQ2 allele in the severity of mucosal damage (Table 3).

Discussion

Celiac disease is a systemic immune mediated disorder caused by the intolerance of gluten containing grains in genetically susceptible person [23]. It was found that there is a significant relation between the wheat consumption and the frequency of HLA alleles DQ2 and DQ8 worldwide [24]. The history of CD is backed to the spreading of wheat cultivation after the agricultural revolution.

The pathogenesis of CD is dependent on the presence of HLA class II genes: HLA- DQ2 (DQA1*05-DQB1*02) and HLA-DQ8 (HLA-DQA1*0301-DQB1*0302) which are specific to gluten [25]. In contrast, the absence of either HLA-DQ2 or HLA-DQ8 has a negative predictive value of nearly 100% in excluding the diagnosis of celiac [8].

This study demonstrated that, among 49 Syrian children patients from the Children's Hospital, Damascus, Syria there were 77.6% carried the DQB1*0201 allele and 10.2% carrying the DQB1*0302 allele. All patients studied that carried two DQ2 or DQ8 alleles had a common severe symptoms (fatigue, weight loss, stunted growth, iron deficiency anemia and chronic abdominal pain) and they had

Table 2 Distribution of HLA-DQ genotypes in patients with celiac disease and control

HLA Genotype	Patient (*n* = 49)		Control (*n* = 58)		Odds ratio	95% CL	Relative risk	*P*-value
	n	Fr (%)	*n*	Fr (%)				
DQ2.5/DQ8	5	10.2	1	1.7	6.48	0.73–57.46	1/10	0.09
DQ2.5/DQ2.5	24	49	6	10.3	8.32	3.02–22.93	1/12.5	< 0.01
DQ2.5/DQ2.2	5	10.2	2	3.4	3.18	0.59–17.19	1/20	0.18
DQ8/DQX	4	8.2	2	3.4	2.49	0.44–14.21	1/25	0.31
DQ2.5/DQ7	8	16.3	4	6.9	2.63	0.74–9.35	1/25	0.13
DQ2.2/DQ8	1	2	1	1.7	1.19	0.07–19.92	1/50	0.90
DQ2.2/DQ2.2	2	4.1	3	5.2	0.78	0.13–4.87	1/100	0.79
DQ2.x	0	0	4	6.9	0.12	0.01–2.33	0	0.16
DQX/DQX	0	0	35	60.3	0.01	0.00–0.11	0	< 0.01

n number of the patients or the control, *Fr* frequency. Odds ratio and *P*-values have been calculated on the total data set comparing CD patients versus the control genotypes. Relative risk of developing disease for specific genotypes were calculated as a ratio of specific HLA-DQ genotype proportion in CD patients and control by taking into account the prevalence of the CD (0.016) in Syrian population

high value of anti-transglutaminase antibody, and most of them had classified according to the March classification and villous atrophy of variable severity [26].

Our results indicated a presence of high significant association between DQB1*02;01 allele and CD development, while, it was a borderline significant association with DQB1*03:02 allele. The results also shown that 87.8% of CD patients carried at least one of DQB1*02:01 or DQB1*03:02 alleles. All these results indicated that there were a high statistically significant association between these two alleles and the Syrians CD patients. This data is in concordance with the results obtained for CD patients from several Arab countries regarding HLA-DQ2 variants: in Egyptian (77.42%); Gaza strip patients (84.6%); Jordanian (100%) and Moroccan CD patients (45.2%) [27–30]. In the other hand, this HLA-DQ2 variants had also high frequented in French (87%), Italian (84%), and in UK (88%) CD patients [31].

We have evaluated the relative risk for different HLA genotypes (Table 2). The highest HLA-DQ genotype relative risk for CD in our patients was associated with DQ2.5/DQ8 genotype carriers (1/10). Also, carriers of DQ2.5/DQ2.5 genotype were in group with high relative risk (1/12.5). Recent published studies also confirmed that DQ2.5/DQ2.5 genotype conferred the highest risk for CD [32–34]. In the other hands, in our group, the patients carried DQ2.5/DQ2.2 or DQ8/DQX or DQ2.5/DQ7 genotypes showed medium risks for CD (1/20 and 1/25) respectively. The lowest risk was detected in patients of DQ2.2/DQ8 or DQ2.2/DQ2.2 genotype carriers. So, patients with a one dose or double dose of HLA-DQ2.5 have high risk for CD, this data is largely consistent with published data about the dose effect for DQB1*02 allele for development of CD [12].

Table 3 Distribution of HLA-DQ2 and DQ8 alleles according to severity of mucosal damage

Marsh classification	Patient (*n* = 42)				*P*-value
	DQ2		DQ8		
	n	Fr (%)	*n*	Fr (%)	
Marsh I	4	9.5	0	0	0.04
Marsh II	10	23.8	2	4.8	0.01
Marsh III	22	52.4	4	9.5	< 0.01

n number of the patients, *Fr* frequency

In our study, the frequency of CD patients with Marsh I and Marsh II carried DQ2 allele was 9.5 and 23.8% respectively, while, it reached 4.8% in the CD patients carried DQ8. In the other hand, Marsh III score was given more than fivefold higher in the CD patients carried DQ2 (52.4%) in compare with CD patients carried DQ8 (9.5%). These results presenting high positive association of DQ2 allele with Marsh III of CD patients. Several previous studies have demonstrated the role of the DQ2 allele in the severity of mucosal damage [35, 36], where, Zamani et al., revealed that 02:01 allele had a significant association with Marsh IIIc patients (pc: 0.02, OR: 14.55) and it represented involvement of this allele in the severity of mucosal damage [34].

Conclusion

We studied for the first time the distribution of HLA-DQ genotypes in the children celiac patients and we estimated the risk for CD development. The significant differences in the frequency of HLA-DQ2 and HLA-DQ8 alleles in Syrian patients compared with controls demonstrated the importance role of these alleles in the development of CD and support the possibility of using HLA-DQ typing in confirmation of the disease.

Abbreviations

Anti-TG2: Anti-tissue transglutaminase; CD: Celiac disease; EMA: Endomysial antibody; HLA: Human leukocyte antigen; SSP-PCR: Single Specific Primer-Polymerase Chain Reaction

Acknowledgments
We would like to thank Prof. Ibrahim Othman, the Director General of AECS, and the head of Molecular Biology & Biotechnology department, for their support. And we would like also to thanks Dr. Mahmoud Bozo and Dr. Jamal Jaradat for this helping in patients sample collection.

Authors' contributions
HM, BJ and IK worked on this manuscript and did all of the researching groundwork. DO and LK collect the blood samples and drafted the manuscript. All authors read and approved the final manuscript.

Competing interests
The authors declare that they have no competing interests.

Author details
[1]Molecular Biology and Biotechnology Department, Human Genetics Division, Atomic Energy Commission of Syria, P.O. Box 6091, Damascus, Syria. [2]Children's hospital, Damascus, Syria.

References
1. Kurppa K, Taavela J, Saavalainen P, Kaukinen K, Lindfors K. Novel diagnostic techniques for celiac disease. Expert Rev Gastroenterol Hepatol. 2016;10: 795–805.
2. Holopainen P. Genetic susceptibility to celiac disease: HLA-unlinked candidate genes: University of Helsinki, Faculty of Science, Department of Biosciences. Helsinki: 2005.
3. Villanacci V, Ceppa P, Tavani E, Vindigni C, Volta U. Coeliac disease: the histology report. Dig Liver Dis. 2011;43(Suppl 4):S385–95.
4. Tucci F, Astarita L, Abkari A, Abu-Zekry M, Attard T, Ben Hariz M, Bilbao JR, Boudraa G, Boukthir S, Costa S, et al. Celiac disease in the Mediterranean area. BMC Gastroenterol. 2014;14:24.
5. Greco L, Timpone L, Abkari A, Abu-Zekry M, Attard T, Bouguerra F, Cullufi P, Kansu A, Micetic-Turk D, Misak Z, et al. Burden of celiac disease in the Mediterranean area. World J Gastroenterol. 2011;17:4971–8.
6. Schuppan D. Current concepts of celiac disease pathogenesis. Gastroenterology. 2000;119:234–42.
7. Schuppan D, Junker Y, Barisani D. Celiac disease: from pathogenesis to novel therapies. Gastroenterology. 2009;137:1912–33.
8. Green PH, Lebwohl B, Greywoode R. Celiac disease. J Allergy Clin Immunol. 2015;135:1099–106. quiz 1107
9. Sollid LM. The roles of MHC class II genes and post-translational modification in celiac disease. Immunogenetics. 2017;69:605–16.
10. Romanos J, Wijmenga C. Predicting susceptibility to celiac disease by genetic risk profiling. Ann Gastroenterol Hepatol. 2010;1(1):1–8.
11. Fallang LE, Bergseng E, Hotta K, Berg-Larsen A, Kim CY, Sollid LM. Differences in the risk of celiac disease associated with HLA-DQ2.5 or HLA-DQ2.2 are related to sustained gluten antigen presentation. Nat Immunol. 2009;10:1096–101.
12. Vader W, Stepniak D, Kooy Y, Mearin L, Thompson A, van Rood JJ, Spaenij L, Koning F. The HLA-DQ2 gene dose effect in celiac disease is directly related to the magnitude and breadth of gluten-specific T cell responses. Proc Natl Acad Sci U S A. 2003;100:12390–5.
13. Congia M, Cucca F, Frau F, Lampis R, Melis L, Clemente MG, Cao A, De Virgiliis SA. Gene dosage effect of the DQA1*0501/DQB1*0201 allelic combination influences the clinical heterogeneity of celiac disease. Hum Immunol. 1994;40:138–42.
14. Husby S, Koletzko S, Korponay-Szabo IR, Mearin ML, Phillips A, Shamir R, Troncone R, Giersiepen K, Branski D, Catassi C, et al. European Society for Pediatric Gastroenterology, hepatology, and nutrition guidelines for the diagnosis of coeliac disease. J Pediatr Gastroenterol Nutr. 2012;54:136–60.
15. Ribes-Koninckx C, Mearin ML, Korponay-Szabo IR, Shamir R, Husby S, Ventura A, Branski D, Catassi C, Koletzko S, Maki M, et al. Coeliac disease diagnosis: ESPGHAN 1990 criteria or need for a change? Results of a questionnaire. J Pediatr Gastroenterol Nutr. 2012;54:15–9.
16. Cummins AG, Roberts-Thomson IC. Prevalence of celiac disease in the Asia-Pacific region. J Gastroenterol Hepatol. 2009;24:1347–51.
17. Challar MH, Jouma M, Sitzmann FC, Seferian V, Shahin E. Prevalence of asymptomatic celiac disease in a Syrian population sample. JABMS. 2004;6:155–160E.
18. Marsh MN. Gluten, major histocompatibility complex, and the small intestine. A molecular and immunobiologic approach to the spectrum of gluten sensitivity ('celiac sprue'). Gastroenterology. 1992;102:330–54.
19. Miller SA, Dykes DD, Polesky HFA. Simple salting out procedure for extracting DNA from human nucleated cells. Nucleic Acids Res. 1988;16:1215.
20. Bunce M, O'Neill CM, Barnardo MC, Krausa P, Browning MJ, Morris PJ, Welsh KI. Phototyping: comprehensive DNA typing for HLA-A, B, C, DRB1, DRB3, DRB4, DRB5 & DQB1 by PCR with 144 primer mixes utilizing sequence-specific primers (PCR-SSP). Tissue Antigens. 1995;46:355–67.
21. Scola L, Lio D, Candore G, Forte GI, Crivello A, Colonna-Romano G, Pes MG, Carru C, Ferrucci L, Deiana L, et al. Analysis of HLA-DRB1, DQA1, DQB1 haplotypes in Sardinian centenarians. Exp Gerontol. 2008;43:114–8.
22. Megiorni F, Mora B, Bonamico M, Barbato M, Nenna R, Maiella G, Lulli P, Mazzilli MC. HLA-DQ and risk gradient for celiac disease. Hum Immunol. 2009;70:55–9.
23. Leonard MM, Sapone A, Catassi C, Fasano A. Celiac disease and nonceliac gluten sensitivity: a review. JAMA. 2017;318:647–56.
24. Lionetti E, Gatti S, Pulvirenti A, Catassi C. Celiac disease from a global perspective. Best Pract Res Clin Gastroenterol. 2015;29:365–79.
25. Megiorni F, Pizzuti A. HLA-DQA1 and HLA-DQB1 in celiac disease predisposition: practical implications of the HLA molecular typing. J Biomed Sci. 2012;19:88.
26. Malamut G, Cellier C. Complications of coeliac disease. Best Pract Res Clin Gastroenterol. 2015;29:451–8.
27. Mohammed MA, Omar NM, Shebl AM, Mansour AH, Elmasry E, Othman G. Celiac disease prevalence and its HLA-genotypic profile in Egyptian patients with type 1 diabetes mellitus. Trends in Medical Research. 2014;9:81–97.
28. Ayesh BM, Zaqout EK, Yassin MM. HLA-DQ2 and -DQ8 haplotypes frequency and diagnostic utility in celiac disease patients of Gaza strip, Palestine. Auto Immun Highlights. 2017;8:11.
29. El-Akawi ZJ, Al-Hattab DM, Migdady MA. Frequency of HLA-DQA1*0501 and DQB1*0201 alleles in patients with coeliac disease, their first-degree relatives and controls in Jordan. Ann Trop Paediatr. 2010;30:305–9.
30. Piancatelli D, Ben El Barhdadi I, Oumhani K, Sebastiani P, Colanardi A, Essaid A. HLA typing and celiac disease in Moroccans. Med Sci (Basel). 2017;5:1–11.
31. Margaritte-Jeannin P, Babron MC, Bourgey M, Louka AS, Clot F, Percopo S, Coto I, Hugot JP, Ascher H, Sollid LM, et al. HLA-DQ relative risks for coeliac disease in European populations: a study of the European genetics cluster on coeliac disease. Tissue Antigens. 2004;63:562–7.
32. Liu E, Lee HS, Aronsson CA, Hagopian WA, Koletzko S, Rewers MJ, Eisenbarth GS, Bingley PJ, Bonifacio E, Simell V, et al. Risk of pediatric celiac disease according to HLA haplotype and country. N Engl J Med. 2014;371:42–9.
33. Stankovic B, Radlovic N, Lekovic Z, Ristic D, Radlovic V, Nikcevic G, Kotur N, Vucicevic K, Kostic T, Pavlovic S, Zukic B. HLA genotyping in pediatric celiac disease patients. Bosn J Basic Med Sci. 2014;14:171–6.
34. Zamani M, Modares-Sadegi M, Shirvani F, Zamani H, Emami MH. The involvement of the HLA-DQB1 alleles in the risk and the severity of Iranian coeliac disease patients. Int J Immunogenet. 2014;41:312–7.
35. Murray JA, Moore SB, Van Dyke CT, Lahr BD, Dierkhising RA, Zinsmeister AR, Melton LJ 3rd, Kroning CM, El-Youssef M, Czaja AJ. HLA DQ gene dosage and risk and severity of celiac disease. Clin Gastroenterol Hepatol. 2007;5: 1406–12.
36. Hernandez-Charro B, Donat E, Miner I, Aranburu E, Sanchez-Valverde F, Ramos-Arroyo MA. Modifying effect of HLA haplotypes located trans to DQB1*02-DRB1*03 in celiac patients of southern Europe. Tissue Antigens. 2008;71:213–8.

25

One-day oral polyethylene glycol based cleanout is effective for pre-colonoscopy preparation in children

Ashwath S. Kumar[1], Brooke L. Beutler[2] and Thomas M. Attard[1,2*]

Abstract

Background: The adequacy of pre-procedure preparation is the principal determinant of the quality of colonoscopy in pediatric as in adult patients. There is a lack of consensus, among providers on a standard pre-procedure regimen. Professional society guidelines include the use of Polyethylene glycol (PEG). Herein we report on the provider-assessed adequacy of a one day, age-categorized dosing, PEG based cleanout regimen in children undergoing colonoscopy in a tertiary institution.

Methods: The standard bowel preparation regime at our institution includes an age dependent minimum PEG dosing regimen in addition to clear liquids the day prior to the procedure. We retrospectively abstracted relevant indices including patient demographics, prep quality, procedure impairment, duration and completion from an institutional quality monitoring survey tool between 2015 and 2016 and similarly abstracted prospectively recorded indices that included the dataset above as well as additional fields for procedure deviations and additional laxative use.

Results: A total of 642 procedures (mean age 12.2 years; F: 380) were accrued, nonadherence to the cleanout regimen (7.3%) and additional laxative use (3.1%) were observed in a small proportion of the prospective dataset subjects, adequate cleanout defined as thin or thick liquid but no solids present was reported in 79. 5% and 15.8% of cases and impaired study from inadequate cleanout was reported in 11.8% of studies albeit the cecum was reached and the terminal ileum was intubated in 97.8 and 93.6% of studies. The duration of the study was significantly longer with the presence of a fellow trainee assisting in the procedure. Patient age and gender did not correlate with prep adequacy or cecal and ileal intubation rates, inadequate cleanout was significantly associated with impairment and incomplete studies.

Conclusion: A one day, single agent, osmotic laxative (Polyethylene glycol) based cleanout regimen is effective in routine pre-procedure cleanout for standard colonoscopy in pediatric age range patients.

Keywords: Pediatric, Colonoscopy, Preparation, Cleanout, Quality, Polyethylene glycol

Background

The adequacy of colon cleansing before colonoscopy is a principal determinant of the quality of colonoscopy in the pediatric as in the adult population. Of the several determinants of bowel prep including regimen, timing, diet, co-morbidities, and patient characteristics, preparation regimen is by far the most important predictor of successful procedure outcomes [1]. Among the many preparation regimens available, Poly-Ethylene-Glycol (PEG), an osmotic laxative, is the primary choice for bowel prep, with demonstrated safety and efficacy in children [2, 3] However, with several other regimens reporting comparable efficacy, no standard protocol exists for pediatric bowel prep.

A common alternative to PEG monotherapy for bowel prep is dual therapy with a stimulant (bisacodyl, senna) or combined stimulant–osmotic (Magnesium Citrate) laxative, which directly affects nerve, smooth muscle, and epithelial cells in the intestine to alter mucosal

* Correspondence: tmattard@cmh.edu
[1]University of Missouri-Kansas City School of Medicine, Kansas City, MO, USA
[2]Children's Mercy Hospital, Kansas City, USA

electrolyte transport [4]. A 2014 review by NASPHGHAN found that while PEG was the regimen of choice for monotherapy, dual therapy with PEG and stimulant laxative was used by between 36% (age 2–5 cohort) and 61% (age 12+ cohort) of physicians [5].

Stimulant laxatives, when used in the context of colonoscopy preparation are often associated with adverse outcomes including bloating, cramps and abdominal discomfort [4], and are even contraindicated in certain patient populations, including patients with renal disease, bowel obstruction, and those at risk for dehydration or electrolyte imbalance [6]. In the treatment of pediatric constipation, stimulant laxatives are recommended as a second-line therapy if a PEG-only regimen fails [7]. Despite these important caveats, stimulant laxatives remain a popular choice for dual-therapy bowel prep in pediatric colonoscopy.

The purpose of this study is to report the experience with a one day PEG-only bowel prep regimen in a pediatric cohort of patients studied at a tertiary pediatric gastroenterology service.

Methods

Children's Mercy Hospital in Kansas City MO, is tertiary, urban, standalone children's hospital with dedicated inpatient and ambulatory gastroenterology services. Standard bowel prep protocol for all patients undergoing elective outpatient colonoscopy during the study period at this institution involved a one day age-based graduated dosing schedule of PEG3550 (Miralax©; 17 g/240 mL/dose) Patients were instructed to take 1 dose every hour for a minimum of 6 ($\leq$ 4 years) – 10 doses, with additional doses as needed to return clear stool free of particulate matter. Dietary recommendations included clear liquids including electrolyte rich and non-red colored liquids through 2 - 4 hours pre-procedure all day or after breakfast ($\leq$ 4 years age) the day before the scheduled procedure. All colonoscopies are tracked with an institutional ethical practice review approved survey instrument completed by the endoscopy staff, including providers immediately following the procedure. The survey includes patient demographics, prep quality, impairment, duration, and completion. A single abstractor reviewed data from all pediatric patients (age 0 – 20) who presented to our GI outpatient clinic for colonoscopy from September 2015 – September 2016 and were given standard PEG monotherapy. Cases in which > 1 of three primary outcomes measures (procedure duration, completion, impairment) were absent were excluded from the final sample.

Additionally, prospective data was collected on patients who presented to the GI outpatient clinic from October 2016 – January 2017 with otherwise identical inclusion and exclusion criteria using a slightly modified abstraction form. Prospective data included an additional field to record procedure deviations where secondary stimulant laxative was added. To characterize outcomes in PEG-only prep, deviations from prep protocol, including the use of additional laxatives and patient non-compliance, were excluded from the final analysis.

Outcomes of interest included quality of prep, procedure impairment, completion, and duration (defined as scope-in to scope-out). Quality of prep was categorized as; thin liquid, thick liquid, and solid matter. Impairment was recorded as a binary variable, based on physician assessment of bowel prep. Completion was measured as a binary variable for two levels – reaching cecum and terminal ileum when ordered. Additionally, retrospective data included a binary variable for the presence of GI Fellows. All binary variables were compared using Chi-Square Test. Procedure duration was compared between procedures performed by attending physicians and fellows using a Fischer Exact Test. Additionally, procedure duration was compared between first, second and third year fellows using a one-way ANOVA. *P*-value of 0.05 was used as a threshold of significance.

Results

Retrospective data is summarized in Table 1. A total of 519 cases met all inclusion and exclusion criteria. Average age was 12.1 ± 4.2 years, with a male to female ratio of 0.64:1. Since cases were only excluded if > 1 primary outcome data field was missing, the total number of cases in each field represents those for which a response was submitted. There were no significant differences between age groups in terms of thin liquid ($p = 0.241$), thick liquid ($p = 0.913$), impairment ($p = 0.783$), reaching cecum ($p = 0.485$), or duration ($p = 0.243$). Significant differences were found in solids ($p = 0.001$) and reaching TI ($p = 002$).

Prospective data is summarized in Table 2. A total of 137 cases met inclusion criteria. 10 subjects were non-compliant with bowel prep regimen, while 4 other,-required additional stimulant laxatives due to perceived poor prep. These cases were excluded from the final analysis. Table 3 summarizes the differences in procedure metrics based on prep quality, and found significant differences in procedure impairment ($p < 0.001$), reaching cecum (< 0.001), reaching TI (< 0.001), and procedure duration (0.011).

A summary of Fellow procedure duration is provided in Table 4. Of a total of 439 recorded cases, 299 were performed by attending physician only, while 140 were performed by a GI fellow with an attending physician present. Table 3 also summarizes differences in procedure duration between first, second and third year trainee fellows. The p value for both comparisons was < 0.0001.

Table 1 Quality of cleanout by age at the time of endoscopy: retrospective cohort

Age	Total	Sex (M)	Quality				Completion		Duration (Mean ± SD)
			Thin Liquid	Thick Liquid	Solid	Impairment	Cecum Reached	TI Reached	
1–5	47	21 (44.7%)	27 (57.4%)	5 (10.6%)	7 (14.9%)	6 (12.8%)	42 (89.4%)	33 (100.0%)	21.6 ± 10.2
6–9	96	38 (39.6%)	68 (70.8%)	14 (14.6%)	3 (3.1%)	8 (8.3%)	93 (96.9%)	85 (96.6%)	21.4 ± 10.3
10–13	136	61 (44.9%)	102 (75%)	20 (14.7%)	2 (1.5%)	13 (9.6%)	129 (94.9%)	123 (94.6%)	24.6 ± 12.1
14–16	172	51 (29.7%)	121 (70.3%)	26 (15.1%)	9 (5.2%)	22 (12.8%)	162 (94.2%)	157 (94.0%)	23.4 ± 11.8
17–20	68	31 (45.6%)	50 (73.5%)	8 (11.8%)	1 (1.5%)	8 (11.8%)	64 (94.1%)	57 (95.0%)	23.0 ± 10.7
p value		0.038	0.241	0.913	0.001	0.783	0.485	0.002	0.243
Measured	519	202	368	73	22	57	490	455	23.5 ± 11.9
Total	519	519	463	463	463	482	501	486	439
Percent	100.00%	38.90%	79.50%	15.80%	4.80%	11.80%	97.80%	93.60%	NA

Discussion

The purpose of this study was to characterize outcomes in a 1-Day PEG-only bowel prep in a pediatric population; pediatric gastroenterologists are generally split in their preference for PEG monotherapy or PEG-stimulant laxative dual therapy for colonoscopy preparation (5). The results of this study support the implementation of a one day PEG-only regimen with high adherence rates and good quality preparation and excellent colonoscopy completion rates.

The choice of a prep strategy in children has to balance between the conflicting desire toward a pristine cleanout with the disadvantages inherent to complex regimens including poor adherence, discomfort from dietary restrictions and poor adherence with complex instructions. This equation in turn needs to be refocused within the goals of colonoscopy in children which rarely, if ever, include detection of small lesions or polyps as in colon cancer surveillance and standard of care reliance on biopsy based diagnosis which decreases the onus for macroscopic assessment and high quality preparation.

Table 2 Quality of cleanout by age at the time of endoscopy: prospective cohort

	Measured	Total	Percent
Total	123	123	100%
Demographics			
Age (Mean ± SD)	13.0 ± 3.7	123	NA
Gender (M)	60	123	48.78%
Outcomes			
Pre- procedure reported constipation	8	123	6.50%
Non-Compliant	10	[137]	7.30%
Additional Laxative	4	[127]	3.10%
Impairment	6	123	4.88%
Completion			
TI Reached	121	123	98.37%
Duration			
Duration/minutes (Mean ± SD)	27 ± 11.5	123	NA

Quality of prep with PEG-only prep was excellent. Solids found in colon during procedure is generally associated with poor prep, while the presence of only thin or thick liquids is considered adequate prep [8] . In our retrospective data, thin liquids were found in 79.48% of cases, thick liquids were found in 15.77% of all cases, and solids were found in only 4.75% of recorded cases, indicating overall adequate prep in > 95% of cases. Physician-determined impairment due to poor prep was noted in 11.8% of retrospective cases. Retrospective data included cases with patient deviation from protocol and additional stimulant laxative, and likely reflects expected prep impairment in a practice setting. In the prospective data, which included only protocol-adherent cases, prep-related impairment was only 4.88%, again indicating adequate prep in > 95% of cases. Only 4 cases (3.1%) required an alternative regimen. In all 4 cases, a parent directly contacted GI clinic staff after partial completion of the PEG regimen requesting additional laxative due to perceived ineffectiveness. In a similar comparison of regimens for constipation in children, 18% of patients given PEG monotherapy required additional laxatives [9].

Cleanout efficacy in our data is comparable to that of other studies of PEG-only regimen, which found cleanout efficacy rates as high as 89% and 95% [10, 11]. Notably, these other studies utilized a 4-day PEG prep of 1.5 g/Kg, a significantly longer and more intrusive protocol. Achieving similar cleanout rates with a lower-dose, one-day regimen is encouraging and significant. Additionally, patient adherence with regimen was also high; with 7.3% of patients being non-compliant with the assigned regimen. Decreased non-adherence rates compares favorably with other studies in which low volume PEG prep was used, in contrast to higher non-adherence found in studies using high volume PEG preparation, which ranged from 38 to 46% [12, 13].

Table 3 Impairment, completion of procedure and duration by quality of cleanout

Quality	Total	Impairment	Cecum	TI	Duration (Mean ± SD)
Thin Liquid	368	10/349 (2.9%)	352/355 (99.2%)	331/347 (95.4%)	22.2 ± 11.4
Thick Liquid	73	25/68 (36.8%)	70/71 (98.6%)	60/67 (89.6%)	26.4 ± 11.4
Solid	22	13/19 (68.4%)	15/21 (71.4%)	13/19 (68.4%)	24.8 ± 6.9
P value		< 0.001	< 0.001	< 0.001	0.011

Completion rates were also quite high, with cecum and terminal ileum visualization in 97.80% and 93.60%, respectively, in retrospective data, and terminal ileum visualization at 98.37% in the prospective group, comparable to results in similar studies using larger volume PEG prep solutions [12]. The results of this study are significant in showing comparable quality, impairment, compliance, and completion of prep in 1-day PEG bowel prep and high-volume, multi-day prep. A number of past studies have highlighted the contrast between superior efficacy of high-volume PEG solution and low patient tolerance and adherence to a multi-day, high-volume PEG prep [2, 12, 14]. Other groups have attempted to address this issue by exploring alternate delivery models such as split-dosing and low-volume PEG with added stimulant laxative [15–17].

Although the dominant alternative that has emerged to high-volume PEG monotherapy is low-dose PEG with stimulant laxative dual therapy, our observations suggest that high volume PEG limited to one day pre-procedure is effective and well tolerated. Further research is required to compare one day monotherapy with dual therapy in terms of safety, outcome based quality of prep, adherence and tolerability [5].

There are several limitations to this study. Our study focuses on an ambulatory care setting and our observations cannot be extrapolated to the inpatient setting. In the retrospective data set, deviations from the standard 1-day PEG regimen were not consistently recorded, including introduction of another cleansing agent or completion of the minimum 10-doses. Given the identical cleanout protocol,patient and provider population, we can extrapolate from the prospective cohort data that the likelihood of stimulant laxative administration, which is at least partially due to ineffective cleanout is approximately 3% and this should be factored with documented poor cleanout. Additionally, there were significant differences between retrospective and prospective data in terms of mean procedure time. We can partially attribute this discrepancy to differences in fellow participation in the two cohorts. Evaluation of impairment and poor prep due to cleanout protocol were ultimately subjective assessments made by the attending physician at the time of procedure. This may lead to significant variation in assessing impairment between providers, as well as overestimation of impairment due to providers attributing non-completion to prep quality rather than other factors such as technique. Another potential limitation is the lack of safety data in the cleanout forms. While this may be a significant exclusion, procedure nursing staff in our institution recall no incidences of medical or surgical adverse events related to cleanout protocol.

Table 4 Effect of fellow participation on procedure duration

	# of Cases	Duration/minutes (Mean ± SD)
Total	439	23.5 ± 11.9
Attending Only	299	22 ± 11.1
Fellow	140	27.1 ± 12.6
p value		< 0.0001
Fellow Yr1	69	30.2 ± 13.5
Fellow Yr2	64	21.8 ± 9.0
Fellow Yr3	22	31.0 ± 14.0
p value		< 0.0001

As an academic institution with an accredited pediatric fellowship program, we had the opportunity to analyze the impact of fellow participation on the duration of the procedure. Procedures performed by fellows were significantly longer (27.1 ± 12.6 min) than procedures performed by attending physicians only (22 ± 11.1 min), with a $p < 0.0001$. This discrepancy can be attributed to several factors including the normal progression in technical expertise, the impact of direct supervision and discussion during the case as well as the increased likelihood of fellows who are more advanced in their training to gravitate toward participating in more complex cases in order to meet their training requirements as well as out of interest. There was, in fact a significant difference in procedure duration between PGY 4 (30.2 ± 13.5 min), PGY 5 (21.8 ± 9.0 min), and PGY 6 (31.0 ± 14.0) fellows($p < 0.0001$).

Conclusion

1-Day PEG monotherapy appears to be an adequate bowel prep regimen for colonoscopy in the pediatric population. Based on the comparable levels prep quality, compliance, completion, of 1-Day prep with high-volume, multi-day PEG prep and other combined laxative solutions, we do not see the need for additional stimulant laxative to be added to the bowel prep regimen.

Abbreviations

NASPGHAN: North American Society for Pediatric Gastroenterology Hepatology and Nutrition; PEG: Polyethylene Glycol

Acknowledgements

Not applicable.

Funding

This study had internal departmental support and no external funding.

Authors' contributions

TMA and AK conceptualized and defined the research question, AK summarized the existent literature, TMA obtained support and obtained institutional review committee approval, BB tracked survey instrument responses, collected responses, abstracted and summarized results (acquisition of data), AK and TMA analyzed results and wrote the corresponding manuscript. All authors have read and approved the manuscript.

Competing interests

The authors declare that they have no competing interests.

References

1. Voiosu T, Tanțău A, Voiosu A, Benguş A, Mocanu C, Smarandache B, Mateescu B. Preparation regimen is more important than patient-related factors: a randomized trial comparing a standard bowel preparation before colonoscopy with an individualized approach. Rom J Intern Med. 2017;55: 36–43.
2. Barrish JO, Gilger MA. Colon cleanout preparations in children and adolescents. Gastroenterol Nurs. 1993;16:106–9.
3. Sahn B, Chen-Lim ML, Ciavardone D, Farace L, Jannelli F, Nieberle M, et al. Safety of a 1-day polyethylene glycol 3350 bowel preparation for colonoscopy in children. J Pediatr Gastroenterol Nutr. 2016;2016(63):19–24.
4. Siegel JD, Di Palma JA. Medical treatment of constipation. Clin Colon Rectal Surg. 2005;18:76–80.
5. Pall H, Zacur GM, Kramer RE, Lirio RA, Manfredi M, Shah M, Stephen TC, Tucker N, Gibbons TE, Sahn B, McOmber M, Friedlander J, Quiros JA, Fishman DS, Mamula P. Bowel preparation for pediatric colonoscopy: report of the NASPGHAN endoscopy and procedures committee. J Pediatr Gastroenterol Nutr. 2014;59:409–16.
6. Turner D, Levine A, Weiss B, Hirsh A, Shamir R, Shaoul R, Israeli Society of Pediatric Gastroenterology and Nutrition (ISPGAN), Berkowitz D, Bujanover Y, Cohen S, Eshach-Adiv O, Jamal G, Kori M, Lerner A, On A, Rachman L, Rosenbach Y, Shamaly H, Shteyer E, Silbermintz A, Yerushalmi B. Evidence-based recommendations for bowel cleansing before colonoscopy in children: a report from a national working group. Endoscopy. 2010;42:1063–70.
7. Nurko S, Zimmerman. Evaluation and treatment of constipation in children and adolescents. Am Fam Physician. 2014;90:82–90.
8. Kim HG, Jeon SR, Kim MY, Lee TH, Cho J-H, Ko BM, et al. How to predict adequate bowel preparation before colonoscopy using conventional polyethylene glycol: prospective observational study based on survey. Dig Endosc. 2015;27(1):87–94.
9. Gordon M, MacDonald JK, Parker CE, Akobeng AK, Thomas AG. Osmotic and stimulant laxatives for the management of childhood constipation. Cochrane Database Syst Rev. 2016;2016:CD009118.
10. Pashankar DS, Uc A, Bishop WP. Polyethylene glycol 3350 without electrolytes: a new safe, effective, and palatable bowel preparation for colonoscopy in children. J Pediatr. 2004;144:358–62.
11. Safder S, Demintieva Y, Rewalt M, Elitsur Y. Stool consistency and stool frequency are excellent clinical markers for adequate colon preparation after polyethylene glycol 3350 cleansing protocol: a prospective clinical study in children. Gastrointest Endosc. 2008;68:1131–5.
12. Dahshan A, Lin CH, Peters J, Thomas R, Tolia V. A randomized, prospective study to evaluate the efficacy and acceptance of three bowel preparations for colonoscopy in children. Am J Gastroenterol. 1999;94:3497–501.
13. Hookey LC, Depew WT, Vanner SJ. Combined low volume polyethylene glycol solution plus stimulant laxatives versus standard volume polyethylene glycol solution: a prospective, randomized study of colon cleansing before colonoscopy. Can J Gastroenterol. 2006;20:101–5.
14. Landreneau SW, Palma JAD. Update on preparation for colonoscopy. Curr Gastroenterol Rep. 2010;12:366–73.
15. Cohen B, Tang RS, Groessl E, Herrin A, Ho SB. Effectiveness of a simplified "patient friendly" split dose polyethylene glycol colonoscopy prep in veterans health administration patients. J Interv Gastroenterol. 2012;2:177–82.
16. Kang SH, Jeen YT, Lee JH, Yoo IK, Lee JM, Kim SH, et al. Comparison of a split-dose bowel preparation with 2L polyethylene glycol plus ascorbic acid and 1L polyethylene glycol plus ascorbic acid and bisacodyl before colonoscopy. Gastrointest Endosc. 2017;86:343–8.
17. Kelly NM, Rodgers C, Patterson N, Jacob SG, Mainie I. A prospective audit of the efficacy, safety, and acceptability of low-volume polyethylene glycol (2 L) versus standard volume polyethylene glycol (4 L) versus magnesium citrate plus stimulant laxative as bowel preparation for colonoscopy. J Clin Gastroenterol. 2012;46:595–601.

Bleeding in patients who underwent scheduled second-look endoscopy 5 days after endoscopic submucosal dissection for gastric lesions

Koichi Izumikawa[1], Masaya Iwamuro[2*], Tomoki Inaba[1], Shigenao Ishikawa[1], Kenji Kuwaki[3], Ichiro Sakakihara[1], Kumiko Yamamoto[1], Sakuma Takahashi[1], Shigetomi Tanaka[1], Masaki Wato[1] and Hiroyuki Okada[2]

Abstract

Background: Bleeding after endoscopic submucosal dissection (ESD) in antithrombotic drug users is still one of the important issues to be solved. We performed scheduled second-look endoscopy (SLE) 5 days after ESD, when the resumption of antithrombotic agents is assumed to have achieved a steady state, rather than on the day after ESD. We investigated bleeding incidence and the status of ulcers.

Methods: A total of 299 lesions in 299 patients subjected to ESD for gastric neoplasms were enrolled. A double dose of proton pump inhibitors was administered after ESD. SLE was planned 5 days after ESD. Post-ESD bleeding occurring before SLE was defined as early phase post-ESD bleeding, whereas bleeding after SLE was defined as later phase post-ESD bleeding. Forrest IIa and IIb ulcers are defined as high-risk ulcers requiring prophylactic hemostasis. We investigated risk factors for post-ESD bleeding, particularly focusing on the use of antithrombotic agents and the presence of high-risk ulcers requiring prophylactic hemostasis during SLE.

Results: Under a double dose of proton pump inhibitors, early phase post-ESD bleeding occurred in 2.3% of non-users (5/218) and 6.2% of users of antithrombotic agents (5/81). High-risk ulcers were found in 19.0% of the cases during scheduled SLE (55/289). Later phase bleeding occurred in 5.5% of cases [2.8% of non-users (6/213) and 13.2% of users of antithrombotic agents (10/76)]. Cox regression analysis revealed that the risk factor for post-ESD bleeding was antithrombotic treatment (HR: 3.56; 95% CI: 1.63–8.02, $p = 0.002$) alone. Among patients with high-risk ulcers, a statistically significant increase in bleeding was observed in the later phase in patients under antithrombotic therapy, compared to those not receiving any antithrombotic agents ($p = 0.001$).

Conclusions: Antithrombotic treatment is a risk factor for post-ESD bleeding despite SLE being scheduled 5 days after ESD. Later phase post-ESD bleeding was observed in 13.2% of the patients under antithrombotic treatment even after prophylactic hemostasis for high-risk ulcers.

Keywords: Antithrombotic treatment, Gastric neoplasms, Gastric ulcer, Second-look endoscopy, Prophylactic hemostasis

* Correspondence: iwamuromasaya@yahoo.co.jp
[2]Department of Gastroenterology and Hepatology, Okayama University Graduate School of Medicine, Dentistry and Pharmaceutical Sciences, 2-5-1 Shikata-cho, Kita-ku, Okayama, Okayama 700-8558, Japan
Full list of author information is available at the end of the article

Background

Although endoscopic submucosal dissection (ESD) has been established as a standard treatment for gastric neoplasms [1–3], post-ESD bleeding remains one of the various procedure-related adverse events that should not be overlooked [4, 5]. Known factors affecting the incidence of post-ESD bleeding include ESD technique, drugs administered prior to ESD (such as antiplatelet and anticoagulant drugs), gastric acid suppressing agents, and second-look endoscopy (SLE) [6–9]. In a recent study, we reported that vonoprazan, a potassium-competitive acid blocker, is superior to proton pump inhibitors (PPIs) in preventing post-ESD bleeding, based on a faster, stronger, and longer inhibition of gastric acid secretion than PPIs [10]. There is an increasing number of patients who are on antithrombotic agents and require ESD, since antithrombotic drugs are widely used for the treatment and prevention of thromboembolism. Thus, post-ESD bleeding in antithrombotic drug users is still one of the important issues to be solved.

For peptic ulcers with active bleeding, previous studies have revealed that SLE after initial endoscopic hemostasis improves mortality [11, 12]. SLE has been empirically performed after ESD with the expectation that it would be effective in reducing frequency of bleeding from ESD-induced ulcers as well as from peptic ulcers. SLE is typically performed on the day after ESD as post-procedural bleeding most frequently occurs within 24 h of ESD [5]. However, a consensus on the proper time of performing SLE has yet to be reached.

Currently, no evidence is available to support the usefulness of routine SLE in patients with hemorrhagic peptic ulcers, owing to recent improvements in endoscopic hemostatic devices and the introduction of PPIs [13]. Moreover there is accumulating evidence that SLE performed on the day after ESD does not help to decrease delayed bleeding from ESD-induced ulcers [14, 15]. However, the relationship between post-ESD bleeding incidence and high-risk ulcers that require prophylactic hemostasis, in antithrombotic drug users has not yet been fully investigated. In order to establish an appropriate strategy for management during the post-ESD period, further studies are required to address the role of specific interventions, such as the time of performing SLE, use of prophylactic hemostasis, and administration of acid-suppressing agents. It is important to accumulate data regarding post-ESD bleeding from manifold aspects.

It has been reported that suppression of platelet aggregation is stabilized 5 days after the administration of antiplatelet therapy such as low dose aspirin or clopidogrel, and anticoagulant therapy such as warfarin [16–18]. In our institution, we do not perform SLE on the day after ESD. Instead, we schedule SLE 5 days after ESD, when the antithrombotic effect is expected to be exhibited after resumption of antithrombotic drugs. The purposes of this study were i) to investigate the bleeding incidence and status of post-ESD ulcers and ii) to investigate risk factors for post-ESD bleeding.

Methods

Participants

Patients who underwent ESD for gastric neoplasm between January 2011 and March 2014 at Kagawa Prefectural Central Hospital, were retrospectively reviewed. In patients who underwent ESD more than twice, we analyzed only the initial lesions. Patient exclusion criteria for this study included the following: (i) patients in whom en bloc resection was not performed endoscopically; (ii) patients in whom endoscopic snare resection was performed; (iii) patients with a remnant stomach; (iv) patients who underwent ESD for lesions located in more than two regions of the stomach [upper (U), middle (M) or lower (L)] on the same day; and (v) patients in whom SLE was not performed 5 days after ESD. All patients enrolled in this study provided written informed consent before undergoing ESD. The association between post-ESD bleeding, state of ulcers during SLE according to Forrest classification, use of antithrombotic agents, and other clinical backgrounds was examined.

Management of patients taking anticoagulants

Antithrombotic agents used in the study subjects were classified into antiplatelet agents (low-dose aspirin, cilostazol, ticlopidine, clopidogrel, icosapentate, sarpogrelate hydrochloride, beraprost sodium, limaprost alfadex, and dipyridamole) and anticoagulants (warfarin). Drug cessation periods before the ESD procedure were 5 days for low-dose aspirin, 7 days for thienopyridine derivatives (ticlopidine and clopidogrel), and 1 day for other antiplatelet agents. Warfarin was discontinued 3 days before ESD and heparin replacement was introduced. Unfractionated heparin (10,000 units/day) was administered and then discontinued 2 h before ESD. All antithrombotic agents were restarted 2 days after ESD, except in cases with post-ESD bleeding. Heparin replacement was discontinued when the prothrombin time-international normalized ratio reached to 1.50. SLE and prophylactic hemostasis were performed while on complete anticoagulant therapy.

Patients were divided into two groups according to their antithrombotic therapy at baseline: (1) the antithrombotic group, which included 81 lesions in patients who had been using antithrombotic agents before undergoing ESD; and (2) the non-antithrombotic group, comprising 218 lesions in patients who had not used antithrombotic agents.

ESD procedures

ESD was conducted as one of the treatment options for lesions with a preoperative diagnosis of either a gastric adenoma or a possible node-negative early gastric cancer, based on the criteria proposed by Gotoda et al. [1, 19]. ESD was performed by one of the two board-certified endoscopists who had previously performed ESDs in > 200 gastric neoplasm cases. ESD was performed according to the standard ESD procedure, which consisted of the following: (i) marking a circumferential region around the lesion; (ii) submucosal injection of solution outside the marked region; (iii) mucosal incision outside the marked region; (iv) additional injection of 0. 4% sodium hyaluronate with 0.1% epinephrine and 1% indigo carmine dye into the submucosa underneath the lesion; (v) submucosal dissection with insulated-tip knife-2 (KD-611 L, Olympus Medical Systems, Co., Tokyo. Japan); (vi) hemostasis of active bleeding and prophylactic coagulation of visible vessels on the mucosal defect performed with hemostatic forceps (Coagrasper®; Olympus Optical Co., Tokyo, Japan) in soft coagulation mode, both during submucosal dissection and at the final step of ESD; and finally (vii) retrieval of the specimen. An electrosurgical current was applied using an electrosurgical generator (VIO 300D; ERBE, Tübingen, Germany). The resected specimens were stretched, pinned flat on a corkboard, and measured.

Management after ESD

A total of 40 mg/day omeprazole was intravenously infused into the patients on the day of ESD (day 0) and on the following day (day 1). Blood tests were performed 2 h after ESD and on day 0. Dietary intake was initiated and 20 mg/day of rabeprazole was administered daily, from day 2 in cases with no evidence of bleeding. Polaprezinc, which is commonly used in Japan for treating peptic ulcers [20, 21], was also administered from day 2. Blood tests and SLE were planned for day 5. Patients without post-ESD bleeding were discharged on that day. Rabeprazole and polaprezinc were administered to all patients until day 51 or day 52.

Post-ESD bleeding was defined as an episode of hematemesis and/or melena, or a decline in hemoglobin levels of ≥2 g/dL. Emergency endoscopy and endoscopic hemostasis were performed in patients with post-ESD bleeding. Post-ESD bleeding that occurred before SLE was defined as early phase post-ESD bleeding, whereas bleeding that occurred after SLE was defined as later phase post-ESD bleeding.

Emergency endoscopy was performed by board-certified endoscopists. Ulcers were classified according to the Forrest classification [22]. When adherent clots (IIb) were observed on the post-ESD ulcer during SLE, the endoscopist carefully checked whether non-bleeding visible vessels (IIa) existed after removing the clots [23]. When active bleeding (Ia and Ib) was observed on the post-ESD ulcer, endoscopic hemostasis with hemostatic forceps (Coagrasper®) in soft coagulation mode or argon plasma coagulation was performed.

SLE

Patients were generally under strict supervision during the hospital stay after ESD and could be immediately treated for overt post-ESD bleeding. In addition, there was no available evidence regarding actual time of performing SLE and usefulness of prophylactic hemostasis for post-ESD ulcers for the prevention of post-ESD bleeding. Therefore, in accordance with the management strategy after endoscopic hemostasis of hemorrhagic peptic ulcers, we did not perform SLE on the day after ESD. Alternatively, we performed SLE on day 5 when the resumption of antithrombotic agents is assumed to achieve a steady state [16–18]. During SLE, post-ESD ulcers were classified according to the Forrest classification. Endoscopic treatment was performed with hemostatic forceps in soft coagulation mode or argon plasma coagulation for Forrest IIa and IIb ulcers, since these ulcers were considered to be at high risk of delayed bleeding. Therefore, Forrest IIa and IIb ulcers were defined as high-risk ulcers and Forrest IIc and III ulcers were classified as low-risk ulcers. The treatment for Forrest IIa and IIb ulcers during SLE, was prophylactic hemostasis. Forrest IIc and III ulcers were not treated during SLE.

Analysis of gastric lesions

The morphology of the lesion was endoscopically classified as an elevated, flat, or depressed lesion. In cases wherein two resected lesions existed in the same region of the stomach, the lesion diameter was calculated as the sum of the diameters of the two lesions, and the morphology of the larger lesion alone was used for analysis. The depth of the lesion, and the presence or absence of ulcer scar within the lesion were pathologically diagnosed.

Statistical analysis and ethical considerations

Continuous variables were expressed as the mean ± standard deviation. For statistical analysis, the chi square test was used for categorical data. Residual analysis was used to analyze the differences between the antithrombotic drugs. Univariate analysis was performed with the log-rank test. Cox regression analyses were performed for factors having statistical significance in univariate analysis. A Kaplan–Meier curve was generated, and a log-rank test was used to compare post-ESD bleeding incidences between groups. Differences with a P-value of < 0.05 were considered statistically significant. JMP Pro ver.10 (SAS

Institute, Cary, NC, USA) software was used for statistical computations.

The present study was approved by the Clinical Ethics Committee of Kagawa Prefectural Central Hospital in accordance with the Helsinki Declaration, and was registered in the UMIN Clinical Trials Registry System (000023306).

Results

Gastric ESD was performed for 403 lesions in 364 patients between January 2011 and March 2014. En bloc resection was achieved for 398 lesions (98.8%). Endoscopic snare resection was performed for 19 lesions, and 8 lesions were in patients with a remnant stomach. Twenty-four lesions were excluded from this study, since these lesions were resected during a second or third ESD. We further excluded 27 lesions, including two perforated lesions, which existed in more than two regions of the stomach. SLE was not performed 5 days after ESD for these lesions, because of ESD-related adverse events such as perforation (N = 2) and pneumonia (N = 2), and because day 5 was a non-working day of our hospital (N = 19). Among patients in whom SLE was not performed on day 5, 6 patients who were not on antithrombotic agents experienced post-ESD bleeding (two patients on day 6, three on day 7, one on day 8). Overall, we retrospectively analyzed 299 lesions in 299 patients in the present study.

Patients' backgrounds are summarized in Table 1. Patients included 225 males and 74 females, with an average age of 71.6 ± 9.1 years. The 299 lesions consisted of 51 adenomas and 248 adenocarcinomas. The antithrombotic group included 81 lesions (27.1%), whereas the non-antithrombotic group was comprised of 218 lesions (72.9%). In the antithrombotic group, patients received a single antiplatelet agent (52 lesions), two or more antiplatelet agents (11 lesions), a single anticoagulant agent (12 lesions), or antiplatelet plus anticoagulant agents (6 lesions). One patient was on hemodialysis for chronic renal failure.

Early phase post-ESD bleeding occurred in 10 lesions, 5 lesions were under antithrombotic treatment and the remaining 5 lesions were not under antithrombotic treatment. Later phase post-ESD bleeding occurred in 16 lesions, including 10 lesions under antithrombotic treatment. Consequently, post-ESD bleeding was detected in 26 lesions (8.7%; Fig. 1). Figure 2 shows the time points and cumulative incidence of post-operative bleeding. There were no instances of bleeding on day 21 or later.

Scheduled SLE was performed in 213 lesions in patients who were not receiving antithrombotic treatment and in 76 lesions in patients under antithrombotic treatment. Antithrombotic treatment included single antiplatelet treatment (N = 50, 65.8%), dual or more antiplatelet treatment (N = 11, 14.5%), single anticoagulant treatment (N = 12, 15.8%), and a combination of antiplatelet and anticoagulant treatment (N = 3, 3.9%). During SLE, the majority of the ESD-induced ulcers were Forrest IIc or III (N = 234, 81.0%). A total of 27 lesions (9.3%) were graded as Forrest IIa, while 28 lesions were classified as Forrest IIb (9.7%). Consequently, prophylactic hemostasis was performed for 55 lesions with high-risk ulcers (Forrest IIa and IIb ulcers, 19.0%). Procedures used for prophylactic hemostasis was argon plasma coagulation (N = 41) and coagulation by using hemostatic forceps (N = 14).

In high-risk ulcers, the ulcer diameter was ≥40 mm in 24/55 lesions (43.6%), compared with ≥40 mm diameter

Table 1 Clinical characteristics of the gastric lesions

	Number	Percent
Total no. of gastric lesions	299	
Age (years, mean ± SD)	71.6 ± 9.1	
Sex		
Male	225	(75.3)
Female	74	(24.7)
Under antithrombotic therapy	81	(27.1)
Single antiplatelet agent	52	
≥ 2 antiplatelet agents	11	
Single anticoagulant agent	12	
Antiplatelet(s) plus anticoagulant	6	
On hemodialysis	1	(0.3)
Tumor location		
Upper third	47	(15.7)
Middle third	142	(47.5)
Lower third	110	(36.8)
Length of the resected specimen (mm, mean ± SD)	36.4 ± 15.3	
Morphology		
Elevated	174	(58.2)
Flat or depressed	125	(41.8)
Pathology		
Adenoma	51	(17.1)
Adenocarcinoma, differentiated type	231	(77.3)
Adenocarcinoma, undifferentiated type	17	(5.7)
Depth of invasion		
M	263	(88.0)
SM, ≤ 500 mm (micrometer)	16	(5.4)
SM, > 500 mm (micrometer)	20	(6.7)
Ulcer scar within the lesion	16	(5.4)
Curative resection by ESD	266	(89.0)

SD standard deviation, *M* mucosal layer, *SM* submucosal layer, *ESD* endoscopic submucosal dissection

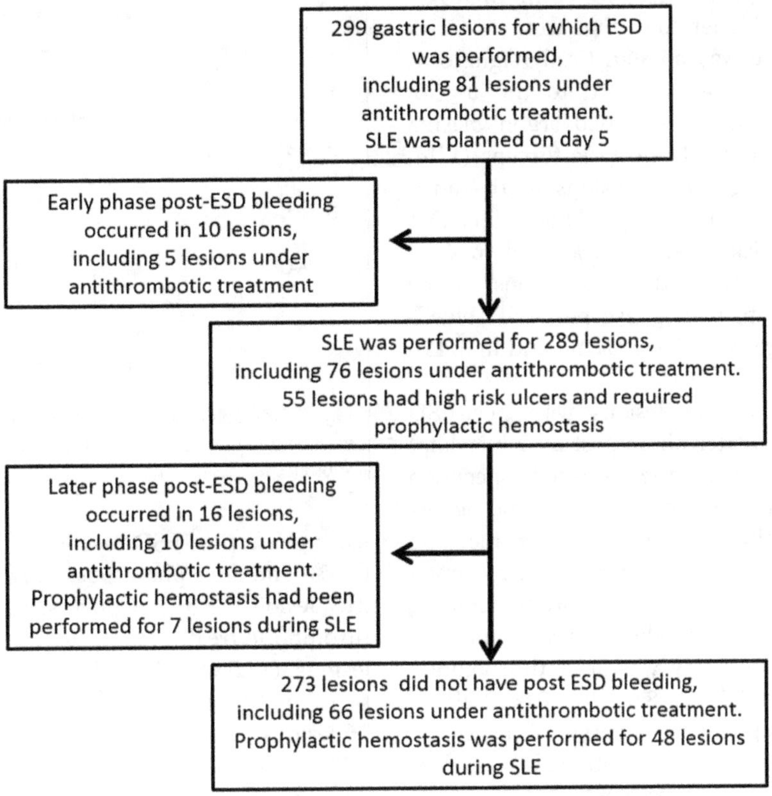

Fig. 1 Flow chart of patients through the study. ESD, endoscopic submucosal dissection; SLE, second-look endoscopy

in 65/234 lesions (27.8%) with low-risk ulcers. The difference was statistically significant between the two groups with regard to the prevalence of ulcers measuring ≥40 mm ($p < 0.034$). Among the 55 patients with high-risk ulcers, 18 (32.7%) were under antithrombotic treatment, while among the 234 patients with low-risk ulcers, 58 (24.8%) were receiving treatment. The difference in the prevalence of antithrombotic treatment between the two groups was not statistically significant ($p = 0.237$) (Table 2).

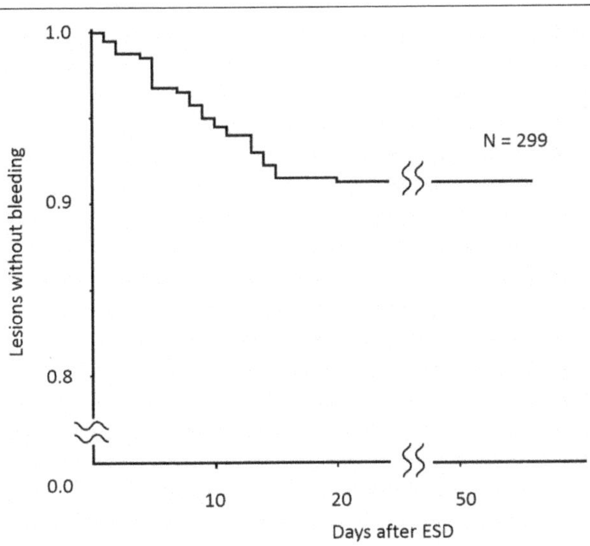

Fig. 2 Time points and cumulative incidence of post-ESD bleeding. ESD, endoscopic submucosal dissection

Later phase post-ESD bleeding was observed in 16 lesions; 6/213 lesions without antithrombotic treatment (2.8%); 5/50 lesions under single antiplatelet treatment (10.0%); 2/11 lesions under dual or more antiplatelet treatment (18.2%); 1/12 lesion under single anticoagulant treatment (8.3%); and 2/3 lesions under a combination of antiplatelet and anticoagulant treatment (66.7%). Despite prophylactic hemostasis, overall 7/55 high-risk ulcers bled in the later phase (12.7%), compared to 9/234 low-risk ulcers that bled in the later phase (3.8%).

Table 2 Ulcer status during second-look endoscopy according to the Forrest classification

	IIa + IIb ($N = 55$)	IIc + III ($N = 234$)	P^* values
Diameter of the resected specimen			
< 40 mm	31 (56.4%)	169 (72.2%)	0.034
≥ 40 mm	24 (43.6%)	65 (27.8%)	
Antithrombotic agents			
Non-user	37 (67.3%)	176 (75.2%)	0.237
User	18 (32.7%)	58 (24.8%)	

The incidence of later phase bleeding from high-risk ulcers was significantly higher than that from low risk ulcers ($P = 0.018$). There was no statistically significant difference between lesions with regard to the use of prophylactic hemostasis, which included argon plasma coagulation (6/41, 14.6%) and hemostatic forceps (1/14, 7.1%) ($p = 0.664$). Among the 76 lesions in the antithrombotic group, later phase post-ESD bleeding occurred in 6/18 high-risk ulcers (33.3%) and in 4/58 low-risk ulcers (6.9%). Among the 213 lesions in the non-antithrombotic group, later phase post-ESD bleeding occurred in 1/37 high-risk ulcers (2.7%) and in 5/176 low-risk ulcers (2.8%).

Univariate analysis of all 26 lesions with post-ESD bleeding (early phase plus later phase post-ESD bleeding) revealed that a diameter of the resected specimen ≥40 mm ($p = 0.036$) and use of antithrombotic agents ($p < 0.001$) were statistically significant factors for bleeding (Table 3). We used the diameter of the resected specimen ≥40 mm and antithrombotic treatment before undergoing ESD in Cox regression analysis, which revealed that the risk factor for post-ESD bleeding was an antithrombotic treatment (HR: 3.56; 95% CI: 1.6–8.02; $p = 0.002$) alone. Figure 3 shows the Kaplan-Meier curve of post-ESD bleeding in patients under antithrombotic treatment and patients without antithrombotic treatment.

Post-ESD bleeding was observed in 11/218 lesions without antithrombotic treatment (5.0%). Among them, early phase post-ESD bleeding occurred in 5/218 lesions (2.3%) and later phase post-ESD bleeding occurred in 6/213 lesions (2.8%). Conversely, in lesions under antithrombotic treatment, post-ESD bleeding arose in 15/81 lesions (18.5%); where bleeding occurred in the early phase in 5/81 lesions (6.2%) and in the later phase in 10/76 lesions (13.2%).

Figure 4 shows the time points when post-ESD bleeding was detected, according to user or non-user of antithrombotic agents and presence or absence of prophylactic hemostasis. Non-scheduled endoscopic

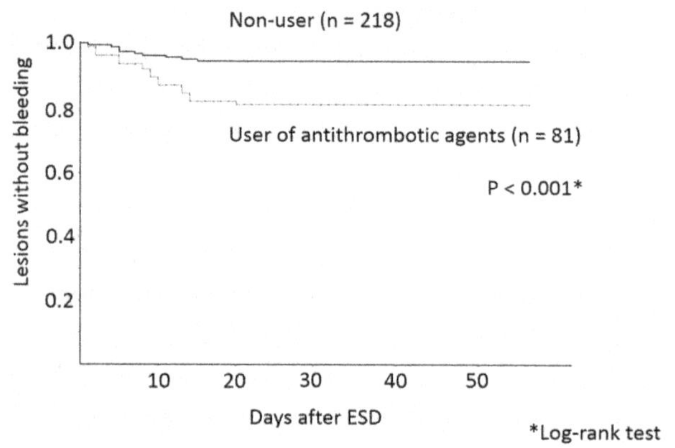

Fig. 3 Time points and cumulative incidence of post-ESD bleeding in users and non-users of antithrombotic agents. ESD, endoscopic submucosal dissection

Table 3 Univariate analyses of post-ESD bleeding risk

	Early phase post-ESD bleeding				Later phase post-ESD bleeding				Total instances of post-ESD bleeding				
	Bleeding		Non-bleeding		Bleeding		Non-bleeding		Bleeding		Non-bleeding		*P*-value
No. of lesions	10		289		16		273		26		273		
Aged ≥65 years	9	90.0%	231	79.9%	13	81.3%	218	79.9%	22	84.6%	218	79.9%	0.539
Male sex	9	90.0%	216	74.7%	14	87.5%	202	74.0%	23	88.5%	202	74.0%	0.103
Tumor location													
Upper third	4	40.0%	43	14.9%	2	12.5%	41	15.0%	6	23.1%	41	15.0%	0.259
Middle third	3	30.0%	139	48.1%	10	62.5%	129	47.3%	13	50.0%	129	47.3%	0.809
Lower third	3	30.0%	107	37.0%	4	25.0%	103	37.7%	7	26.9%	103	37.7%	0.277
Length of the resected specimen ≥40 mm	6	60.0%	89	30.8%	7	43.8%	82	30.0%	13	50.0%	82	30.0%	0.036
Elevated type morphology	6	60.0%	168	58.1%	9	56.3%	159	58.2%	15	57.7%	159	58.2%	0.949
Depth of invasion													
M	8	80.0%	255	88.2%	13	81.3%	242	88.6%	21	80.8%	242	88.6%	0.230
SM, ≤500 uL	1	10.0%	15	5.2%	1	6.3%	14	5.1%	2	7.7%	14	5.1%	0.562
SM, > 500 uL	1	10.0%	19	6.6%	2	12.5%	17	6.2%	3	11.5%	17	6.2%	0.297
Ulcer scar within the lesion	0	0.0%	16	5.5%	0	0.0%	16	5.9%	0	0.0%	16	5.9%	0.214
Use of antithrombotic agents	5	50.0%	76	26.3%	10	62.5%	66	24.2%	15	57.7%	66	24.2%	0.0002
Forrest IIa + IIb ulcers requiring prophylactic hemostasis	–		–		7	43.8%	48	17.6%	7	26.9%	48	17.6%	0.275

ESD endoscopic submucosal dissection, *CI* confidence interval, *M* mucosal layer, *SM* submucosal layer

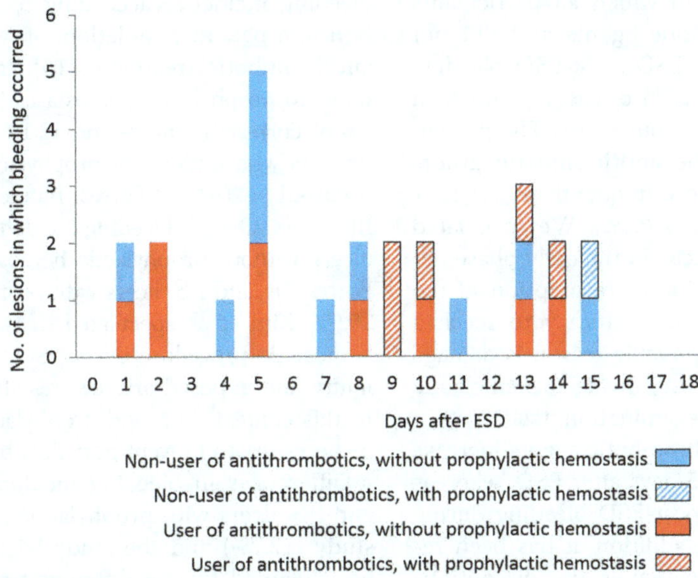

Fig. 4 Schematic diagram showing the number of patients with post-ESD bleeding and the time elapsed since their ESD procedure

examinations were performed in 10 patients with early phase post-ESD bleeding, in whom Forrest Ia (N = 2), Ib (N = 5), IIa (N = 1), and III (N = 2) ulcers were identified. Hemostasis was performed for Forrest Ia and Ib ulcers with hemostatic forceps. Argon plasma coagulation was used for Forrest IIa ulcers. No endoscopic procedure was done for Forrest III ulcers. These patients were excluded from the analysis for scheduled SLE. Two patients exhibited melena and three patients showed a decline in hemoglobin levels by ≥2 g/dL, 5 days after ESD. These patients were classified as early phase post-ESD bleeding. There were approximately equal proportions of early phase post-ESD bleeding (10/299, 3.3%) and later phase post-ESD bleeding complications (16/289, 5.5%).

Log-rank tests revealed that bleeding incidence after SLE was higher in high-risk ulcers in the antithrombotic group, compared with those in the non-antithrombotic group. The result was statistically significant (p = 0.001) (Fig. 5).

Later phase post-ESD bleeding occurred in seven high-risk ulcers. Emergency endoscopy and endoscopic hemostasis were performed in 5/7 high-risk ulcers with later phase post-ESD bleeding. The remaining two patients were treated with medication only, as they rejected emergency endoscopic examination. In four of five bleeding high-risk ulcers, bleeding was observed from the sites where prophylactic hemostasis was performed during SLE. In this study, all patients with post-ESD bleeding recovered and were discharged from our hospital.

Discussion

Although the reported frequency of post-ESD bleeding varies depending on the definition of "bleeding", it has been reported as ~ 5%, provided that post-ESD bleeding is defined as an episode of hematemesis/melena, or a decline in hemoglobin levels by ≥2 mg/dL, as seen in the present study [4, 8]. In this study, post-ESD bleeding was observed in 8.7% of lesions, which was relatively higher than the reported incidence. In this study, 27.1% of the lesions (81/299 lesions) had been treated with antithrombotic agents before undergoing ESD. Therefore as compared to other studies (8.0-16.3%), the relatively higher number of patients under antithrombotic therapy enrolled for this study may have resulted in a higher incidence of post-procedural bleeding.

In this study, the incidence of post-ESD bleeding in the early and later phase were 2.3 and 2.8%, respectively, in the non-antithrombotic group, and 6.2 and 13.2%, respectively, in the antithrombotic group. In a previous

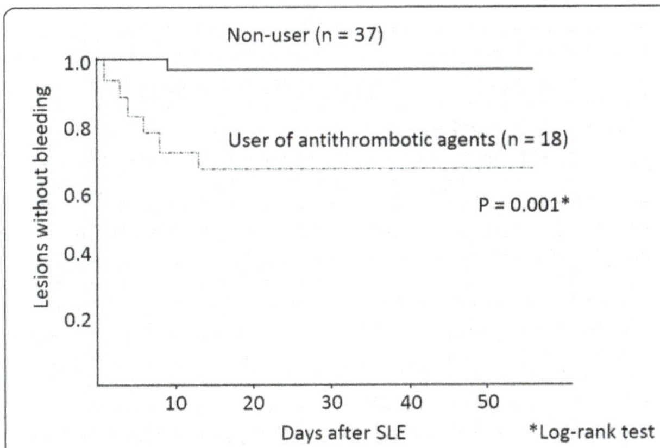

Fig. 5 Time points and cumulative incidence of later phase post-ESD bleeding that occurred after prophylactic hemostasis in patients with high-risk ulcers (Forrest IIa and IIb ulcers). ESD, endoscopic submucosal dissection; SLE, second-look endoscopy

randomized controlled study, in which all participants were non-users of antithrombotic agents and did not undergo SLE on the day after ESD, post-ESD bleeding occurred in the early phase in 2.3% of cases [24], which is similar to the incidence rate in our study. The present study also revealed that in the antithrombotic group, post-ESD bleeding occurred more frequently in the later phase than early phase (13.2% vs 6.2%). We speculated that bleeding is less likely to occur in the early phase because several days are required after resumption of the antithrombotic agents for the drug efficacy to reach a steady state [16–18]. Another possible reason is damage to the post-ESD ulcer during SLE, owing to hemostatic procedures and/or endoscopic examination itself.

Koh et al. reported that antithrombotic agents increase post-ESD bleeding incidence ≥5 days after ESD, whereas these agents did not increase post-ESD bleeding during the 0–4 days after ESD [7]. In addition, it has been reported that heparin replacement after the discontinuation of antithrombotic agents is a risk factor for post-ESD bleeding ≥5 days after ESD [25].

Recent studies comparing between patients undergoing prophylactic hemostasis and patients without prophylactic hemostasis during SLE performed on the day after ESD reported that although there was no statistical difference, post-ESD bleeding incidence relatively increased in the former patient group [15, 24], suggesting the possibility that prophylactic hemostasis did not prevent post-ESD bleeding. Mochizuki et al. speculated that prophylactic hemostasis itself causes additional damage to the vessels within the ESD-induced ulcer and may induce hemorrhage [24]. We were unable to evaluate role of prophylactic hemostasis in this study, as it was applied for all high-risk ulcers (Forrest IIa and IIb ulcers).

Coagulation is used as a hemostatic procedure to prevent bleeding during both ESD and SLE. Argon plasma coagulation and hemostatic forceps were used in this study. The safety of these procedures during ESD has been previously reported [8, 26]. However, thermal injury from argon plasma coagulation increases depending on the energy output [27]. For example, application of argon plasma coagulation for intact colon mucosa can contribute to muscle layer damage [28]. During SLE, thermal damage by argon plasma coagulation and hemostatic forceps followed by exposure to gastric acid may injure the arteries. This hypothesis is supported by the present results, which indicated that later phase bleeding in high-risk ulcers occurred where prophylactic hemostasis was performed.

Typically, endoscopic hemostasis is performed for Forrest IIa and IIb ulcers. Therefore, the true incidence rate of hemorrhage from Forrest IIa and IIb ulcers has not been revealed till date. Kim et al. performed scheduled SLE on the day after ESD and investigated post-ESD bleeding incidence according to each Forrest classification in a patient population, of which 11.2% were under antithrombotic treatment [15]. In patients who did not undergo prophylactic hemostasis, bleeding occurred in 11.1% of Forrest IIa ulcers and 12.1% of Forrest IIb ulcers. In patients who underwent prophylactic hemostasis, bleeding occurred in 20.0% of Forrest IIa ulcers and 21.4% of Forrest IIb ulcers. Overall bleeding incidence in Forrest IIa and IIb ulcers without prophylactic hemostasis was 11.8%, and in Forrest IIa and IIb ulcers with prophylactic hemostasis was 20.5%. Kim et al. speculated that air insufflations and the hemostatic procedure during SLE may have caused tissue injury and exposed arteries, resulting in delayed bleeding. In this context, SLE and prophylactic hemostasis may not be necessary to prevent post-ESD bleeding.

Differences in bleeding incidence rates of Forrest IIa and IIb ulcers with prophylactic hemostasis between our study (12.7%) and the study by Kim et al. (20.5%) may be explained by the different times of performing SLE and prophylactic hemostasis. Kim et al. performed SLE on the day after of ESD, whereas SLE was performed on day 5 in the present study. ESD-induced gastric ulcers are reported easier and faster to heal, compared with peptic ulcers [29]. Therefore, since the healing process of ulcers is likely to progress by day 5, hemostatic procedure may be less harmful for post-ESD ulcers when SLE is performed on day 5.

A recent meta-analysis has reported that delayed post-ESD bleeding was more frequent in patients who underwent prophylactic hemostasis than in those who did not [30]. However, previous studies were single-arm studies, in which prophylactic hemostasis was intended for all high-risk ulcers, and the relationship between antithrombotic agents and prophylactic hemostatic procedure has never been taken into consideration.

The bleeding incidence and the status of post-ESD ulcers have never been investigated in users and non-users of antithrombotic agents, who do not undergo SLE on the day after ESD. The present study revealed that under a double dose of PPIs, early phase post-ESD bleeding occurs in 2.3% of non-users and in 6.2% of users of antithrombotic agents. We also demonstrated that high-risk ulcers were found in 19.0% of the cases during scheduled SLE, 5 days after ESD.

We consider that a possible alternative of SLE may be only to perform emergency endoscopic examination in patients exhibiting post-ESD bleeding. Administration of vonoprazan may be another alternative of SLE, which enables stronger and faster suppression of gastric acid secretion [10].

This study had several limitations. First, the sample size was relatively small. Second, this study was retrospectively conducted in a single institution. Third, in cases with two lesions resected by ESD, although the resected areas of the two lesions were close to each other, the actual diameter of the post-ESD ulcer created by ESD was not identical to the calculated value as the sum of the diameters of the two lesions. Fourth, there mights have been technical disparities in the endoscopic hemostatic procedures conducted by the endoscopists. Fifth, none of the included patients were on newer anti-coagulant agents, that is, direct oral anticoagulant. Thus, further multi-centered studies with larger sample sizes are required.

Conclusions

In conclusion, we performed SLE 5 days after ESD, when the resumption of antithrombotic agents is assumed to achieve a steady state, rather than on the day after ESD. We investigated the bleeding incidence and the status of ulcers, and the results revealed that the (i) use of antithrombotic agents before ESD was a risk factor for post-ESD bleeding, (ii) post-ESD bleeding occurred in 3.3% of cases during the early phase (2.3% of non-users and 6.2% of users of antithrombotic agents), (iii) high risk ulcers were found in 19% of the cases during scheduled SLE, and (iv) even after prophylactic hemostasis for a high-risk ulcer (Forrest IIa or IIb ulcer), bleeding occurred in 5.5% of cases during the later phase (2.8% of non-users and 13.2% of users of antithrombotic agents). Consequently, healthcare providers must be particularly aware of bleeding from high-risk ulcers in patients under antithrombotic treatment, irrespective of prophylactic hemostasis during ESD. The data obtained in this study will serve as useful reference for future research.

Abbreviations

ESD: Endoscopic submucosal dissection; PPIs: Proton pump inhibitors; SLE: Second-look endoscopy

Funding

No funding to declare.

Authors' contributions

KI, SI, IS, KY, S Takahashi, S Tanaka, and MW collected the data; KI and TI analyzed the data; KI and MI drafted the manuscript; KK provided analytical oversight; TI designed and supervised the study; HO revised the manuscript for important intellectual content. All authors have read and approved the final version to be published.

Authors' information

Koichi Izumikawa, M.D., Tomoki Inaba, M.D., Shigenao Ishikawa, M.D., Ichiro Sakakihara, M.D., Kumiko Yamamoto, M.D., Sakuma Takahashi, M.D., Shigetomi Tanaka, M.D., and Masaki Wato, M.D.; Department of Gastroenterology, Kagawa Prefectural Central Hospital, 1–2-2 Asahi-machi, Takamatsu, Kagawa 760–8557, Japan. Masaya Iwamuro, M.D. and Hiroyuki Okada, M.D.; Department of Gastroenterology and Hepatology, Okayama University Graduate School of Medicine, Dentistry and Pharmaceutical Sciences, 2–5-1 Shikata-cho, Kita-ku, Okayama, Okayama 700–8558, Japan. Kenji Kuwaki, M.D.; Department of Internal Medicine, Fukuyama City Hospital, 5–23-1 Zao--cho, Fukuyama, Hiroshima 721–8511, Japan.

Competing interests

The authors declare that they have no competing interests.

Author details

[1]Department of Gastroenterology, Kagawa Prefectural Central Hospital, 1-2-2 Asahi-machi, Takamatsu, Kagawa 760-8557, Japan. [2]Department of Gastroenterology and Hepatology, Okayama University Graduate School of Medicine, Dentistry and Pharmaceutical Sciences, 2-5-1 Shikata-cho, Kita-ku, Okayama, Okayama 700-8558, Japan. [3]Department of Internal Medicine, Fukuyama City Hospital, 5-23-1 Zao-cho, Fukuyama, Hiroshima 721-8511, Japan.

References

1. Gotoda T, Yanagisawa A, Sasako M, Ono H, Nakanishi Y, Shimoda T, et al. Incidence of lymph node metastasis from early gastric cancer: estimation with a large number of cases at two large centers. Gastric Cancer. 2000;3:219–25.
2. Ono H, Yao K, Fujishiro M, Oda I, Nimura S, Yahagi N, et al. Guidelines for endoscopic submucosal dissection and endoscopic mucosal resection for early gastric cancer. Dig Endosc. 2016;28:3–15.
3. Fernández-Esparrach G, Calderón A, de la Peña J, Díaz Tasende JB, Esteban JM, Gimeno-García AZ, et al. Endoscopic submucosal dissection. Endoscopy. 2014;46:361–70.
4. Toyokawa T, Inaba T, Omote S, Okamoto A, Miyasaka R, Watanabe K, et al. Risk factor for perforation and delayed bleeding associated with endoscopic submucosal dissection for early gastric neoplasms: analysis of 1123 lesions. J Gastroenterol Hepatol. 2012;27:907–12.
5. Goto O, Fujishiro M, Oda I, Kakushima N, Yamamoto Y, Tsuji Y, et al. A multicenter survey of the management after gastric endoscopic submucosal dissection related to postoperative bleeding. Dig Dis Sci. 2012;57:435–9.
6. Takeuchi T, Ota K, Harada S, Edogawa S, Kojima Y, Tokioka S, et al. The postoperative bleeding rate and its risk factors in patients on antithrombotic therapy who undergo gastric endoscopic submucosal dissection. BMC Gastroenterol. 2013;13:136.
7. Koh R, Hirasawa K, Yahara S, Oka H, Sugimori K, Morimoto M, et al. Antithrombotic drugs are risk factors for delayed postoperative bleeding after endoscopic submucosal dissection for gastric neoplasms. Gastrointest Endosc. 2013;78:476–83.
8. Takizawa K, Oda I, Gotoda T, Yokoi C, Matsuda T, Saito Y, et al. Routine coagulation of visible vessels may prevent delayed bleeding after endoscopic submucosal dissection–an analysis of risk factors. Endoscopy. 2008;40:179–83.
9. Uedo N, Takeuchi Y, Yamada T, Ishihara R, Ogiyama H, Yamamoto S, et al. Effect of a proton pump inhibitor or an H2-receptor antagonist on prevention of bleeding from ulcer after endoscopic submucosal dissection of early gastric cancer: a prospective randomized controlled trial. Am J Gastroenterol. 2007;102:1610–6.
10. Kagawa T, Iwamuro M, Ishikawa S, Ishida M, Kuraoka S, Sasaki K, et al. Vonoprazan prevents bleeding from endoscopic submucosal dissection-induced gastric ulcers. Aliment Pharmacol Ther. 2016;44:583–91.
11. Marmo R, Rotondano G, Bianco MA, Piscopo R, Prisco A, Cipolletta L. Outcome of endoscopic treatment for peptic ulcer bleeding: is a second look necessary? A meta-analysis. Gastrointest Endosc. 2003;57:62–7.
12. Calvet X, Vergara M, Brullet E, Gisbert JP, Campo R. Addition of a second endoscopic treatment following epinephrine injection improves outcome in high-risk bleeding ulcers. Gastroenterology. 2004;126:441–50.
13. El Ouali S, Barkun AN, Wyse J, Romagnuolo J, Sung JJ, Gralnek IM, et al. Is routine second-look endoscopy effective after endoscopic hemostasis in acute peptic ulcer bleeding? A meta-analysis. Gastrointest Endosc. 2012;76:283–92.
14. Takahashi F, Yoshitake N, Akima T, Kino H, Nakano M, Tsuchida C, et al. A second-look endoscopy may not reduce the bleeding after endoscopic submucosal dissection for gastric epithelial neoplasm. BMC Gastroenterol. 2014;14:152.
15. Kim DS, Jung Y, Rhee HS, Lee SJ, Jo YG, Kim JH, et al. Usefulness of the forrest classification to predict artificial ulcer rebleeding during second-look endoscopy after endoscopic submucosal dissection. Clin Endosc. 2016;49:273–81.
16. Jakubowski JA, Stampfer MJ, Vaillancourt R, Deykin D. Cumulative antiplatelet effect of low-dose enteric coated aspirin. Br J Haematol. 1985;60:635–42.

17. Jakubowski JA, Matsushima N, Asai F, Naganuma H, Brandt JT, Hirota T, et al. A multiple dose study of prasugrel (CS-747), a novel thienopyridine P2Y12 inhibitor, compared with clopidogrel in healthy humans. Br J Clin Pharmacol. 2007;63:421–30.
18. Hirsh J, Dalen JE, Anderson DR, Poller L, Bussey H, Ansell J, et al. Oral anticoagulants: mechanism of action, clinical effectiveness, and optimal therapeutic range. Chest. 1998;114:445S–69S.
19. Gotoda T, Iwasaki M, Kusano C, Seewald S, Oda I. Endoscopic resection of early gastric cancer treated by guideline and expanded National Cancer Centre criteria. Br J Surg. 2010;97:868–71.
20. Arakawa T, Satoh H, Nakamura A, Nebiki H, Fukuda T, Sakuma H, et al. Effect of zinc L-carnosine on gastric mucosal and cell damage caused by ethanol in rats. Dig Dis Sci. 1990;35:3140–6.
21. Watanabe S, Wang XE, Hirose M, Kivilioto T, Osada T, Miwa H, et al. Insulin-like growth factor I plays a role in gastric wound healing: evidence using a zinc derivative, polaprezinc, and an in vitro rabbit wound repair model. Aliment Pharmacol Ther. 1998;12:1131–8.
22. Forrest JA, Finlayson ND, Shearman DJ. Endoscopy in gastrointestinal bleeding. Lancet. 1974;2:394–7.
23. Heldwein W, Schreiner J, Pedrazzoli J, Lehnert P. Is the Forrest classification a useful tool for planning endoscopic therapy of bleeding peptic ulcers? Endoscopy. 1989;21:258–62.
24. Mochizuki S, Uedo N, Oda I, Yamamoto Y, Yamashina T, Suzuki H, et al. Scheduled second-look endoscopy is not recommended after endoscopic submucosal dissection for gastric neoplasms (the SAFE trial): a multicentre prospective randomised controlled non-inferiority trial. Gut. 2015;64:397–405.
25. Matsumura T, Arai M, Maruoka D, Okimoto K, Minemura S, Ishigami H, et al. Risk factors for early and delayed post-operative bleeding after endoscopic submucosal dissection of gastric neoplasms, including patients with continued use of antithrombotic agents. BMC Gastroenterol. 2014;14:172.
26. Fujishiro M, Yahagi N, Nakamura M, Kakushima N, Kodashima S, Ono S, et al. Safety of argon plasma coagulation for hemostasis during endoscopic mucosal resection. Surg Laparosc Endosc Percutan Tech. 2006;16:137–40.
27. Garrido T, Baba ER, Wodak S, Sakai P, Cecconello I, Maluf-Filho F. Histology assessment of bipolar coagulation and argon plasma coagulation on digestive tract. World J Gastrointest Endosc. 2014;6:304–11.
28. Norton ID, Wang L, Levine SA, Burgart LJ, Hofmeister EK, Yacavone RF, et al. In vivo characterization of colonic thermal injury caused by argon plasma coagulation. Gastrointest Endosc. 2002;55:631–6.
29. Kakushima N, Yahagi N, Fujishiro M. The healing process of gastric artificial ulcers after endoscopic submucosal dissection. Dig Endosc. 2004;16:327–31.
30. Kim EH, Park SW, Nam E, Eun CS, Han DS, Park CH. Role of second-look endoscopy and prophylactic hemostasis after gastric endoscopic submucosal dissection: a systematic review and meta-analysis. J Gastroenterol Hepatol. 2017;32:756–68.

Epidemiology of gastrointestinal symptoms in young and middle-aged Swiss adults: prevalences and comorbidities in a longitudinal population cohort over 28 years

Maria Avramidou[1*], Felix Angst[1], Jules Angst[2], André Aeschlimann[1], Wulf Rössler[2,3,4] and Ulrich Schnyder[5]

Abstract

Background: Although subacute and chronic gastrointestinal symptoms are very common in primary care, epidemiological date are sparse. The aim of the study was to examine and quantify the prevalence of subacute and chronic gastrointestinal symptoms and their associations with somatic and mental disorders in the general population.

Methods: Data were collected prospectively between 1981 (age m = 22, f = 23) and 2008 (age 49/50) from the Zurich Cohort Study (n = 292 men, 299 women), a representative general population survey. The participants were assessed using a semi-structured interview, the "Structured Psychopathological Interview and Rating of the Social Consequences of Psychological Disturbances for Epidemiology" (SPIKE). Prevalence rates were computed to be representative of the general population aged 22–50. Associations were quantified by odds ratios (ORs) and their 99% confidence intervals (CI).

Results: The prevalences of intestinal and of gastric symptoms were significantly higher among women in all categories examined. For example, any gastric symptoms: f. 26.4% vs m.15.2%; any intestinal symptoms: 27.6% vs 14.6%; nausea/vomitus: 19.1% vs 4.5%; constipation: 15.8% vs 6.5% (all $p < 0.001$). Strong associations (all $p < 0.0001$) were found between fatigue (1 month) and chronic stomach (OR = 9.96, 99%-CI: 5.53–17.94) and chronic intestinal symptoms (OR = 9.02, 99%-CI: 4.92–16.54). Panic attacks were associated with subacute intestinal symptoms (OR = 4.00, 99%-CI: 2.43–6.59). Anxiety was more strongly associated with subacute intestinal symptoms (OR = 3.37, 99%-CI: 2.23–5.08) than with subacute stomach symptoms (OR = 1.85, 1.20–2.86). Bipolar disorders were associated with subacute stomach symptoms (OR = 1.83, 1.18–2.17) and unipolar depression with subacute intestinal symptoms (OR = 2.05, 1.34–3.15).

Conclusions: Remarkably high prevalence rates of gastric and intestinal complaints were observed in women (over 1/4; men 1/7). Fatigue/neurasthenia was the strongest co-factor in both conditions. Various syndromes related to anxiety, phobia, and panic disorders showed further significant associations. The integration of psychiatric and/or psychological treatment could help address the functional part of gastric and intestinal syndromes.

Keywords: Epidemiology, Prevalence, General population survey, Associations, Odds ratios, Gastrointestinal, Functional

* Correspondence: avramidmar@gmail.com
[1]Research Department, Rehabilitation Clinic ("RehaClinic"), Quellenstrasse 34, 5330 Bad Zurzach, Switzerland
Full list of author information is available at the end of the article

Background

Gastrointestinal (GI) symptoms are widespread and carry heavy economic and social consequences. It is estimated that in the United States 11% of the population suffer from a chronic digestive disease, with a prevalence rate as high as 35% for those 65 years and over [1]. In 2010 alone, a reported 60 to 70 million people in the United States suffered from a digestive disease [2]. Although subacute and chronic gastrointestinal symptoms are very common, there has so far been no thorough investigation of the relevant Swiss epidemiological data, including the possible associations of gastrointestinal symptoms with somatic and psychiatric disorders in the general population.

Functional gastrointestinal disorders (FGIDs), represented by functional dyspepsia (FD) and irritable bowel syndrome (IBS), include variable combinations of chronic or acute gastrointestinal symptoms not explained by structural or biochemical abnormalities [3–5]. Worldwide the prevalence rates in the general population of dyspepsia/FD and IBS according to Rome III diagnostic criteria are 5.3–20.4% and 1.1–29.2%, respectively. Recent reports on Rome III FD and IBS indicate a female predominance [6, 7]. The prevalence of IBS subtypes is characterised by a male predominance for IBS with diarrhoea, and a female predominance for IBS with constipation. Genetic and environmental factors play an important role in the development of FGIDs. Gene polymorphisms are involved in the development of FGIDs. The prevalence of FGIDs differs across races and geographical areas. Food may also affect their development, but the causal relationships are not conclusive [8].

Psychosomatic concepts have long been postulated to account for irritable bowel syndrome in the absence of other objective aetiology and biomarkers, and it is common knowledge that many chronic conditions are associated with psychological disorders. It is worth noting that ulcerative colitis was interpreted by psychosomatic theory until the discovery of immune dysregulation [9].

In general, causal relationships are hard to establish. Clinical and population-based studies worldwide have found that some types of somatoform disorders (e.g., somatisation disorder, somatic-symptom-index (SSI) 4.6, and pain disorder) frequently co-occur with anxiety and depressive disorders. These findings could suggest either a causal relationship between those disorders or that they share certain aetiological factors. Irritable bowel syndrome occurs most frequently in young adults in response to emotional and other factors [10].

The aim of our analysis was to quantify the prevalence of gastrointestinal symptoms in Swiss adults between the ages of 22 (m)/23 (f) and 49/50 years, i.e. over a 28-year period, stratified by duration into subacute (1 week) and chronic (3 months, diarrhoea: 1 month). In addition, their associations with a range of somatic and psychiatric disorders were examined (see Methods section below).

Based on the current literature [7], our first hypothesis was that gastric and intestinal symptoms, especially chronic symptoms, are more prevalent in women than in men. Our second hypothesis was that there is a statistically significant association between gastrointestinal symptoms and certain psychiatric disorders, especially anxiety, suggesting that some GI symptoms are partially non-organic in nature.

Methods

Setting and data sampling

This study analyses data from the Zurich Study, an age cohort representative of the general population of the canton of Zurich, which accounts for approximately one sixth of the total Swiss population. The design was prospective, longitudinal, long-term, and naturalistic. The Zurich Study comprised a cohort of 4547 subjects (2201 men, 2346 women) representative of the canton of Zurich in Switzerland, who were screened in 1978 with the Symptom Checklist (SCL-90R), when the men were 19 and the women 20 years old. Male and female participants were sampled using different approaches. In Switzerland every male person undergoes military screening at the age of 19. With the consent of the military authorities but independently of their procedure, 50% of all male conscripts on the recruiting lists were randomly screened. Of these, 99.7% were included (n = 2201) (refusal rate 0.3%). The female sample was based on the complete population registers (civil status registers) of the canton of Zurich, from which 50% of the women born in 1958 were randomly selected. They were mailed questionnaires, to which n = 2346 (75%) responded. Because of the lower response rate of women with poorer educational levels, the interview sample was corrected for this bias. Written informed consent was obtained from all participants.

For economic reasons and in the interest of the long-term design of the study, in the second stage, a stratified sample of 591 subjects (292 men, 299 women) was selected for interview. The interview sample was enriched with persons reporting high levels of psychopathological symptoms and distress and therefore at risk for the development of psychiatric syndromes. Thus two thirds (n = 394) of the final interview sample consisted of randomly selected "high scorers" (defined by the 85th percentile or more on the Global Severity Index (GSI) of the SCL-90-R) and the remaining third (n = 197) of low scorers (<85th percentile). A detailed description of the Zurich Study design and method was published previously [11].

The use of such a two-phase method, consisting of initial screening and subsequent interview with a subsample stratified to enrich the sample with individuals of specific interest, was recommended in epidemiology [12]. Altogether, seven interview waves were carried out, when the participants were aged 20(m)/21(f) to 49/50: in 1979 (n = 591), 1981 (n = 456), 1986 (n = 457), 1988 (n = 424), 1993 (n = 407), 1999 (n = 367), and 2008 (n = 335, reflecting a 56.9% retention rate). Details of the interview waves and the drop-out rates and characteristics are published elsewhere [11]. The initial ratio of high-scorers to low-scorers (two thirds: one third) did not change significantly over the 30 years of the study; the sample therefore remained representative of the general population. The interview sample during the period 1981–2008 comprised 490 participants, who, weighted for stratified sampling, represent 2342 subjects (1141 men, 1201 women).

Data from the year 1979 were not included in the current analysis, because at that interview the assessment of symptom duration was limited to 1 month. In all subsequent interview waves a symptom duration up to 12 months was assessed, thus allowing the definition of chronic gastrointestinal problems (see below). We accordingly included the 490 subjects who took part in the interviews between 1981 and 2008. For each interview, all members of the initial sample of 1979 (n = 591) were followed up. In order to be included in our analysis, a participant had to have been interviewed at least once between 1981 and 2008. Because of the varying response rates the number of participants happened to be slightly higher in 1986 (n = 457) than in 1981 (n = 456).

Instruments and measures

The instruments used comprised the Structured Psychopathological Interview and Rating of the Social Consequences of Psychological Disturbances for Epidemiology (SPIKE) [13], a clinical syndrome list (SL), the revised 90-item symptom check list (SCL-90R), a life-event inventory, and scales measuring coping behaviour and dissimulation. The interviews were conducted in the subjects' homes by specially trained psychologists or psychiatrists and focused mainly on the past year in order to minimise forgetting.

The SPIKE is a semi-structured interview specifically developed for epidemiological surveys in psychiatric research. It assesses socio-demography, psychopathology, substance use, medication, health service use, impairment, and social activity. Data on its reliability and validity have been published previously [14]. Unlike other diagnostic interviews, which apply DSM (diagnostic and statistical manual) diagnoses using a top-down approach with multiple cut-offs, the SPIKE uses a bottom-up approach, assessing the past-year presence of about 14 somatic (including gastrointestinal) and 15 psychiatric syndromes, for each of which it checks symptoms, duration, frequency of episodes, distress, impairment and treatment.

The interviewers collected data on a total of 26 comorbid conditions: repeated panic attacks, anxiety (≥1 month Generalised Anxiety Disorder (GAD)), major depression (unipolar depression), bipolar depression, simple phobia, specific phobia, social phobia, agoraphobia, obsessive-compulsive disorder, suicidality, drug dependence, sedative/ tranquilliser dependence, alcohol dependence, smoking, bulimia, obesity, fatigue, sexual problems, sleep disorders, hypertension, hypotension, back pain, headache, other pain (not classified), cardiovascular symptoms and asthma spectrum conditions.

Interviewees were asked about specific gastrointestinal symptoms, for example: pain in the stomach, burning in the stomach, pressure in the stomach, nausea, vomitus, constipation, diarrhoea, intestinal pain, bloating, blood in the stool. Assessment on this pure symptom level provides obvious face and content validity. We defined as stomach symptoms, those symptoms perceived in the upper abdominal region (pain, burn, pressure, nausea, vomitus). Intestinal symptoms were defined as those located in the lower abdominal region (constipation, diarrhoea, pain, pressure, bloating). Participants were only asked about their symptoms; the cause of the symptoms was not evaluated. Consequently, liver and pancreas disorders could also cause gastrointestinal symptoms of the upper and lower gastrointestinal tract.

Participants were also specifically questioned about the duration and the intensity of their symptoms, in particular to specify the number of days they had experienced gastrointestinal symptoms over the past 12 months [11]. We defined as subacute, gastrointestinal symptoms lasting more than 1 week but less than 3 months: 1 week<= subacute<=3 months. Chronic symptoms that lasted 3 months or more: chronic≥3 months. An exception was made for diarrhoea: 1 week≤subacute< 1 month and chronic, which was defined as subacute if lasting 1 week or more but less than 1 month and as chronic ≥1 month. Acute gastrointestinal symptoms (< 1 week = 7 days) were excluded, because of the high probability that they were caused by a viral or bacterial infection. The intensity of the gastrointestinal symptoms/suffering experienced was subjectively quantified on a 0–100 mm "thermometer" scale: 0 = no distress/symptoms, 100 = maximum distress/symptoms [15]. The degree of distress/subjective suffering associated with a condition is an individual's most important measure of their state of health and the primary reason for seeking help.

The main outcome was measured on the symptom level, for example, nausea, pressure, constipation, etc. The concomitant comorbidities were classified on the syndrome/disorder level, for example, major depression, specific phobia, asthma, etc.

Analysis

The analysis of prevalence was limited to the period 1981–2008. All participants in at least one interview were included and analysed by weighting for stratified sampling. Descriptive statistics consisted of means (M) and standard deviations (SD) if the frequency distribution was approximately symmetrical, and of medians and quartiles (q1 and q3) if it was not. All data on prevalence were weighted back to the composition of the original, representative, population-based age cohort, comprising women born in 1958 and men born in 1959 living in the canton Zurich; quantification was in percentages (%) [13, 14].

Associations of gastrointestinal symptoms (present/absent as dependent variable) with psychiatric conditions were analysed by stepwise multivariate logistic regression to various comorbid conditions as independent variables, adjusting for sex and education level (confounding co-variates) in the interview sample of $n = 490$. We used backward stepwise regression, i.e., after each step the least significant variable was excluded. The observation period of the Zurich age cohort ended in 2008; thus associations were not confounded by age. The associations were expressed as odds ratios (ORs) with corresponding intervals of 99% confidence (99% CI). A type I error of 1% was chosen because the logistic models were stepwise determined after a maximum of 5 steps, which leads to a Bonferroni correction of 0.05/5. The OR quantifies the relative frequency (often also termed "risk") of gastrointestinal symptoms if a given characteristic is present or not. All analyses were performed using SAS 9.3 for Windows (SAS Inc., Cary, NC, USA).

Results

Prevalences

Over the period 1981–2008 prevalence rates for any (subacute and chronic) stomach symptoms was 20.9% and for any intestinal symptoms 21.3%. (Tables 1 and 2).

Among the gastric symptoms (Table 1), overall pain/burn/pressure was more common (18.1%) than nausea/vomitus (11.0%). For subacute stomach pain, burn (reflux), pressure the prevalence rate was 10.8% in women and 7.9% in men. The rates by gender for the corresponding chronic symptoms were 13.2 and 4.1%. Indeed, the prevalence rates for all examined symptom groups were consistently higher in women, with the differences being statistically highly significant except in the subgroup of any subacute symptoms. The widest gender difference was 10.1% vs 0.6% for chronic nausea, vomitus. Overall, there was a female preponderance (26.4% vs 15.2%) for any (subacute + chronic) gastric/stomach symptoms.

The prevalence rates in every group of intestinal symptoms examined were also higher in women (Table 2). With the exception of diarrhoea, the gender differences were statistically highly significant: constipation subacute 7.7% vs 3.4%, chronic 8.1% vs 3.1%; pain/pressure/bloating subacute 11.3% vs 5.7%, chronic 11.4% vs 4.6%. Overall, the female preponderance was 27.6% to 14.6% for any (subacute + chronic) intestinal symptoms. Pain/pressure/bloating was the most prevalent intestinal syndrome (16.7%).

Distress (scale 0–100)

The highest distress levels were found in 54 subjects with chronic gastric symptoms, with a mean of 67.9 (standard deviation: 24.0), followed by 76 subjects with subacute gastric symptoms with a mean of 55.4

Table 1 Numbers and weighted prevalence rates (%) of stomach symptoms by gender

		N	M + F%	M%	F%	*p*
Pain, burn, pressure	subacute≥1 week	65	9.3	7.9	10.8	0.012
	chronic≥3 months	51	8.8	4.1	13.2	< 0.001
	subacute+chronic	116	18.1	12.0	24.0	< 0.001
Nausea, vomitus	subacute≥1 week	36	7.0	4.8	9.0	< 0.001
	chronic≥3 months	40	5.5	0.6	10.1	< 0.001
	subacute+chronic	76	11.0	4.5	19.1	< 0.001
Pain, burn, pressure with nausea, vomitus	subacute≥1 week	35	4.9	2.9	7.1	< 0.001
	chronic≥3 months	33	5.0	0.6	9.0	< 0.001
	subacute+chronic	68	9.9	3.5	16.1	< 0.001
Any symptoms	subacute≥1 week	54	11.6	11.0	12.2	0.385
	chronic≥3 months	76	9.3	4.2	14.2	< 0.001
	subacute+chronic	130	20.9	15.2	26.4	< 0.001

Legend: n = number in the sample, prevalences: rates, back-weighted to the general population, M = male, F = female, p = type I error that the prevalences of m and f are different (two-sided)

Table 2 Numbers and weighted prevalence rates (%) of intestinal symptoms by gender

		N	M + F%	M%	F%	p
Constipation	subacute≥1 week	39	5.6	3.4	7.7	< 0.001
	chronic≥3 months	51	5.7	3.1	8.1	< 0.001
	subacute+chronic	90	11.3	6.5	15.8	< 0.001
Diarrhoea	subacute≥1 week	42	4.9	4.2	5.5	0.133
	chronic≥1 month	57	7.7	6.7	8.7	0.068
	subacute+chronic	99	12.6	10.9	14.2	0.013
Pain, pressure, bloating	subacute≥1 week	47	8.6	5.7	11.3	< 0.001
	chronic≥3 months	66	8.1	4.6	11.4	< 0.001
	subacute+chronic	113	16.7	10.4	22.7	< 0.001
Any symptoms	subacute≥1 week	57	9.0	6.3	11.7	< 0.001
	chronic≥1 or 3 months	91	12.2	8.3	16.0	< 0.001
	subacute+chronic	148	21.3	14.6	27.6	< 0.001

Legend: *n* = number in the sample, prevalences: rates, back-weighted to the general population, M = male, F = female, *p* = type I error that the prevalences of m and f are different (two-sided)

(standard deviation: 26.3). There were no significant distress-related gender differences (Table 3).

Comorbid conditions

Stepwise logistic regression modelling selected all conditions having significant associations with gastrointestinal symptoms, adjusting for sex and level of education; no adjustment for age was necessary, since all interviewees had the same age per assessment time point.

Subacute stomach symptoms (Fig. 1) were found to be moderately associated with anxiety (OR = 1.85, 99%-CI: 1.20–2.86), bipolar disorder (1.83, 1.18–2.82) and back pain (1.48, 1.01–2.17). An inverse (protective) association was found between subacute stomach symptoms and obesity (0.41, 0.19–0.88).

Chronic stomach symptoms (Fig. 2) were strongly associated with fatigue (OR = 9.96, 99%-CI: 5.53–17.94) and moderately with high blood pressure (4.67, 2.80–7.78), social phobia (3.00, 1.70–5.27) and anxiety (2.64, 1.60–4.36). An inverse association was found with bulimia/binge eating (0.20, 0.09–0.45).

Subacute intestinal symptoms (Fig. 3) were strongly associated with panic attacks (OR = 4.00, 99%-CI: 2.43–6.59), bulimia/binge eating (3.97, 2.30–6.82), anxiety (3.37, 2.23–5.08) and moderately with unipolar major depression (2.05, 1.34–3.15). Inverse associations were documented for sleep disorders (0.45, 0.29–0.71), alcohol dependence (0.42, 0.27–0.65) and agoraphobia (0.34, 0.14–0.82).

Chronic intestinal symptoms (Fig. 4) were very strongly associated with fatigue (OR = 9.02, 99%-CI: 4.92–16.54), social phobia (4.77, 2.66–8.54) and bulimia (4.76). A moderate association was found with bipolar disorder (3.07, 1.69–5.57). Inverse (protective) associations were documented for obesity (0.20, 0.09–0.46), specific/simple phobia (0.28, 0.15–0.52) and anxiety (0.21, 0.09–0.52).

Table 3 Distress levels of any symptoms (0 = no to 100 = maximum distress)

Gastric	N	mean	sd	Intestinal	n	mean	sd
subacute all	76	55.4	26.3	subacute all	57	50.9	28.1
subacute m	33	52.5	26.5	subacute m	20	46.0	26.4
subacute f	43	57.6	26.2	subacute f	37	53.5	28.9
p (m vs f)		0.399				0.330	
chronic all	54	67.9	24.0	chronic all	91	51.9	30.3
chronic m	17	69.3	23.9	chronic m	33	50.5	32.8
chronic f	37	67.3	24.3	chronic f	58	52.7	29.1
p (m vs f)		0.776				0.733	

Legend: *n* = number in the sample, m = male, f = female, mean = arithmetic mean, sd = standard deviation, *p* = type I error that the distress of m and f are different (two-sided)

Discussion

This study provides new insights into the longitudinal epidemiology of functional gastrointestinal symptoms in Switzerland. In our sample of 490 participants, male and female, one in five complained of subacute or chronic stomach symptoms and of subacute or chronic intestinal symptoms. Stomach symptoms were defined as symptoms of the upper gastrointestinal tract (pain, burn, pressure, nausea, vomitus) and intestinal symptoms as symptoms of the lower gastrointestinal tract (constipation, diarrhoea, pain, pressure, bloating). Pain and pressure were most prevalent among the gastric as well the intestinal symptom groups. For both sexes, the prevalences of subacute and chronic complaints were comparable in most of the symptom groups.

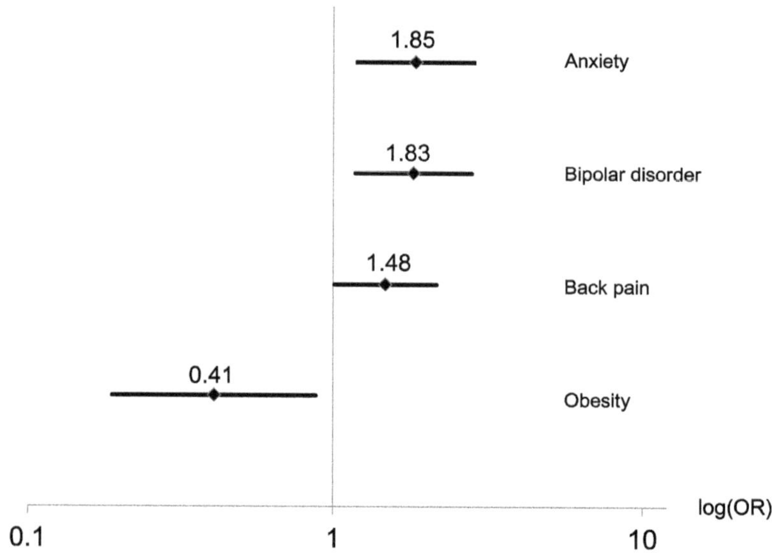

Fig. 1 Associations with subacute stomach symptoms (n = 76 with, n = 410 without symptoms): Odds ratios (OR), 99% CI, adjusted for sex and education level. Explained variance: 15.7%. Legend: Odds ratios (OR), 99% CI, adjusted for sex and education level

In a review of the prevalence of functional dyspepsia, two studies could be found that were comparable to ours [16]. A British study of a randomly selected sample of 20% of patients registered at two health centre practices who were examined by endoscopy to exclude organic disease reported an estimated prevalence of functional gastrointestinal symptoms of 11.5%. A carefully designed endoscopy study of the inhabitants of a Norwegian community (Sørreisa) aged 20–69 found a prevalence of functional gastrointestinal disorders of 14.7%. Comparing those results (11.5% and 14.7%) to our own prevalence rates of around 20% of any gastric symptoms, it may be concluded that 1/2 to 3/4 of the gastric symptoms are functional in our sample.

Our analysis focused on gastrointestinal (GI) symptoms of at least 1 week's duration, which excludes acute infections but covers most of the functional syndromes. People with functional GIs suffer by definition from disorders without somatic background, which can be very difficult to understand and to accept. The symptoms, which cause shame and embarrassment, tend to isolate the sufferer and impact heavily on their working and social lives. It may thus be assumed that there is a bidirectional relationship between functional GI symptoms and psychiatric

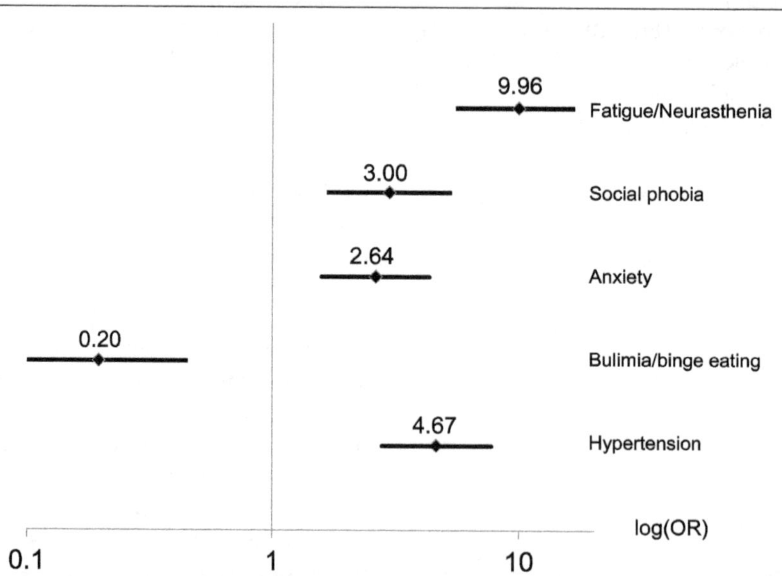

Fig. 2 Associations with chronic stomach symptoms (n = 54 with, n = 372 without symptoms): Odds ratios (OR), 99% CI, adjusted for sex and education level. Explained variance: 52.4%. Legend: Odds ratios (OR), 99% CI, adjusted for sex and education level

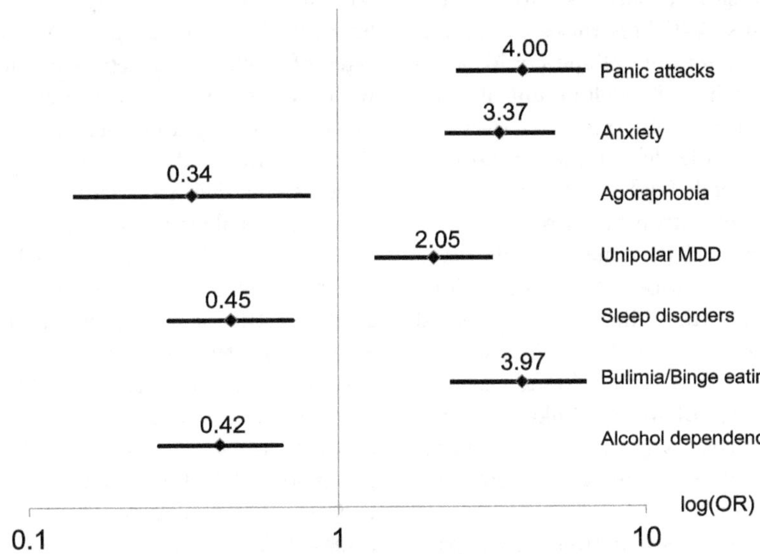

Fig. 3 Associations with subacute intestinal symptoms (n = 78 with, n = 345 without symptoms): Odds ratios (OR), 99% CI, adjusted for sex and education level. Explained variance: 38.2%. Legend: Odds ratios (OR), 99% CI, adjusted for sex and education level

disorders, with the latter being both partial cause and frequent product of the former, creating a vicious circle.

We found the highest distress levels in subjects with chronic followed by subacute gastric symptoms. The correlation between chronic symptoms and higher distress levels might be explained by exhaustion (fatigue/neurasthenic syndrome) as discussed later. Women and men were equally distressed by subacute and chronic gastrointestinal symptoms although more women had GI illnesses.

As initially hypothesised, our study found higher female prevalence rates in all subgroups of gastrointestinal syndromes examined. Our findings are in line with earlier studies. In Smith's epidemiological study of 1978 women with IBS outnumbered men by a ratio of 2.3:1 [1]. However, a recent Japanese report showed a male predominance for the IBS-subtype with diarrhoea and a female predominance for the IBS-subtype with constipation, the overall prevalence of IBS being assessed at 13.1%, 15.5% for females and 10.7% for males [8].

In our study the strongest associations overall were found between fatigue and chronic stomach and chronic intestinal symptoms. This finding is compatible with the results of a recent study showing a strong association

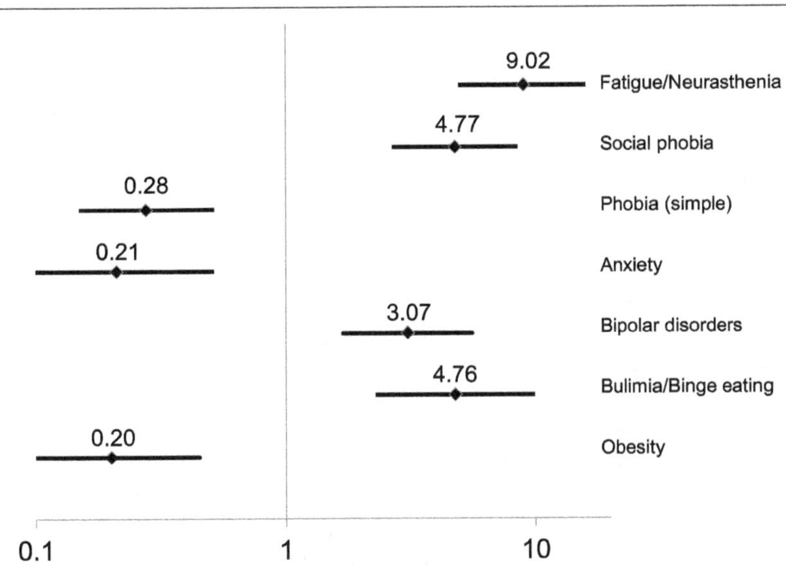

Fig. 4 Associations with chronic intestinal symptoms (n = 76 with, n = 345 without symptoms): Odds ratios (OR), 99% CI, adjusted for sex and education level. Explained variance: 45.7%. Legend: Odds ratios (OR), 99% CI, adjusted for sex and education level

between fatigue and depression in patients with Crohn's disease and ulcerative colitis [17]. This raises the perennial question of "cause or effect", as fatigue could be an important aetiological factor in the development of functional gastrointestinal symptoms but also the result of those symptoms. The key role of fatigue in chronic gastrointestinal symptoms needs further research.

Hypertension was relatively strongly associated with chronic stomach symptoms. Hypertension could be a primary or secondary manifestation of rhythm disturbances or angina, which are thought to be associated with gastrointestinal symptoms. This hypothesis is supported by an interesting review, which found associations between rhythm disturbances, linked angina pectoris and oesophageal diseases [18]. Further, inflammatory large bowel disorders, were associated with hypotension and hypertension.

We found a moderate association between back pain and subacute stomach symptoms. Interestingly, obesity was inversely correlated with subacute stomach and chronic intestinal symptoms. Or rather, conversely, it is possible that people who do not suffer from stomach or intestinal problems are more prone to obesity than those who do; this may be due to the fact that gastrointestinal problems limit food intake. Bulimia and binge eating, however, had a fourfold higher association with subacute and chronic intestinal symptoms but an inverse association with chronic stomach symptoms. To the best of our knowledge there is no literature that elucidates these relationships.

In line with our initial hypothesis that GI symptoms correlate with psychiatric disorders, we found that some anxiety states (social phobia, anxiety ≥1 month Generalised Anxiety Disorder – GAD) tended to be associated to varying degrees with every subgroup of gastrointestinal disorders (Figs. 1, 2, 3 and 4). An exception was specific phobia, which was negatively associated with chronic intestinal symptoms.

In our study major mood disorders were also varyingly associated with GI symptoms: bipolar disorder with subacute stomach and chronic intestinal symptoms, and major depression with subacute intestinal symptoms but not with the chronic forms.

There is ample literature on the role of emotional factors in functional gastrointestinal symptoms. An early study by Young et al. reported a "psychiatric illness" in 72% of a group of participants with irritable bowel syndrome (IBS), compared to 18% in the control group [19]. The prevalence of depression and anxiety in patients with IBS and ulcerative colitis (UC) has been reported in three studies. Hartono et al. found an excess prevalence of depression and anxiety of 38.7% and 6.5% respectively in IBS patients relative to healthy patients [20]. Uz et al. reported an excess prevalence of depression or anxiety of 34% and 2% in patients with IBS in comparison to healthy controls [21]. Shah et al. conducted a systematic review on prevalence rates of anxiety and depression in patients with IBS and with UC. In addition to the above-mentioned prevalence rates for anxiety and depression in IBS patients, the authors documented an excess prevalence of anxiety in UC patients relative to healthy controls of 41.7% (22.2% baseline prevalence in healthy controls) based on a State-Trait Anxiety Inventory (STAI) score greater than 40. Excess depression of 38.9%, with a baseline prevalence of 11.1% in the healthy population, was evaluated with a Zung Depression Scale (ZDS) score greater than 49. The authors concluded that both IBS and UC are associated with psychological disorders versus healthy controls and that the association between irritable bowel syndrome and psychological factors might be attributed to the psychological suffering caused by this chronic and debilitating disease [9].

Further studies have confirmed associations between GI symptoms and syndromes and anxiety and depression. A Canadian study of 2015 showed an association between irritable bowel syndrome and general anxiety [22]. Other recent studies have reported an association between gastrointestinal reflux disease and visceral anxiety [23]. An American study, which focused on correlations of anxiety disorders and physical health conditions in elderly Americans, found a statistically significant association between certain anxiety forms and gastrointestinal disease [24]. A study of 2016 showed a clear association of gastrointestinal reflux disease with anxiety and depression in Australian men [25].

Our findings are compatible with the above studies as regards a significant association between gastrointestinal symptoms and anxiety. However, the association with depressive syndromes in our data was limited to subacute intestinal symptoms only.

The significant associations found between GIs and other somatic and psychiatric disorders, could suggest the need to modify the clinical approach and treatment in the field. In particular, the evaluation and treatment of patients with gastrointestinal symptoms would benefit from the integration of psychiatric and/or psychological aspects, broadening the perspective on the pathophysiological mechanisms involved.

The most important strengths of the Zurich Cohort Study are its long-term longitudinal and comprehensive design covering all relevant psychiatric and somatic issues. The study greatly benefited from the continued large number of participants and from the multiple follow-ups conducted over decades. The multivariate logistic models attained high variances, i.e. explained a large proportion of the characteristics of gastrointestinal symptoms, indicating that the assessment of the determining factors was comprehensive. Furthermore, the logistic regression models were adjusted for sex and level of education, which were both kept in the model irrespective of their significance and which are well-known important confounders.

The study also has limitations: by virtue of its longitudinal design the participation rate fluctuated across the six interviews (1981–2008). Furthermore, the associations were examined over the whole observation period and no time-linked cause-effect relationships were analysed. No causal conclusions can therefore be drawn from our association data. Finally all data are interview based without physical examination.

Conclusions

This study provides new insights into the epidemiology of gastric and intestinal symptoms in young and middle-aged persons in the general population.

Functional gastric and intestinal symptoms are remarkably common in the general population, especially in women. We found very strong associations between fatigue/neurasthenia and both conditions and significant associations with various somatic and mental (especially anxiety-related) syndromes. Since there can be no early clarification of the "cause or effect" relationship between GI symptoms and accompanying psychiatric syndromes, screening of functional GI patients followed by the integration of appropriate psychiatric and/or psychological treatment could be an important tool in addressing effectively the functional part of their condition.

More research is needed to clarify the role of fatigue, anxiety disorders and major mood disorders as primary cause or secondary expression of gastrointestinal symptoms.

Abbreviations

CI: Confidence interval; DSM: Diagnostic and Statistical Manual; FD: Functional dyspepsia; FDIG: Functional gastrointestinal disorder; GAD: Generalised anxiety disorder; GI: Gastrointestinal; GSI: Global Severity Index; IBS: Irritable bowel syndrome; M: Mean; OR: Odds ratio; SCL-90R: Revised 90-item Symptom Check List; SD: Standard deviations; SL: Syndrome list; SPIKE: Structured Psychopathological Interview and Rating of the Social Consequences of Psychological Disturbances for Epidemiology; SSI: Somatic-Symptom-Index; STAI: State-Trait Anxiety Inventory; UC: Ulcerative colitis; ZDS: Zung Depression Scale

Acknowledgements

We gratefully thank all the psychologists involved in conducting the comprehensive interviews over the 30 years of the study, and Ms. Elizabeth Kyrke for the English editing.

Funding

This work was supported by Grant numbers 3200–050881.97/1 and 32–50881.97 of the Swiss National Science Foundation. The present study was further supported by the Zurzach Rehabilitation Foundation SPA, Bad Zurzach, Switzerland.

Authors' contributions

MA, with help of US, planned the present study's content and analysis, interpreted the data and wrote the paper. FA helped in the conception of the study's aim and content, together with JA and MA analysed the data, helped to interpret the findings and to write the article. JA initiated and performed the whole survey until 1993, analysed the data and helped to interpret the findings and to write the paper. WR performed the follow-ups of 1999 and 2008 and helped to interpret the findings and to write the paper. AA and US ensured the availability of personal and time resources for the present study and helped to interpret the findings and to write the paper. All authors have read and approved the final manuscript.

Competing interests

The authors declare that they have no competing interests.

Author details

[1]Research Department, Rehabilitation Clinic ("RehaClinic"), Quellenstrasse 34, 5330 Bad Zurzach, Switzerland. [2]Department of Psychiatry, Psychotherapy and Psychosomatics, Psychiatric Hospital, University of Zurich, Zurich, Switzerland. [3]Institute of Psychiatry, Laboratory of Neuroscience (LIM 27), University of São Paulo, São Paulo, Brazil. [4]Department of Psychiatry and Psychotherapy, Charité University Medicine, Berlin, Germany. [5]Department of Psychiatry und Psychotherapy, University Hospital Zurich, University of Zurich, Zurich, Switzerland.

References

1. Smith ER. Epidemiology of gastrointestinal disorders. Can Fam Phys. 1978; 24:1007–11.
2. Peery AF, Dellon ES, Lund J, Crockett SD, McGowan CE, Bulsiewicz WJ, et al. Burden of gastrointestinal disease in the United States: 2012 update. Gastroenterol. 2012;143(5):1179–87.
3. Wessely S, Nimnuan C, Sharpe M. Functional somatic syndromes: one or many? Lancet. 1999;354(9182):936–9.
4. Henningsen P, Zipfel S, Herzog W. Management of functional somatic syndromes. Lancet. 2007;369(9565):946–55.
5. Hungin AP, Whorwell PJ, Tack J, Mearin F. The prevalence, patterns and impact of irritable bowel syndrome: an international survey of 40,000 subjects. Aliment Pharmacol Ther. 2003;17(5):643–50.
6. Nakajima S, Takahashi K, Sato J, Fukuda M, Yamamoto K, Inoue T, et al. Spectra of functional gastrointestinal disorders diagnosed by Rome III integrative questionnaire in a Japanese outpatient office and the impact of overlapping. J Gastroenterol Hepatol. 2010;25(1):138–43.
7. Heitkemper MM, Chang L. Do fluctuations in ovarian hormones affect gastrointestinal symptoms in women with irritable bowel syndrome? Gend Med. 2009;6(2):152–67.
8. Tadayuki O, Hiroto M. Epidemiology of functional gastrointestinal disorders in Japan and in the world. J Neurogastroenterol Motil. 2015;21(3):320–9.
9. Shah E, Rezaie A, Riddle M, Pimentel M. Psychological disorders in gastrointestinal disease: epiphenomenon, cause or consequence? Ann Gastroenterol. 2014;27:224–30.
10. Lieb R, Meinlschmidt G, Araya R. Epidemiology of the association between somatoform disorders and anxiety and depressive disorders: an update. Psychosom Med. 2007;69(9):860–3.
11. Angst J, Dobler-Mikola A, Binder. The Zurich study - a prospective epidemiological study of depressive, neurotic and psychosomatic syndromes. I. Problem, methodology. Eur Arch Psychiatr Neurol Sci. 1984; 234:13–20.
12. Dunn G, Pickles A, Tansella M, Vazquez-Barquero J-L. Two-phase epidemiological surveys in psychiatry. Br J Psychiatry. 1999;174:95–100.
13. Angst J, Paksarian D, Cui L, Merikangas KR, Hengartner MP, Ajdacic-Gross V, Rössler W. The epidemiology of common mental disorders from age 20 to 50: results from the prospective Zurich cohort study. Epidemiol Psychiatr Sci. 2016;25(1):24 32.
14. Angst J, Gamma A, Neuenschwander M, Adjacic-Gross V, Eich D, Rössler W, Merikangas KR. Prevalence of mental disorders in the Zurich cohort study: a twenty year prospective study. Epidemiol Psichiatr Soc. 2005;14:68–76.
15. Angst J, Gamma A, Clarke D, Ajdacic-Gross V, Rössler W, Regier D. Subjective

distress predicts treatment seeking for depression, bipolar, anxiety, panic, neurasthenia and insomnia severity spectra. Acta Psychiatr Scand. 2010;122: 488–98.

16. El-Serag HB, Talley NJ. Systematic review: the prevalence and clinical course of functional dyspepsia. Aliment Pharmacol Ther. 2004;19:643–54.
17. Cohen BL, Zogea H, Shah SA, LeLeiko N, Lidofsky S, Bright R, et al. Fatigue is highly associated with poor health-related quality of life, disability and depression in newly-diagnosed patients with inflammatory bowel disease, independent of disease activity. Aliment Pharmacol Ther. 2014;39(8):811–22.
18. Manisty C, Hughes-Roberts Y, Kaddoura S. Cardiac manifestations and sequelae of gastrointestinal disorders. Br J Cardiol. 2009;16:175–80.
19. Young SJ, Alpers DH, Norland CC, Woodruff RA. Psychiatric illness and irritable bowel syndrome; practical implication for the primary physician. Gastroenterol. 1976;70(2):162–6.
20. Hartono JL, Mahadeva S, Goh KL. Anxiety and depression in various functional gastrointestinal disorders: do differences exist? J Dig Dis. 2012;13: 252–7.
21. Uz E, Türkay C, Aytac S, Bavbek N. Risk factors for irritable bowel syndrome in Turkish population: role of food allergy. J Clin Gastroenterol. 2007;41:380–3.
22. Fuller-Thomson E, Lateef R, Sulman J. Robust association between inflammatory bowel disease and generalized anxiety disorder: Findings from a nationally representative Canadian study. Inflamm Bowel Dis. 2015;21(10): 2341–8.
23. Cohen E, Bolus R, Khanna D, Hays RD, Chang L, Melmed GY, et al. GERD symptoms in the general population: prevalence and severity versus care-seeking patients. Dig Dis Sci. 2014;59(10):2488–96.
24. El-Gabalawy R, Mackenzie CS, Pietrzak RH, Sareen J. A longitudinal examination of anxiety disorders and physical health conditions in a nationally representative sample of U.S. older adults. Exp Gerontol. 2014;60: 46–56.
25. On ZX, Grant J, Shi Z, Taylor AW, Wittert GA, Tully PJ, et al. The association between gastroesophageal reflux disease with sleep quality, depression and anxiety in a cohort study of Australian men. J Gastroenterol Hepatol. 2017; 32(6):1170–7.

Permissions

All chapters in this book were first published in GASTROENTEROLOGY, by BioMed Central; hereby published with permission under the Creative Commons Attribution License or equivalent. Every chapter published in this book has been scrutinized by our experts. Their significance has been extensively debated. The topics covered herein carry significant findings which will fuel the growth of the discipline. They may even be implemented as practical applications or may be referred to as a beginning point for another development.

The contributors of this book come from diverse backgrounds, making this book a truly international effort. This book will bring forth new frontiers with its revolutionizing research information and detailed analysis of the nascent developments around the world.

We would like to thank all the contributing authors for lending their expertise to make the book truly unique. They have played a crucial role in the development of this book. Without their invaluable contributions this book wouldn't have been possible. They have made vital efforts to compile up to date information on the varied aspects of this subject to make this book a valuable addition to the collection of many professionals and students.

This book was conceptualized with the vision of imparting up-to-date information and advanced data in this field. To ensure the same, a matchless editorial board was set up. Every individual on the board went through rigorous rounds of assessment to prove their worth. After which they invested a large part of their time researching and compiling the most relevant data for our readers.

The editorial board has been involved in producing this book since its inception. They have spent rigorous hours researching and exploring the diverse topics which have resulted in the successful publishing of this book. They have passed on their knowledge of decades through this book. To expedite this challenging task, the publisher supported the team at every step. A small team of assistant editors was also appointed to further simplify the editing procedure and attain best results for the readers.

Apart from the editorial board, the designing team has also invested a significant amount of their time in understanding the subject and creating the most relevant covers. They scrutinized every image to scout for the most suitable representation of the subject and create an appropriate cover for the book.

The publishing team has been an ardent support to the editorial, designing and production team. Their endless efforts to recruit the best for this project, has resulted in the accomplishment of this book. They are a veteran in the field of academics and their pool of knowledge is as vast as their experience in printing. Their expertise and guidance has proved useful at every step. Their uncompromising quality standards have made this book an exceptional effort. Their encouragement from time to time has been an inspiration for everyone.

The publisher and the editorial board hope that this book will prove to be a valuable piece of knowledge for researchers, students, practitioners and scholars across the globe.

List of Contributors

Per G. Farup and Knut Hestad
Department of Research, Innlandet Hospital Trust, N-2381 Brumunddal, Norway

Per G. Farup
Unit for Applied Clinical Research, Department of Cancer Research and Molecular Medicine, Faculty of Medicine, Norwegian University of Science and Technology, N-7491 Trondheim, Norway

Knut Rudi
Department of Chemistry, Biotechnology and Food Science, Norwegian University of Life Sciences, Norway

Knut Hestad
Department of Psychology, Faculty of Social Sciences and Technology Management, Norwegian University of Science and Technology, N-7491 Trondheim, Norway
Department of Public Health, Hedmark University College, N-2418 Elverum, Norway

Masakazu Nagahori and Mamoru Watanabe
Department of Gastroenterology, Tokyo Medical and Dental University, 1-5-45, Yushima, Bunkyoku, Tokyo 113-8519, Japan

Shuji Kochi
Division of Gastroenterology, Matsuyama Red Cross Hospital, 1 Bunkyocho, Matsuyama Ehime, Japan

Hiroyuki Hanai
Center for Gastroenterology and Inflammatory Bowel Disease Research, Hamamatsu South Hospital, 26 Shirowacho, Minamiku, Hamamatsu, Shizuoka, Japan

Takayuki Yamamoto
Inflammatory Bowel Disease Center, Yokkaichi Hazu Medical Center, 10-8 Hazuyamacho, Yokkaichi, Mie, Japan

Shiro Nakamura
Department of Inflammatory Bowel Disease, Division of Internal Medicine, Hyogo College of Medicine, 1-1 Mukogawacho, Nishinomiya, Hyogo, Japan

Soji Omuro
Medical Affairs, Clinical Development Center, Kyorin Pharmaceutical Co., Ltd. 4-6 Kanda Surugadai, Chiyodaku, Tokyo, Japan

Toshifumi Hibi
Center for Advanced IBD Research and Treatment, Kitasato Institute Hospital, Kitasato University, 5-9-1 Shirokane, Minatoku, Tokyo, Japan

Bernardette Bonello, Alex Ghanouni, Harriet L. Bowyer, Jane Wardle and Christian von Wagner
Health Behaviour Research Centre, Department of Epidemiology and Public Health, University College London, 1-19 Torrington Place, London WC1E 7HB, UK

Eilidh MacRae and Wendy Atkin
Department of Surgery and Cancer, Imperial College London, London, UK

Stephen P. Halloran
NHS Bowel Cancer Screening Southern Programme Hub, Guildford, Surrey, UK
Royal Surrey County Hospital NHS Foundation Trust and University of Surrey, Guildford, Surrey, UK

Francesca Uberti, Claudio Bardelli, Vera Morsanuto, Sabrina Ghirlanda and Claudio Molinari
Laboratory of Physiology, Department of Translational Medicine, University of Piemonte Orientale, via Solaroli 17, Novara 28100, Italy

Rohan Chaminda Siriwardana, Rajapaksha Walimuni Mudiyanselage Anuradha Lokubandara, Dona Subani Priyangika Jayatunge and Chandika Anuradha Habarakada Liyanage
Department of Surgery, Faculty of Medicine, University of Kelaniya, Ragama, Sri Lanka

Shivanthi Janaki De Silva Hewavisenthi and Saumya Kumuduni Liyanage
Department of Pathology, Faculty of Medicine, University of Kelaniya, Ragama, Sri Lanka
Thiago Gagliano-Jucá and Gilberto De Nucci
Institute of Biophysics Carlos Chagas Filho, Federal University of Rio de Janeiro (UFRJ), 21941-902 Rio de Janeiro, Brazil

Ronilson A. Moreno
Galeno Research Unit, Campinas, Brazil; Faculty of Medical Sciences, Metropolitan University of Santos, Santos, Brazil

Tiago Zaminelli and Gilberto De Nucci
Department of Pharmacology, Faculty of Medical Sciences, State University of Campinas (UNICAMP), Campinas, Brazil

Mauro Napolitano
Department of Pharmacology, ICB - University of Sao Paulo (USP), 05508-900 Sao Paulo, Brazil

Miriam S. Trevisan and Antônio Frederico N. Magalhães
Department of Gastroenterology, Faculty of Medical Sciences, State University of Campinas (UNICAMP), Campinas, Brazil

Aloísio Carvalhaes
Brazilian Society for Digestive Endoscopy (SOBED), Sao Paulo, Brazil

John L. Wallace and Gilberto De Nucci
Unicastelo Medical School, University Camilo Castelo Branco (UNICASTELO), Fernandopolis, Brazil

Gilberto De Nucci
Department of Pharmacology, ICB - University of Sao Paulo (USP), Sao Paulo, Brazil

Stephanie Wong, Ilmars Lidums and Wendy Uylaki
Department of Gastroenterology, The Queen Elizabeth Hospital, Woodville South 5011, Adelaide, South Australia, Australia

Christophe Rosty
Envoi Specialist Pathologists, Kelvin Grove 4059, Brisbane, QLD, Australia
School of Medicine, University of Queensland, Herston 4006, Brisbane, QLD, Australia
Department of Pathology, Colorectal Oncogenomics Group, Genetic Epidemiology Laboratory, The University of Melbourne, Parkville 3010, Melbourne, VIC, Australia

Andrew Ruszkiewicz
Division of Anatomical Pathology, SA Pathology, Adelaide 5000, South Australia, Australia

Andrew Ruszkiewicz
Centre for Cancer Biology, University of South Australia, Adelaide 5000, South Australia, Australia

Susan Parry
Familial GI Cancer Service and Ministry of Health Bowel Cancer Programme, Auckland City Hospital, Auckland, New Zealand

Aung Ko Win
Centre for Epidemiology and Biostatistics, Melbourne School of Population and Global Health, The University of Melbourne, Parkville 3010, Melbourne, VIC, Australia

Yoko Tomita, Amanda Townsend, Jennifer E. Hardingham, Eric Smith, Wendy Uylaki, Timothy J. Price and Joanne P. Young
Department of Haematology and Oncology, The Queen Elizabeth Hospital, Woodville South 5011, Adelaide, South Australia, Australia

Sina Vatandoust and Dainik Patel
Flinders Medical Centre, Bedford Park 5042, Adelaide, South Australia, Australia

Jennifer E. Hardingham, Eric Smith, Daniel L. Worthley, Timothy J. Price and Joanne P. Young
School of Medicine, University of Adelaide, Adelaide 5000, South Australia, Australia

David Roder
Cancer Epidemiology and Population Health, University of South Australia, Adelaide 5000, South Australia, Australia

Paul Drew
School of Nursing and Midwifery, Flinders University, Bedford Park 5042, Adelaide, South Australia, Australia
Basil Hetzel Institute, The Queen Elizabeth Hospital, Woodville South 5011, Adelaide, South Australia, Australia

Julie Marker
Cancer Voices SA, Kensington Park 5068, Adelaide, South Australia, Australia

Peter Hewett
University of Adelaide Department of Surgery, The Queen Elizabeth Hospital, Woodville South 5011, Adelaide, South Australia, Australia

Daniel L. Worthley
Cancer Theme, South Australian Health and Medical Research Institute, Adelaide 5000, South Australia, Australia

Erin Symonds and Graeme P. Young
Flinders Centre for Innovation in Cancer, Flinders University, Bedford Park 5042, Adelaide, South Australia, Australia

Erin Symonds
Bowel Health Service, Repatriation General Hospital, Daw Park 5041, Adelaide, South Australia, Australia

Timothy J. Price and Joanne P. Young
SAHMRI Colorectal Node, Basil Hetzel Institute, Woodville South, Adelaide, South Australia 5011, Australia

Sena Bluemel, Oliver Goetze, Michael Fried, Werner Schwizer, Mark Fox and Andreas Steingoetter
Division of Gastroenterology and Hepatology, University Hospital Zurich, Raemistrasse 100, CH-8091 Zurich, Switzerland

Andreas Steingoetter
Institute for Biomedical Engineering, University and ETH Zurich, Zurich, Switzerland

Dieter Menne
Menne Biomed Consulting, Tuebingen, Germany

Gabriella Milos
Psychiatric Department, University Hospital Zurich, Zurich, Switzerland

Michael Fried, Werner Schwizer and Mark Fox
Zurich Centre for Integrative Human Physiology (ZIHP), University of Zurich, Zurich, Switzerland

Andrew Mitchell and Tony Petrella
Department of Anatomical Pathology and Cytology, Maisonneuve-Rosemont Hospital, 5415 Boulevard de L'Assomption, Montreal, Quebec H1T 2M4, Canada

Michelle Shui Yee Lau, Peter D. Mooney, William L. White and David S. Sanders
Academic Department of Gastroenterology, Royal Hallamshire Hospital, Sheffield Teaching Hospitals, Sheffield, UK

Victoria Appleby and Sulleman Moreea
Department of Gastroenterology, Bradford Royal Infirmary, Bradford, UK

Ismail Haythem and Sami Hoque
Department of Gastroenterology, Whipps Cross University Hospital, London, UK

Joshua E. Elias, Kiran Bundhoo and Gareth D. Corbett
Department of Gastroenterology, Addenbrooke's Hospital, Cambridge, UK

Liam Wong and Her Hsin Tsai
Department of Gastroenterology, Hull Royal Infirmary, Hull, UK

Simon S. Cross
Academic Unit of Pathology, Department of Neuroscience, Faculty of Medicine, Dentistry and Health, The University of Sheffield, Sheffield, UK

John M. Hebden
Department of Gastroenterology, Northern General Hospital, Sheffield Teaching Hospitals, Sheffield, UK

Qiongzhen Li
Department of Anesthesia, Shanghai Chest Hospital, Shanghai Jiao Tong University, Shanghai, China

Qinghe Zhou, Wangpin Xiao and Hongmei Zhou
Department of Anesthesia, Second Hospital, Jiaxing Medical College, No. 1518, North Huancheng Road, Jianshe Street, Nanhu District, Jiaxing 314000, Zhejiang, China

Jonathan Barontini, Marco Antinucci, Sergio Tofanelli, Maurizio Cammalleri, Massimo Dal Monte, Federica Gemignani, Roberto Marangoni, Roberto Barale, Stefano Landi and Daniele Campa
Department of Biology, University of Pisa, Via Derna 1, 56100 Pisa, Italy

Pavel Vodicka, Ludmila Vodickova and Veronika Vymetalkova
Department of Molecular Biology of Cancer, Institute of Experimental Medicine, Academy of Science of Czech Republic, Prague, Czech Republic
Institute of Biology and Medical Genetics, 1st Medical Faculty, Charles University, Prague, Czech Republic

Pavel Vodickab and Ludmila Vodickova
Biomedical Centre, Medical School Pilsen, Charles University in Prague, Pilsen, Czech Republic

Juozas Kupcinskas
Department of Gastroenterology, Lithuanian University of Health Sciences, Kaunas, Lithuania

Asta Forsti
Genomic Epidemiology Group, German Cancer Research Center (DKFZ), Heidelberg, Germany

Federico Canzian and Angelika Stein
Division of Molecular Genetic Epidemiology, German Cancer Research Center (DKFZ), Heidelberg, Germany

Victor Moreno
Cancer Prevention and Control Program, Catalan Institute of Oncology (ICO), IDIBELL, CIBERESP and Department of Clinical Sciences, Faculty of Medicine, University of Barcelona, Barcelona, Spain

Nicola Mastrodonato, Francesca Tavano and Anna Panza
Division of Gastroenterology and Research Laboratory, IRCCS Scientific Institute and Regional General Hospital "Casa Sollievo della Sofferenza", San Giovanni Rotondo, Italy

Hind Mrabti, Mounia Amziren, Ibrahim ElGhissassi, Youssef Bensouda, Narjiss Berrada, Halima Abahssain Saber Boutayeb and Hassan Errihani
Department of Medical Oncology, National Institute of Oncology, University Hospital, Rabat, Morocco

Samira El Fakir and Chakib Nejjari
Department of Epidemiology and Public health, Faculty of Medicine, Fez, Morocco

Abdellatif Benider
Department of Radiotherapy, Ibn Rochd University Hospital, Casablanca, Morocco

Nawfel Mellas and Omar El Mesbahi
Department of Medical Oncology, Hassan II University Hospital, Fez, Morocco

Maria Bennani, Rachid Bekkali and Ahmed Zidouh
Lalla Salma Foundation-Prevention and Treatment of Cancers, Rabat, Morocco

Yuki Ohta, Tatsuo Kanda, Tatsuro Katsuno, Shin Yasui, Yuki Haga, Reina Sasaki, Masato Nakamura, Shuang Wu, Makoto Arai and Osamu Yokosuka
Department of Gastroenterology and Nephrology, Chiba University, Graduate School of Medicine, 1-8-1 Inohana, Chuo-ku, Chiba 260-8670, Japan

Shingo Nakamoto
Department of Molecular Virology, Chiba University, Graduate School of Medicine, 1-8-1 Inohana, Chuo-ku, Chiba 260-8670, Japan

Ke-ke Qi, Jia-jia Lv, Jie Wu and Zi-wei Xu
Institute of Animal Science, Zhejiang Academy of Agricultural Sciences, 198 Shiqiao Road, Jianggan, Hangzhou 310021, China

Craig A. Friesen and John M. Rosen
Division of Gastroenterology, Hepatology, and Nutrition, Children's Mercy Kansas City, 2401 Gillham Road, Kansas City, MO 64108, USA

Jennifer V. Schurman
Division of Developmental and Behavioral Sciences, Children's Mercy Kansas City, 2401 Gillham Road, Kansas City, MO 64108, USA

Dalyong Kim, Sun Young Kim, Yong Sang Hong, Jeong Eun Kim, Kyu-pyo Kim, Young-Kwang Yoon and Tae Won Kim
Department of Oncology, Asan Medical Center, University of Ulsan College of Medicine, 88, Olympic-ro 43-gil, Songpa-gu, Seoul 05505, Republic of Korea

Ji Sung Lee, Young-Kwang Yoon and Tae Won Kim
Clinical Research Center, Asan Institute for Life Sciences, Asan Medical Center, University of Ulsan College of Medicine, Seoul, South Korea

Jihun Kim and Se Jin Jang
Department of Pathology, Asan Medical Center, University of Ulsan College of Medicine, Seoul, South Korea

Dalyong Kim
Department of Hematology/Oncology, Yuseong Sun Hospital, 93, Bugyuseong-daero, Yuseong-gu, Daejeon 34084, South Korea

Chaoyong Shen, Yuan Yin, Xiaonan Yin, Zhaolun Cai, Bo Zhang and Zhixin Chen
Department of Gastrointestinal Surgery, West China Hospital, Sichuan University, Chengdu 610041, Sichuan, China

Huijiao Chen
Department of Pathology, West China Hospital, Sichuan University, Chengdu 610041, Sichuan, China

Ruixue Wang
State Key Laboratory of Biotherapy and Cancer Center/Collaborative Innovation Center for Biotherapy, West China Hospital, Sichuan University, Chengdu 610041, Sichuan, China

Zongguang Zhou
Institute of Digestive Surgery and State Key Laboratory of Biotherapy, West China Hospital, Sichuan University, Chengdu 610041, Sichuan, China

Paulo C. Soares and Rommel Mario Rodríguez Burbano
Hospital Ophir Loyola, Belém, Pará 66060-281, Brazil

Paulo C. Soares
Universidade do Estado do Pará, Belém, Pará, Brazil

Eliana S. Abdelhay, Luiz Claudio S. Thuler and Luis Felipe Ribeiro Pinto
Instituto Nacional de Câncer, Rio de Janeiro, Brazil

Bruno Moreira Soares and Rommel Mario Rodríguez Burbano
Laboratório de Citogenética Humana, Instituto de Ciências Biológicas, Belém, Pará, Brazil

Gessica Valéria Rocha Ferro, Paulo P. Assumpção and Samia Demachki
Núcleo de Pesquisas em Oncologia, Universidade Federal do Pará, Belém, Pará, Brazil

Leticia Martins Lamarão
Fundação de Hematologia e Hemoterapia do Pará, Belém, Pará, Brazil

Darina Kohoutova and Jan Bures
Charles University, Faculty of Medicine in Hradec Kralove, University Hospital Hradec Kralove, 2nd Department of Internal Medicine - Gastroenterology, Sokolska 581, 500 05 Hradec Kralove, Czech Republic

Jaroslav Pejchal
University of Defence, Faculty of Military Health Sciences, Hradec Kralove, Czech Republic

Jie Yuan
Department of Gastroenterology, Nanjing First Hospital, Nanjing Medical University, 68, Changle Road, Nanjing 210006, China

Lei Gu and Fei Xu
Nanjing Municipal Center for Disease Control and Prevention, Nanjing, China
The School of Public Health, Nanjing Medical University, Nanjing, China

Anne Stine Kvehaugen
Department of Surgery, Innlandet Hospital Trust, Kyrre Greppsgate 11, 2819 Gjøvik, Norway

Dag Tveiten
Lab1 AS, Sandvika, Norway

Per G. Farup
Department of Research, Innlandet Hospital Trust, Brumunddal, Norway
Unit for Applied Clinical Research, Department of Clinical and Molecular Medicine, Faculty of Medicine and Health Sciences, Norway

Xuexue Deng, Ronghua Fang, Jianshu Zhang and Rongqiong Li
Department of General Medicine, West China Hospital, Sichuan University, No. 37 Guoxuexiang, Wuhou District, Chengdu City, Sichuan Province, China

Hossam Murad, Batoul Jazairi and Issam Khansaa
Molecular Biology and Biotechnology Department, Human Genetics Division, Atomic Energy Commission of Syria, Damascus, Syria

Doaa Olabi and Lina Khouri
Children's hospital, Damascus, Syria

Ashwath S. Kumar
University of Missouri-Kansas City School of Medicine, Kansas City, MO, USA

Brooke L. Beutler and Thomas M. Attard
Children's Mercy Hospital, Kansas City, USA

Koichi Izumikawa, Tomoki Inaba, Shigenao Ishikawa, Ichiro Sakakihara, Kumiko Yamamoto, Sakuma Takahashi, Shigetomi Tanaka and Masaki Wato
Department of Gastroenterology, Kagawa Prefectural Central Hospital, 1-2-2 Asahi-machi, Takamatsu, Kagawa 760-8557, Japan

Masaya Iwamuro and Hiroyuki Okada
Department of Gastroenterology and Hepatology, Okayama University Graduate School of Medicine, Dentistry and Pharmaceutical Sciences, 2-5-1 Shikata-cho, Kita-ku, Okayama, Okayama 700-8558, Japan

Kenji Kuwaki
Department of Internal Medicine, Fukuyama City Hospital, 5-23-1 Zao-cho, Fukuyama, Hiroshima 721-8511, Japan

Maria Avramidou, Felix Angst and André Aeschlimann
Research Department, Rehabilitation Clinic ("RehaClinic"), Quellenstrasse 34, 5330 Bad Zurzach, Switzerland

Jules Angst and Wulf Rössler
Department of Psychiatry, Psychotherapy and Psychosomatics, Psychiatric Hospital, University of Zurich, Zurich, Switzerland

Wulf Rössler
Institute of Psychiatry, Laboratory of Neuroscience (LIM 27), University of São Paulo, São Paulo, Brazil
Department of Psychiatry and Psychotherapy, Charité University Medicine, Berlin, Germany

Ulrich Schnyder
Department of Psychiatry und Psychotherapy, University Hospital Zurich, University of Zurich, Zurich, Switzerland

Index

www.ingramcontent.com/pod-product-compliance
Lightning Source LLC
LaVergne TN
LVHW080715210926
848485LV00003B/468